CYTOKINES IN HUMAN REPRODUCTION

CYTOKINES IN HUMAN REPRODUCTION

Edited by
Joseph A. Hill, M.D.

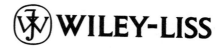

A John Wiley & Sons, Inc., Publication

New York • Chichester • Weinheim • Brisbane • Singapore • Toronto

This book is printed on acid-free paper. ⊚

Copyright © 2000 by Wiley-Liss, Inc. All rights reserved.

Published simultaneously in Canada.

While the authors, editor, and publisher believe that drug selection and dosage and the specification and usage of equipment and devices, as set forth in this book, are in accord with current recommendations and practice at the time of publication, they accept no legal responsibility for any errors or omissions, and make no warranty, express or implied, with respect to material contained herein. In view of ongoing research, equipment modifications, changes in governmental regulations, and the constant flow of information relating to drug therapy, drug reactions, and the use of equipment and devices, the reader is urged to review and evaluate the information provided in the package insert or instructions for each drug, piece of equipment, or device for, among other things, any changes in the instructions or indication of dosage or usage and for added warnings and precautions.

For order and customer service, call 1-800-CALL-WILEY.

Library of Congress Cataloging-in-Publication Data:
Cytokines in human reproduction / edited by Joseph A. Hill.
    p. cm
   Includes index.
   ISBN 0-471-35242-X (alk. paper)
    1. Human reproduction—Immunological aspects.   2. Cytokines—
Physiological effect.   3. Cytokines—Pathophysiology.
   4. Generative organs, Female—Diseases—Molecular aspects.
   I. Hill, Joseph A.
   QP252.5.C96   2000
   612.6—dc21   99-15234

Printed in the United States of America.

10 9 8 7 6 5 4 3 2 1

To my mentors, students, and patients who have taught me that the true meaning of life is the betterment of the human condition and the world in which we live, and especially to Deborah, whose words and deeds exemplify that critical questioning of every insight and assumption enable us to separate the dreams that serve us inadequately from those that serve us well.

Contents

Preface

Cytokines are families of proteins originally isolated from supernatants of activated immune and inflammatory cells. However, cytokines are now known to be secreted by a wide variety of cell types and tissues including endocrinologically responsive tissues. In the broadest context cytokine families encompass not only those proteins secreted by immune and inflammatory cell populations originally described, but also a myriad of growth factors, oncogenes, chemokines, and other soluble factors that affect the growth, differentiation, and viability of cells in a paracrine, autocrine, and juxtacrine manner through binding to their membrane bound receptors.

Cytokine receptors are generally dimers or trimers grouped in families based on the presence of conserved domains and overall structure that either singularly or in receptor complexes bind to their respective ligand. Following ligand–receptor binding, signal transduction occurs, producing a cascade of intracellular signals and effects. There are also naturally occurring soluble forms for many cytokine receptors, which are often, but not invariably, the ligand binding component of the receptor complex. These soluble receptors have been described in many body secretions where they may serve several functions. One such function may be protecting ligands from proteolysis. They may also serve a transport function or act as a reservoir holding cytokines in reserve until they can be presented to surface receptors, thus potentiating cytokine action. Soluble cytokine receptors may also act as antagonists by competing with surface receptor binding of ligand. These enhancing and inhibiting functions are providing insight into the development of novel treatment strategies for maladaptive processes in which too much or too little of an individual cytokine or cytokines may be contributing to disease. As more is learned concerning cytokine involvement with the pathophysiology of disease, cytokines and their receptors will become both obvious targets and vehicles themselves for therapeutic intervention.

Much has been learned over the past decade concerning cytokines in reproduction, yet there is no one source available providing a review of the subject. The objective of this text is not to provide a detailed inventory of the known cytokine and cytokine receptor families, because these descriptions have already been published in other texts. The intent of this text is to have respected investigators in the field of reproductive immunology and cytokine biology synthesize much of the data concerning what is known about cytokines in reproduction into a heretofore unavailable single source of reference. It is also my hope that this book may serve as a catalyst for further investigation by students, basic scientists, clinicians, and others interested in the potential role cytokines play in human reproduction.

I am grateful for the expertise of the authors who have contributed the chapters that make up this text. I would also like to thank Denise Galotti and Bernadette Aidonidis for their secretarial assistance and the individuals of John Wiley and Sons for their patience and cooperation in the preparation of this text. Lastly, but most importantly, I would like to thank my family for making it all worthwhile.

Joseph A. Hill, M.D.
Boston, Massachusetts

Contributors

Deborah J. Anderson, Fearing Research Laboratory, Department of Obstetrics, Gynecology, and Reproductive Biology, Brigham and Women's Hospital, Harvard Medical School, Boston, MA 02115

Aydin Arici, Department of Obstetrics and Gynecology, Yale University School of Medicine, POB 208063, 333 Cedar Street, New Haven, CT 06520-8063

Jonathan S. Berek, Gynecologic Oncology Service, Department of Obstetrics and Gynecology, Jonsson Comprehensive Cancer Center, UCLA School of Medicine, 10833 LeConte Avenue, Los Angeles, CA 90095-1740

Craig L. Best, Department of Obstetrics and Gynecology, Carney Hospital, 2100 Dorchester Ave., Boston, MA 02120

Celeste M. Brabec, Department of Obstetrics and Gynecology, Creighton University, Omaha, NE 68154

Nasser Chegini, Department of Obstetrics and Gynecology, University of Florida, Gainesville, FL 32610

Oliver Dorigo, Gynecologic Oncology Service, Department of Obstetrics and Gynecology, Jonsson Comprehensive Cancer Center, UCLA School of Medicine, 10833 LeConte Avenue, Los Angeles, CA 90095-1740

Donald J. Dudley, School of Medicine, University of Texas at San Antonio, San Antonio, TX

Raina N. Fichorova, Fearing Research Laboratory, Department of Obstetrics, Gynecology, and Reproductive Biology, Brigham and Women's Hospital, Harvard Medical School, Boston, MA 02115

Florina Haimovici, Harvard South Shore Psychiatry Residency Program, Boston, MA 02115

Dale Buchanan Hales, Department of Physiology and Biophysics, University of Illinois at Chicago, 835 S Wolcott Ave., Chicago, IL 60612-7342

Joseph A. Hill, Department of Obstetrics, Gynecology, and Reproductive Biology, Brigham and Women's Hospital, Harvard Medical School, 75 Francis Street, Boston, MA 02115

Joan S. Hunt, Department of Anatomy and Cell Biology, University of Kansas Medical Center, 3901 Rainbow Blvd., Kansas City, KS 66160-7400

Ellen S. Moore, Reproductive Endocrinology Center, Department of Obstetrics and Reproductive Sciences, University of California, San Francisco, CA 94143-0556

Isabelle P. Ryan, Reproductive Endocrinology Center, Department of Obstetrics and Reproductive Sciences, University of California, San Francisco, CA 94143-0556

Emre Seli, Department of Obstetrics and Gynecology, Yale University School of Medicine, POB 208063, 333 Cedar Street, New Haven, CT 06520-8063

Robert N. Taylor, Reproductive Endocrinology Center, Department of Obstetrics and Reproductive Sciences, University of California, San Francisco, CA 94143-0556

R. Stan Williams, Department of Obstetrics and Gynecology, University of Florida, Gainesville, FL 32610

CYTOKINES IN HUMAN REPRODUCTION

1

THE ROLE OF PSYCHONEUROENDOCRINE IMMUNOLOGY IN REPRODUCTION

Florina Haimovici and Joseph A. Hill

Brigham and Women's Hospital, Harvard Medical School,
Boston, Massachusetts

The interdisciplinary field of psychoneuroendocrine immunology has undergone explosive growth in recent years. This field deals with the influence of the central nervous system on how thoughts and emotions affect immune and endocrine function. The nervous, endocrine, and immune systems are anatomically and functionally interconnected. These systems express and respond to a large number of regulatory molecules (hormones, cytokines, neuropeptides) in common, and these provide the molecular basis for bidirectional integration. This chapter focuses on these concepts with emphasis on those factors particularly relevant to reproduction.

An estimated 10% of married couples in the United States are involuntarily childless, and an additional 10% have fewer children than they desire (1). The cause of infertility remains unexplained in a significant proportion of these couples. Temporary impaired fertility facilitates energy conversion during times of hardship for the organism. Recent

Cytokines in Human Reproduction, Edited by Joseph A. Hill
ISBN 0-471-35242-X   Copyright © 2000 Wiley-Liss, Inc.

work has investigated the effect of stress on the neurochemistry and morphology of the brain (2) and the rapid and enduring hormonal and immune disturbances produced by stress through its effect on the components of the hypothalamus–pituitary–gonadal axis (HPG) (2). Evidence suggests that stress can affect all three components of the HPG axis and is speculated to result in decreased reproductive function (3, 4). However, little has been done to elucidate pathways and mediators of psychoneuroendocrine actions in the context of both systemic and mucosal immunity.

PSYCHOLOGICAL FACTORS IN MALE REPRODUCTION

The majority of the psychological literature prior to 1970 regarding male fertility was composed of anecdotal case reports and retrospective studies (5). Both chronic and traumatic psychosocial stress have been associated with male infertility (6–11). Anxiety and tension or a tendency to conceal disturbed feelings have been observed in infertile men (8, 12–16). Testicular atrophy has resulted in complete failure of spermatogenesis in men awaiting execution and oligospermia in men awaiting sentencing for rape where pregnancy occurred (15). A number of authors have suggested that negative influences of occupational and familial stress are associated with adverse seminal parameters (sperm count, motility, and morphology) (12, 13, 17, 18). Two studies suggested that testosterone levels and spermatogenesis were affected adversely by stress-induced and behaviorally mediated arousal of the sympathetic nervous system (19, 20). Another study in healthy volunteers reported a negative correlation between stress and both semen volume and the percentage of spermatozoa with normal morphology (21).

Different mechanisms have been proposed to explain the effects of stress on male fertility. Monden et al. reported that testosterone levels were significantly decreased for 3 weeks following major surgery; 17 ketosteroids were also significantly decreased 4–8 weeks after surgery, but corticotropin (adrenocorticotrophic hormone, ACTH) levels were unaffected (22). Schwartz and Kolasky reported no significant difference in plasma testosterone levels between a group of 341 men with sexual dysfunction and a group of 199 fertile men (23). The biologic amines, cathecolamines, and serotonin are involved in stress and may affect reproduction in different ways. Epinephrine and norepinephrine may affect the testis by altering blood flow or through the enzyme monoamine oxidase (MAO), which is known to be involved in testicular maturation (24, 25). Serotonin may affect testicular function by inducing anatomic changes in the testes through vasoconstriction or by influencing testicular metabolism and endocrine activity (26, 27). Urry reported that infertile men had higher levels of serotonin and its metabolite 5-hydroxyindoleacetic acid (5 HIAA), compared with fertile men, and that the levels of 5 HIAA correlated inversely with sperm cell concentration (28).

PSYCHOLOGICAL FACTORS IN FEMALE REPRODUCTION

Over the past four decades much has been written on the psychological profile of women with reproductive dysfunction; whether one causes the other is open to question. Infertile women have been reported to have more psychotic diagnoses than fertile women, but the same number of neurotic diagnoses. Others have reported that infertile women are more neurotic, dependent, and anxious than their counterparts and more likely to have conflicting feelings regarding their femininity and to be fearful of reproduction (29–31).

In another study, comparing women with unexplained infertility to fertile women, women with unexplained infertility were reported to be more introverted, inclined to be more quiet, introspective, and retiring, and preferring to keep their feelings under control; they were also found to be more tense, have more anxiety, and to be more guilt prone than fertile controls (8). The incidence of psychosomatic disorders has also been reported to be increased in infertile compared to fertile women (32). Women with menstrual disturbances, menstrual pains, and acne were also more likely to have clinical depression. Using the Giessen personality test, infertile women appeared significantly more compulsive and depressed and identified themselves more with their mothers than did fertile controls (32).

Wasser et al., studying the effect of psychological stress on fertility, compared women with anatomic abnormalities, women with functional abnormalities of the hypothalamic–pituitary–ovarian axis, and women with unexplained infertility and concluded that women with unexplained infertility had fewer sources of social support, increased conflicts with their fathers, and more hostility, anxiety, phobic anxiety, and evidence of somatic complaints than the other groups (33). Some authors considered psychogenic infertility as a defense mechanism against dangers inherent in reproductive function (34). Others have reported that infertile couples displayed a more ambivalent attitude toward children than fertile couples (35).

There is a general widespread impression that infertile couples who adopt often subsequently have children on their own. Cooper compared conception rates before and after adoption and reported that once arrangements for adoption were under way or, more commonly, following adoption, a previously infertile woman often became pregnant (37). Sandler suggested that adoption facilitated conception by relieving emotional stress in cases where organic factors had been adequately treated (37). The relationship of adoption and subsequent conception has been speculated to represent a reduction in stress and subsequently, alterations in the neuroendocrinologic characteristics of the infertile couple (38).

INFLUENCE OF PSYCHOLOGICAL STRESS ON EARLY PREGNANCY LOSS

The occurrence of chromosomally normal early pregnancy loss has been associated with psychological factors. Women with recurrent pregnancy loss have been characterized, using psychological testing, as having impairment of the ability to plan and anticipate, poor emotional control, emphasis on conformity and compliance with the conventional, stronger feelings of dependency, and greater proneness to guilt feelings (39). Cause versus effect associations are difficult to ascribe because these psychological characteristics may result from recurrent pregnancy loss rather than be the cause. It is clear, however, that recurrent pregnancy loss is associated with significant psychological distress (40). However, several authors have claimed that emotional factors can lead to miscarriage (41–44). Commonly postulated contributing factors include an absent or unsupportive father, repressed anger against a critical mother, representation of the fetus as an aspect of bad self or a bad object, and rejection of motherhood and/or the fetus (41). Others have claimed that women with a history of recurrent spontaneous abortion were more likely not to have a living father and to report childhood neurotic symptoms and a poor relationship in childhood with their mothers (42). In an epidemiologic study reported by Janerich et al., a correlation was found between stress and subsequent spontaneous abortion in the population of a rural village who experienced a flood disaster necessitating evacuation of the inhabitants (43). There was a 30% increase in the miscarriage rate compared to the percentages reported in the years before and after the flood. No etiologic agent was found and there was no increase in the fetal malformation rate. In a case control study using Life Events and Difficulties Schedule, O'Hare and Creed reported that women with recurrent pregnancy loss were more likely to have experienced a "severe life event" ($p < 0.005$), "major social difficulty" ($p < 0.002$), or "life events of severe short-term threat" ($p < 0.002$) within 3 months preceding their miscarriage (44). Other factors significantly associated with miscarriage included maternal childhood separation, poor relationship with partners, and fewer social contacts than women not experiencing pregnancy loss. In another study Neugebauer et al. reported that recent negative life events increased the odds of spontaneous abortion of a chromosomally normal compared to abnormal conceptus. This association held for postconception events and was unaltered by adjustment for smoking, caffeine intake, and alcohol consumption (45).

Studies performed on successful pregnant women and women with threatened abortion who subsequently experienced pregnancy loss suggested that psychological stress significantly correlated with plasma levels of free radical products such as lipoperoxides, and that both stress and free radicals were higher in women who experienced spontaneous fetal loss compared to women who had a successful pregnancy (46). Further work is needed to validate a causal relationship between stress and subsequent pregnancy loss.

PSYCHONEUROENDOCRINE–IMMUNE SYSTEM INTERACTIONS AND REPRODUCTION

There are anatomic and functional interconnections between the nervous, endocrine, and immune systems mediated by hormones, cytokines, and neuropeptides. An important element in psychoneuroendocrine–immune interaction is the concept of stress and the stress response. Stress is defined as a complex dynamic condition in which normal homeostasis, or the steady-state internal milieu, is disturbed or threatened (46, 47). Both physical and emotional stressors above certain thresholds elicit a plethora of physical, mental, and behavioral adaptational responses to counteract the effects of stressors. This complex process of adaptation responses is called the stress system or stress response. Mental and behavioral components of the stress response include the central nervous system, endocrine system and immune system. Any overactive or underactive response to stress is theorized to produce or contribute to disease. According to the *Diagnostic and Statistical Manual of Mental Disorders* (DSM) (49), when major depressions develop after trauma, the diagnosis of major depression should be considered as a separate entity. The activity of the hypothalamic–pituitary axis (HPA) is profoundly affected by the stress response. This includes the hypothalamic/pituitary-prolactin and -growth hormone connections, and the hypothalamic/pituitary-thyroid (HPT) and -gonadal (HPG) axes. Activation of the stress response inhibits the HPG axis at multiple levels. Corticotropin releasing hormone (CRH) is thought to be the coordinator of the stress response (50). Stressful thoughts and emotions may reach the hypothalamus by axons relayed by neurons from the limbic system or from the forebrain. Norepinephrine, serotonin, and acetylcholine are important neurotransmitters that mediate much of the neurogenic stimulation of CRH production (51). CRH suppresses secretion of luteinizing hormone releasing hormone (LHRH) either directly or indirectly via the stimulation of beta-endorphin or corticosteroids. Corticosteroids also directly inhibit pituitary release of luteinizing hormone (LH) and gonadal production of sex steroids (estrogen, progesterone, and testosterone). In addition they can also inhibit the tissue effects of sex steroids (47, 52–55). Sex steroids also modulate HPA activity, creating a bidirectional system.

The concept is emerging that an integrated and coordinated bidirectionally regulated neuroendocrine–immune response occurs to stress. Production of neuropeptides by immune cells is physiologically relevant for both the immune and nervous systems. The common chemical language for the brain and immune and endocrine systems to communicate suggests a plausible way in which sensory information can be conveyed between these systems. Specifically, physical and psychological stimuli may set off patterns of neurotransmitters, hormones, and cytokines, which act via their receptors on immune cells and alter immune function either directly or through the induction of other substances. These converging findings offer a better understanding of the physiological interplay between the traditionally defined immune and neuroendocrine systems. Studies are now under way to elucidate the role of these interactions in the bigger picture of immunologic dysfunction. Dysfunction in the communication between the nervous, endocrine, and immune systems may lead to development of autoimmune disease (reviewed in ref. 56). Whether failure of central nervous system regulation of the immune response is a factor in the etiology of infertility remains speculative. Sustained hyperactivity of the HPA axis has been associated with several psychiatric disorders, most notably, major depression (57). Studies support the view that major depression represents a generalized stress response (57). There is an association between psychological stress and increased susceptibility to infection by downregulating immunity (57). Major depression may be accompanied by significant changes in cell mediated and humoral immunity (58). The "acute phase" (AP) response in depression was suggested by modulation of AP proteins and the most prominent disorders were associated with plasma levels of haptoglobin (Hp). A significant positive relationship was detected between plasma Hp levels and the number of peripheral blood leukocytes, monocytes, neutrophils, and activated T cells, suggesting an immune association with the pathophysiology of the AP response in major depression (59). Impaired immunity in major depression is suggested by increased titers of antinuclear and antiphospholipid antibodies and by B cell proliferation and increased IgG levels in peripheral blood (58). Castle et al. have demonstrated that depression associated with chronic stress is associated with immunomodulation of T cell subsets, altering their number and function (60). Correlations between emotional stress or psychiatric disorders and impairment of the mucosal immune system are being defined. La Via reported a relationship between stress and an increased frequency of upper respiratory tract infections in medical students taking National Board Examinations, patients with generalized anxiety disorders, and patients with panic disorders (61). Functional links between the central nervous system (CNS) and immunologic events at defined mucosal sites has been suggested by studies investigating CNS regulation of mucosal immune cells in gastrointestinal and respiratory tissues (62, 63).

Corticosteroids modulate lymphocyte and macrophage functions, but removal of adrenal function by adrenalectomy or suppression of corticosteroid synthesis with metapyrone eliminates many but not all of the immunosuppressive effects of stress, indicating that other molecules in addition to corticosteroids mediate stress-induced immunologic effects (57). Other substances produced by the brain or immune cells are also regarded as mediators in neuroendocrine–immunologic interactions. Both lymphocytes and macrophages have β_2-adrenergic, growth hormone, and prolactin receptors in addition to receptors for cortisol (51). Goetzl et al. have demonstrated that macrophages possess a high-affinity specific uptake system for serotonin (5-HT) that can be blocked by imipramine and fluoxetine (64). 5-HT has been reported to have modulating activity on immune function (65) and has also been shown to modulate interferon (IFN) induced expression of Ig antigen (66) and to have a biphasic effect on phagocytosis (67). Recent studies have also implicated 5-HT in the modulation of chemotaxis and in the inhibition of lymphocyte proliferation (68).

Interleukin-1 (IL-1), interleukin-6 (IL-6), tumor necrosis factor α (TNF-α), interleukin-2 (IL-2), and interferon-gamma (IFN-γ) function as bidirectional regulators of neuroendocrine–immune function (69, 70). IL-1, IL-2, IL-3, IL-6, IL-10, IFN-γ, TNF-α, and granulocyte macrophage colony stimulating factor (GMCSF) are produced and act on neural and neuroendocrine tissues (65). IL-3 mRNA is found in the medial habenulae, hippocampus, and cerebellum, and IL-10 is present and functional in the HPA axis (71). Neurons and endocrine cells have receptors and receptor mRNA for IL-1, IL-2, IL-3, and IL-6 (72). Major depression with or without melancholia is characterized by higher plasma levels of IL-1-β, IL-6, sIL–6, sIL-2, and transferrin receptor (TfR). IL-1β, IL-6, TNF-α, macrophage colony stimulating factor (MCSF), transforming growth factor (TGF)-β1, and leukemia inhibiting factor (LIF) have been detected in the reproductive tracts of both men and women (73).

The function of the cytokines IL-1 and IL-6 as bidirectional regulators of neuroendocrine communication has been well studied. IL-1 is locally synthesized in the hypothalamus and hippocampus, areas that are involved in regulating responses to stress and coordinating neural and endocrine functions. Both neurons (74) and glial cells (75) are embryologically related to macrophages and are able to synthesize IL-1. Activation of the HPA axis by IL-1 involves CRH and the stress response system (76, 77). IL-1, particularly IL-1ß, inhibits the HPG axis by suppressing gonadotrophins and sex steroid secretion (77, 78). IL-1 receptors on pituitary cells are upregulated by CRH, which may account for CRH mediated sensitization of the pituitary gland to IL-1. This may also represent a pivotal site where interaction occurs between cytokines and releasing hormones. Thus very mild psychological or physical stress could mediate CRH release and profoundly sensitize the pituitary gland to inflammatory cytokines (72). Administration of IL-1 ß into the brain increases circulating IL-6 levels (79, 80). Recent studies suggest that brain derived IL-1 participates in neurochemical and endocrine responses to stressors. Intracerebroventricular and regional IL-1 ß microinjection produce all the aspects of the acute phase response including peripheral changes such as leukocytosis (81). IL-1 has been found to affect in vitro human granulosa cell estradiol but not progesterone production (82), and data from animal models indicate that inhibition of both estradiol and progesterone secretion occurs in response to IL-1 (83). IL-1ß has also been reported to partially inhibit the attachment of blastocysts to fibronectin matrix but significantly enhanced outgrowth of trophoblast cells from attached blastocysts (84). IL-1 can also stimulate proliferation of placental cell lines (85) but may be toxic to embryos at very high concentrations (86).

IL-6 is both produced by folliculostellate cells of the pituitary gland and able to stimulate LH release from cultured pituitary cells. These cells are thought to be of immune cell origin because they resemble macrophages in many respects (87). Soluble (s) IL-6R originates from monocytes, CD4+ and CD8+ T cells, and activated B cells. IL-6 may upregulate the expression of IL-6R mRNA (88). Locally produced IL-6 participates in regulation of ovarian and Sertoli cell functions (89, 90). IL-6 is also produced by the placenta (90). The IL-6/IL-6R system is implicated in various systemic diseases. Increased levels of sIL-6R have also been described in HIV infection (91) and in some patients with systemic lupus erythematosus (88). Increased IL-6 concentrations in blood have been observed in a variety of immune-related disorders such as systemic lupus erythematosus, rheumatoid arthritis, type I diabetes, HIV disease, and multiple myeloma (88, 93). It is also known that psychological stress may cause increased IL-6 production in rodents (94, 95). IL-6 secretion was increased in culture supernatants of mitogen stimulated peripheral blood monocytes from patients with major depression compared to normal controls (88). There is also a significantly increased plasma concentration of soluble IL-6R (sIL-6R) in major depression (57). Therefore, the positive relationship between IL-6 and sIL-6R concentrations observed in major depression, but not in normal controls, suggests that increased secretion of sIL-6R in depression is related to IL-6 hyperproduction (58). Others have reported that levels of sIL-6R and IL-6 were higher in major depressed subjects than in normal controls (88). A positive relationship between plasma concentrations of IL-6 and IL-2R in major depression, but not in normal controls, has also been reported that may be due to IL-6 involvement in T cell activation, because IL-6 induces IL-2R expression on T cells and increases IL-2 responsiveness (96).

IL-2 is the most potent secretagogue for ACTH known, being even more active than the classic ACTH regulator, CRH. IL-2 has been shown to be produced by human corticotropic adenomas and murine pituitary cells. Increased peripheral blood concentrations of soluble IL-2 receptor (sIL-2R), which is a marker of T cell activation, has been reported in depressed patients (57) and in individuals attempting suicide (97). These data are supportive of studies reporting an increased number of activated T cells (CD25+, HLA-DR+) in patients with major depression (58). IL-2 has also been reported to modulate Sertoli cell function in the testis (89, 90).

Interferons (IFNs) were the first cytokines reported to affect neural and endocrine cells, mediating steroidogenesis, melanogenesis, iodine uptake, excitation of neurons, and binding to opiate receptors (72). IFN-γ has also been reported to inhibit estradiol and progesterone biosynthesis of human granulosa cells, and may modulate apoptosis in the ovary (98). IFN-γ has been reported to have adverse effects on sperm motility (99) and may affect adversely pregnancy by interfering with embryo development and implantation (100), trophoblast outgrowth (101, 102), and trophoblast proliferation (85,103).

The macrophage cytokine TNF-α has been reported to induce the release of pituitary hormones and ACTH (57). TNF-α has also been shown to inhibit granulosa cell synthesis of progesterone and estradiol in vitro (98). TNF-α may also play a role in pregnancy. TNF-α has been reported to facilitate (105) and inhibit (86) mouse embryo development, trophoblast outgrowth (101), and trophoblast proliferation (103). TNF-α has also been reported to inhibit sperm motion parameters by some investigators (99). TNF-α modulates Sertoli cell function (89, 90) and ovarian steroidogenesis (104). TNF-α and TGF-ß2 have been implicated in ultrasonic-induced stress in hamsters and correlated with the increased abortion rate observed in these animals (106). A model of stress-triggered abortion in mice has also been proposed where TNF-α production in the decidua is boosted by release of the neurotransmitter substance P, which regulates TGF-ß2-related suppressive activity, allowing increased TNF-α production (105).

Different hypotheses may explain how cytokines modulated by stress/depression may affect the reproductive system. Cytokines produced in the central nervous system may influence gonadal function by changing hormone production and responsiveness within the HPA axis or through brain–gonad connections bypassing the pituitary (80, 107). Central nervous system cytokines may also cause changes in peripheral leukocyte activation and function (108) and may provoke cascades of cytokines produced peripherally that can modulate specific functions related to reproduction. On the other hand, altered neural stimulation in stress/depression may change directly immune cell activity and cytokine/growth factor balance in the gonads, the placenta, or the genital tract mucosa. There is also the possibility that central cytokines may influence peripheral events through systemic (endocrine) action, because increased levels of cytokines have been detected in the peripheral circulation under stress. Very few cytokines have been studied with regard to their potential psychoneuroendocrine–immune interactions. Probably other cytokines and cytokine receptors in the genital tract can be modulated by stress or depression and play a role in reproduction either as direct effectors or through extensive interactions with other cytokines and growth factors (reviewed in ref. 100) (Fig. 1.1).

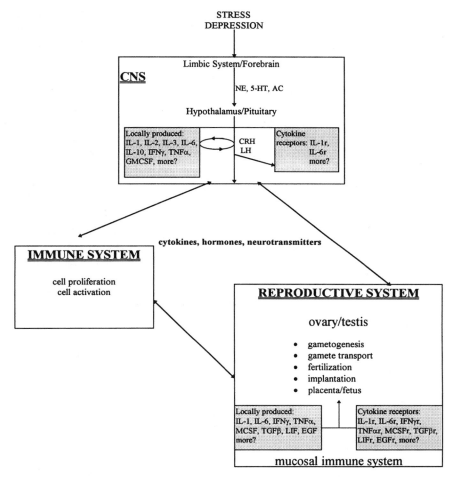

Figure 1.1. A simplified model illustrating psychoneuroendocrine–immune interactions related to reproductive functions. CNS, central nervous system; NE, norepinephrine; 5-HT, serotonin; AC, acetylcholine, CRH; corticotropin releasing hormone; LH, luteinizing hormone.

SUMMARY

The field of reproductive psychopathology is emerging. There are indications of bi-directional communications between the immune, psychoneuroendocrine, and reproductive systems. There is also a considerable amount of controversy associated with this field especially because differentiation between cause and effect phenomena are difficult to define. Whether psychological factors contribute to infertility or merely result from the stress associated with infertility is not known with certainty. Most probably, a circular dynamic exists whereby infertility enhances stress and depression, contributing to further reproductive dysfunction. Correlations between infertility and immune parameters must be studied separately in individuals with defined primary and secondary depression.

CONCLUSION

There is as yet no unified hypothesis that defines clearly the mechanism of how psychological dysfunction is involved with reproduction. Methodological approaches involving research in reproduction are heterogeneous and many studies have lacked proper controls. The term "psychological stress" is generally not well defined. Depending on the author's theoretical or clinical interest, psychological involvement has been called psychogenic (108), psychological (109), idiopathic (8), functional (110), or behavioral (35), or just left unexplained. Methodological differences between studies also make comparisons between results of individual studies difficult. Psychosomatic approaches specifying interactive processes of psychological and biological variables are rarely applied. Animal models involving rodents have most often been used owing to the high cost of the more appropriate primate models. Rodent models are limiting because they may not provide an adequate model of the human condition. The equivalency of psychological stress between rodents and humans is very difficult to define, and both the human male and female genital tracts are anatomically and physiologically different from those of rodents. Adequate methods to obtain objective, valid, and reliable data on psychological and biologic human parameters must be established. Beyond the mechanistic interest, elucidating the role psychoneuroendocrine immunology plays in human reproduction may lead to more effective treatment strategies for restoring normal reproductive function.

REFERENCES

1. Mc Grady AV. Effects of psychological stress on male reproduction: a review. Arch Androl 1984;13:1.
2. McEwen BS, Mendelson S. Effects of stress on the neurochemistry and morphology of the brain: counterregulation versus damage. In: Goldberger L, Bereznitz S, eds. Handbook of Stress: Theoretical and Clinical Aspects. 2nd ed. New York: Free Press, 1993:101–126.
3. Dolan RJ, Calloway SP, Fonngy P, et al. Life events, depression and hypothalamic pituitary adrenal axis function. Br J Psychiatry 1985;147:429–433.
4. Roy A, Picker D, Linnoila M, et al. Cerebrospinal fluid monoamine and monoamire metabolite levels and the dexamethasome suppression tests in depression: relationship to live event. Psychiatry 1986;43:356–360.
5. Bents H. Psychology of male infertility: a literature survey. Int J Androl 1985;8:325.
6. Hochstaedt B, Langer G. Psychoendocrine factors in sterility. Int J Fertil 1959;4:253.
7. McLeod J. Human seminal cytology as sensitive indicator of the germinal epithelium. Int J Fertil 1964;9:281.

8. O'Moore AM, O'Moore RR, Harrison RF, Murphy G, Carruthers ME. Psychosomatic aspects in idiopathic infertility: effects of treatment with autogenic training. J Psychosom Res 1983;27:145.

9. Palti Z. Psychogenic male infertility. Psychosom Med 1969;31:326.

10. Popenoe P. The childless marriage: sexual and marital maladjustments. Fertil Steril 1954;5:168.

11. Sandler B. Emotional stress and infertility. J Psychosom Res 1968; 12:51

12. Agostini R, Patella A, Primiero FM: The endocrine profile in male sterility due to stress. In: Carenza L and Zichella L, eds. Emotions and Reproduction. London: Academic Press, 1979:283.

13. Dominici L, Coghi I, Pancheri P, et al. Psychological evaluation in couples with sterility without apparent cause. In: Carenza L and Zichella L, eds. Emotions and Reproduction. London: Academic Press, 1979:261.

14. Knorre P. Uber das Ausmass korperlicher und psychischer Bbeschwerden steriler Ehepartner. Zbl Gynakol 1981;103:644.

15. Stieve H. Der Einfluss des Nervensystems auf Bau und Tatigkeit der Geschechts-organe des Menschen. Stuttgart: Thieme, 1952.

16. Banks AL, Rutherford RN, Coburn WA. A new medication for the psychogenically infertile couple. West J Surg Obstet Gynecol 1963;71:9.

17. Kaden R. Atiologische faktoren bei fertilitats storungen. Z Haut 1968;43:537.

18. Schuermann H. Uber die Zunahme mannlicher Fertilitatssorungen and uber die Bedeutung psychischer Einflusse fur zentralnervose Regulation der Sermiogenese. Med Klin 1948;43:366.

19. Hellhammer DH, Hubert W, Freischem CW, Nieschlag E. Male infertility: relationship among gonadotrophins, sex steroids, seminal parameters and personality attitudes. Psychosom Med 1985;47:58.

20. Hubert W, Hellhammer DH, Freishem CW. Psychobiological profiles in infertile men. J Psychosom Res 1985;29:161

21. Giblin PT, Poland ML, Moghissi KS. Effects of stress and characteristic adaptability on semen quality in healthy men. Fertil Steril 1988;49:127.

22. Monden Y, Koshiyama K, Tanaka H, Yozumi T, Matsumoto K. Influence of major surgical stress on plasma testosteron, plasma LH and urinary steriods. Acta Endocrinol (copenh) 1972;69:542.

23. Schwartz MF, Kolasky R. Plasmatestosterone levels of sexually functional and disfunctional men. Arch Sex Behav 1980; 9:355.

24. Guyton A. Textbook of Medical Physiology. Philadelphia: Saunders, 1981.

25. Ellis LC, Jaussi AW, Baptista MH et al. Correlation of age changes in monoamine oxidase and androgen synthesis by rat testicular minced and teased-tubular preparation in vitro. Endocrinology 1992;90:1610.

26. Segal S, Sadovsky E, Poeti Z, Pfiefer Y, Polishuk W. Serotonin and 5 HIAA in infertile and subfertile man. Fertil Steril 1975;26:310.

27. Urry RL Pathophysiological principles of male infertility Urol Clin North Am 1981;Feb:3.

28. Urry RL. Stress and infertility In: Cockett ATK, Urry RL, eds. Male Infertility Work-up, Treatment and Research. New York: Grune & Stratton.

29. Ford ESG, Forman I, Wilson JR, Char W, Mixon WT, Scholtz C. A psychodynamic approach to the study of infertility. Fertil Steril 1953;4:456.

30. Morris TA, Sturgis SH. Practical aspects of psychosomatic sterility. Clin Obstet Gynecol 1959;2:890.

31. Sturgis SH, Taymor ML, Morris T. Routine psychiatric interviews in a sterility investigation. Fertil Steril 1957;8:778.

32. Kemeter Peter. Studies on psychosomatic implications of infertility-effects of emotional stress on fertilization and implantation in in-vitro fertilization. Human Reprod 1988;3:341.

33. Wasser SK, Sewall G, Soules MR. Psychosocial stress as a cause of infertility. Fertil Steril 1993;59,3:685.

34. Mozley PD. Psychophysiologic infertility: an overview. Clin Obstet Gynecol 1976;19:407.

35. Mai F, Monday R, Rump E. Psychiatric interview comparisons between infertile and fertile couples. Psychosom Med 1972;34:430.

36. Cooper HC. Psychogenic infertility and adoption. A Afr Med J 1971;45:719

37. Sandler B. Conception after adoption: a comparison of conception rates. Fertil Steril 1965;16:313

38. Seibel MM, Taymor ML. Emotional aspects of infertility. Fertil Steril 1982;37,2:137.

39. Grimm ER. Psychological investigation of habitual abortion. Psychosom Med 1975;57:173.

40. Klock SC, Chang G, Hiley A, Hill JA. Psychological distress among women with recurrent spontaneious abortion. Psychosomatics 1997;38:503–507.

41. Graves WL. Psychological aspects of spontaneous abortion. In: Bennett MJ, Edmonds, DK, eds. Spontaneous and Recurrent Abortion. Oxford: Blackwell Scientific. 1987.

42. Kaij L Mamquist A, Nilsson A. Psychiatric aspects of spontaneous abortion. II. The importance of bereavement attachment and neurosis in early life. J Psychosom Res 1969;13:53.

43. Janerich DT. Stark AD, Greenwald P et al. Increased leukemia, lymphoma and spontaneous abortion in western New York following a flood disaster. Public Health 1981;96:350.

44. O'Hare T, Creed F. Life events and miscarriage. Br J Psychiatr 1995;167:799.

45. Neugebauer R, Kline J, Stein Z, Shrout P, Warburton D, Susser M. Association of stressful life events with chromosomally normal spontaneous abortion. Am J Epidemiol 1996;143:588–596.

46. Scarpellini F, Sbracia M, Scarpellini L. Psychological stress and lipoperoxidation in miscarriage. Ann NY Acad Sci 1994;709:210.

47. Chrousos GP, Gold PW. The concepts of stress and stress system disorders. J Am Med Assoc 1992;267:1244.

48. Sternberg EM, Chrousos GP, Wilder RL, Gold PW The stress response and regulation of inflamatory disease. Ann Intern Med 1992;117:854.

49. Diagnostic and Statistical Manual of Mental Disorders, 4th ed. Washington DC: American Psychiatric Association, 1994:431.

50. Dunn AJ. Stress-related activation of cerebral dopaminergic system. Ann NY Acad Sci 1988;537:188.

51. Black Paul, H. Central nervous system-immune system interactions: Psychoeuroendocrinology of stress and its immune consequences. Antimicrob Agents Chemotherap 1994:38(1):1.

52. Reichlin S. Neuroendocrine interactions. New Engl J Med 1993;329:1246.

53. Vermeulen A. Enviroment, human reproduction, menopause and andropause Environ Health Perspect 1993;101(Suppl. 2):91.

54. Rivier C, Rivest S. Effect of stress on the activity of the hypothalamic-pituitary-gonadal axis: peripheral and central mechanisms. Biol Reprod 1991;45:523.

55. Ferrn M. Neuropeptides, the stress response and hypothalamic-pituitary-gonadal axis in the female rhesus monkey. Ann NY Acad Sci 1993;697:106.

56. Wilder RL Neuroendocrine–immune system interactions and autoimmunity. Ann Rev Immunol 1995;13:307.

57. Black Paul H. Immune system-central nervous system interaction: effect and immunomodulatory consequences of immune system mediators on the brain. Antimicrob Agents Chemotherap 1994:38;1:7.

58. Maes M, Meltzer HY, Bosmans E, Bergmans R, Vandoolaeghe E, Ranjan R, Desnyder R. Increased plasma concentrations if interleukin-6. Soluble interleukin-2 and transferrin receptor in major depression. J Affect Dis 1995;34:301.

59. Maes M, Scharpe S, Meltzer HY, et al. Increased neopterin and interferon–gamma secretion and lower availability of L-tryptophan in major depression: further evidence for an immune response. Psychiatr Res 1994;54:143.

60. Castle S., Wilkins E, Heck K, Tanzy J, Fahey J. Depression in caregivers of demented patients is associated with altered immunity: impaired proliferative capacity, increased CD8+, and a decline in lymphocytes with surface signal transaction molecules (CD38+) and a cytotoxicity marker (CD56+ CD8+). Immunology 1995;101:487.

61. La Via MF, Munno I, Lydiard RB, et al. The influence of stress intrusion on immunodepression in generalized anxiety disorder patients and controls. Psychosom Med 1996;58:138.

62. McKay DM, Bienenstock J. The interaction between mast cells and nerves in the gastrointestinal tract. Immunol Today 1994;15:533.

63. Persoons JH, Schornagel K, Breve J, Berkenbosch F, Kraal G. Acute stress affects cytokines and nitric oxide production by alveolar macrophages differently. Am J Respir Crit Care Med 1995; 152(2):619.

64. Goetzl EJ, Turck CW, Sreedharan SP. Production and recognition of neuropeptides by cells of the immune system. In: Ader R, Felten DL, Cohen N, eds. Psychoneuroimmunology. 2nd ed. San Diego: Academic Press, 1991:263.

65. Smith EM, Ebaugh MJ. Neuroimmunoendocrinology and sexual dimorphism of the immune response. In: Bronson RA, Alexander NJ, Anderson DJ, Branch DW, Kutteh WH, eds. Reproductive Immunology. Cambridge, MA: Blackwell Science, 1996:103.

66. Sternberg EM, Trial J, Parker CW. Effect of serotonin on murine macrophages: suppression on Ig expression by serotonin and its reversal by 5 HT serotonergic receptor antagonists. J Immunol 1986;137:276.

67. Sternberg EM, Wender HJ, Leung MK, Parker CW. Effect on serotonin (5HT) and other monoamines on murine macrophages: modulation of IFN-α induced phagocytosis J Immunol 1987;138:4360.

68. Jackson JC, Walker RF, Brooks WH, Roszman TL. Specific uptake of serotonin by murine macrophages. Life Sci 1988;42:1641.

69. Jones TH, Kennedy RL. Cytokines and hypothalamic-pituitary function. Cytokine 1993;5:531.

70. Imura H, Fukata J-I. Endocrine-paracrine interactions in communication between the immune and endocrine systems. Activation of the hypothalamic-pituitary-adrenal axis in inflammation. Eur J Endocrinol 1994;130:32.

71. Hughes TK, Cadet P, Rady PL, et al. Evidence for the production and action of IL-10 in pituitary cells. Cell Mol Neurobiol 1994;14:59.

72. Blalock JE. The syntax of immune-neuroendocrine communication. Immunol Today 1994;15,11:504.

73. Best CL, Hill AH. Immunology of unexplained infertility. Infertil Reprod Medicine. Clin North Am. 1997

74. Lechan RM, Toni R, Clark BD, et al. Immunoreactive interleukine-1b localization in the rat forebrain. Brain Res. 1990;514:135.

75. Yao J, Keri JE, Taffs RE, Colton CA. Characterization of interleukin-1 production by microglia in culture. Brain Res. 1992;591:88.

76. Breder CD, Dinarello CA, Saper C. Interleukin-1 immunoreactive innervation of the hypothalamus.Science 1988;240:321.

77. Bertini R, Bianci M, Ghezzi P. Adrenectomy sensitizes mice to the lethal effects of IL-1 and tumor necrosis factor. J. Exp Med 1988;167:1708.

78. Rivier C, Vale W. Cytokines act within brain to inhibit luteinizing hormone secretion and ovulation in the rat. Endocrinology 1990;127:849.

79. Rettori V, Gimeno MF, Karara A, Gonzalez MC, McCaan SM. Interleukin-1 inhibits prostaglandin E2 release to suppress pulsatile release of luteinizing hormone, but not follicle stimulating hormone. Proc Natl Acad Sci USA 1991;88:2763.

80. Turnbull A, Rivier C. Brain–periphery connections: do they play a role in mediating the effect of centrally injected interleukin-on gonadal function? Neuroimmunomodulation. 1995;2:224.

81. Morimoto A Watanabe T, Sakata Y, Murakami N. Leukocytosis induced by microinjection of endogenous pyrogen or interleukin-1 into preoptic and anterior hypothalamus. Brain Res 1998;475:345.

82. Best CL, Hill JA. Interleukin-1 alpha and beta modulation of luteinized human granulosa cell estrogen and progesterone biosynthesis. Human Reprod, 1996;10:3206

83. Adashi EY, Resnick CE, Packman JN, et al. Cytokine–mediated regulation of ovarian function: Tumor necrosis factor-α inhibits gonadotropin–supported progesterone accumulation by differentiating and luteinized murine granulosa cells. Am J Obstet Gynecol, 1990;162:889.

84. Haimovici F, Hill JA, Anderson DJ. The effect of soluble products of activated lymphocytes and macrophages on blastocyst implantation events in vitro. Biol Reprod 1991;44:69

85. Hunt JS, Soares MJ, Lei MG, Smith RN, Wheaton D, Atherton RA, Morrison DE. Products of lipopolysaccharide-activated macrophages (tumor necrosis factor-a, transforming growth factor-a) but not lipopolysaccharide modify DNA synthesis by rat trophoblast cells exhibiting the 80-kDa lipopolysaccharide–binding protein. J Immunol 1989;143:1606.

86. Hill JA, Haimovici F, Anderson DJ. Products of activated T-lymphocytes and macrophages inhibit mouse embryo development in vitro. J Immunol 1987;139:2250.

87. Lyson K, McCann SM. The effect of interleukin-6 on pituitary hormone release in vivo and in vitro. Neuroendocrinology 1991;54:262.

88. Bock GR, Marsh J, Widdows K. Polyfunctional Cytokines: IL-6 and LIF. In: 1987 Ciba Foundation Symposium 167. Chichester, UK: John Wiley.

89. Brannstorm M, Norman RJ, Seamark RF, Robertson SA. Rat ovary produces cytokines during ovulation. Biol Reprod 1994;50:88.

90. Brookfor FR, Scwartz LK. Effects of interleukin-6 , interleukin-2 and tumor necrosis factor a on transferrin release from Sertoli cells in culture. Endocrinology 1991;129:256.

91. Kauma SW Herman K, Wang Y, Walsh SW. differential mRNA expression and production of interleukin-6 in placental trophoblast and vilous core compartments. Am J Reprod Med 1993;30:131.

92. Honda M, Yamamoto S, Cheng M, et al. Human soluble IL-6 receptor: its detection and enhanced released by HIV infection. J. Immunol 1992;148:2175.

93. Spronk PE Borg EJ, Limburg PC Kallenberg CGM. Plasma concentration of IL-6 in systemic lupus erythematosus; an indicator of disease activity. Clin Exp Immunol 1992;90:106.

94. Zhou D, Kusnecov AW, Shurin MR, DePaoli M, Rabin BS. Exposure to physical and psychological stressors elevates plasma interleukin-6: relationship to activation of hypothalamic-pituitary-adrenal axis. Endocrinology 1993;133:2523.

95. LeMay LG, Vander AJ, Kluger MJ. The effects of psychological stress on plasma interleukin-6 activity in rats. Physiol Behav1990;47:957.

96. Vink A, Uyttenhove C, Wauters P, Van Snick J. Accessory factors involved in murine T cell activation. Distinct roles of interleukin-6, interleukin-1 and tumor necrosis factor. Eur J Immunol 1990;20:1.

97. Nassberger l, Traskman-Bbendz l. Increased soluble interleukin-II receptor concentrations in suicide attempters. Acta Psychiatr Scand 1993;88:48.

98. Best CL, Griffin PM, Hill JA. Interferon gamma inhibits luteinized human granulosa cell steroid production in vitro. Am J Obstet Gynecol 1995;172:1505

99. Hill JA, Haimovici F, Politch JA, Anderson DJ. Effects of soluble products of activated lymphocytes and macrophages (lymphokines and monokines) on human sperm motion parameters. Fertil Steril 1987;47:460.

    Haimovici F, Anderson DJ. Cytokines and growth factors in implantation. Microsc Res Technol 1993;25:201.

100. Haimovici F, Anderson DJ Effects of growth factors and growth factor–extracellular matrix interaction on mouse trophoblast outgrowth in vitro. Biol Reprod 1993 49:124.

101. Suffys P, Beyaert R, Van RF, Fiers W. TNF in combination with interferon gamma is cytotoxic to normal untransformed mouse and rat embryo fibroblast-like cells. Anticancer Res. 1989;9:167.

102. Berkowitz RS, Hill JA, Kurtz CB, Anderson JA. Effects of products of activated leukocytes (lymphokines and monokines) on the growth of malignant trophoblast cells in vitro. Am J Obstet Gynecol 1988;158:199.

103. Best CL, Pudney J, Anderson DJ, et al. Modulation of human granulosa cell steroid production in vitro by tumor necrosis factor alpha: Implications of white blood cells in culture. Obstet Gynecol, 1994; 84:121.

104. Paria BC, Dey SK. Preimplantation embryo development in vitro: Cooperative interaction among embryos and role of growth factors. Proc Natl Acad Sci USA 1990;87:4756.

105. Ark PC, Merali FS, Manuel J, Chaouat G, Clark DA. Stress-triggered abortion: inhibition of protective suppression and promotion of tumor necrosis factor-a (TNF-a) release as a mechanism triggering resorptions in mice. AJRI 1995;33(1):74.

106. Clark DA, ArkPC, Jalali R, Merali FS, Manuel J, Chaouat G, Underwood JL, Mowbray JF. Psycho–neuro–cytokine/endocrine pathways in immunoregulation during pregnancy. AJRI 1996;35:330

107. Maier SF, Watkins LR. Intracerebroventricular interleukin-1 receptor antagonist blocks the enhancement of fear conditioning and interference with escape produced by inescapable shock. Brain Res 1995;695:279.

108. Rutherford RN, Klemer RH, Banks AL, Coburn WA. Psychogenic infertility from the male viewpoint. Pac Med Surg. 1979;74:131.

109. Carr GD. A psycholosociobiological study of fertile and infertile marriages. Inaug. Diss, USC, Los Angeles 1963.

110. Goldschmidt O, de Boor C. Psychoanal Psyche 1976;30:899.

2

CYTOKINES AND TESTICULAR FUNCTION

Dale Buchanan Hales

University of Illinois at Chicago, Chicago, Illinois

Inflammatory disease has long been known to affect male reproductive function. Inflammatory disease is known to be associated with elevated levels of pro-inflammatory cytokines. There is a mounting body of evidence that demonstrates the importance of cytokines in the regulation of testicular function during pathophysiological states as well as under normal physiological conditions, when cytokines act as growth and differentiation factors. The purpose of this chapter is to examine the role of cytokines in the regulation of steroidogenesis and spermatogenesis during normal and pathophysiological states.

Spermatogenesis is an autonomous process largely under the control of paracrine factors. Growth factors and cytokines that potentially exert effects on spermatogenic cell populations are produced within the seminiferous epithelium and influence post-meiotic stages of spermatogenesis. Although the importance of follicle-stimulating hormone and androgens to the initiation and maintenance of spermatogenesis is clearly documented, the role of paracrine regulatory factors remains to be elucidated. Spermatogenesis is a compartmentalized and continuous process that takes place sequestered within the blood–testis barrier, thus there is a need for regulation by locally produced factors. Androgen production by the Leydig cells takes place in the vascu-

Cytokines in Human Reproduction, Edited by Joseph A. Hill
ISBN 0-471-35242-X   Copyright © 2000 Wiley-Liss, Inc.

larized interstitial tissue of the testis, and testosterone is produced for both the seminiferous tubule compartment and the peripheral circulation for delivery to extratesticular androgen target tissues. Owing to the nature of testicular compartmentalization both anatomically and functionally, regulation of interstitial cell numbers and functions is under the control of both extra- and intratesticularly elaborated factors.

Cytokines are a broadly defined group of polypeptide mediators involved in the communication network of cells of the immune system (1). In addition, cytokines have important activities outside of the immune system. In particular, cytokines are known to regulate testicular steroid hormone production during inflammation. Cytokines have been implicated as novel growth and differentiation factors involved in the regulation of cells in both compartments of the testis. Cytokines are important factors in the integration of the neuro–endocrine–immune network that controls testicular function. Recent reviews have examined the control of testis function by locally produced peptides (2), cell–cell interactions (3, 4) growth factors (5, 6), neuronal signals (7), neuroendocrine mechanisms (8, 9), and inflammatory mediators (10). This chapter presents an overview of the neuroendocrine–immune networks that control testicular functions during inflammation and under normal physiologic conditions.

INFLAMMATION AND REPRODUCTION

It has long been appreciated that chronic inflammation and systemic infection are associated with decreased reproductive capacity (for a review see ref. 8). Men with critical illness, burn trauma, sepsis, and rheumatoid arthritis are reported to have markedly reduced serum testosterone levels (11–21). Experimental adjuvant induced arthritis (22) results in similar dramatic decreases in serum testosterone levels in rodents. Injection of lipopolysaccharide (LPS), an endotoxin derived from the cell walls of gram negative bacteria, results in the inhibition of gonadal steroidogenesis. Studies from Bosmann et al. demonstrated that LPS injected male mice have markedly reduced serum testosterone levels (23). Studies from Sancho-Tello et al. showed that LPS injection resulted in the inhibition of ovarian steroidogenesis in female rats (24). Induction of sepsis in rats with cecal slurry results in a significant decrease in testosterone (25).

Lipopolysaccharide and Endotoxemia

The presence of LPS signals the presence of gram-negative bacteria. Recognition of LPS triggers gene induction by immune and nonimmune cells, principally monocyte/macrophages of myeloid lineage. These inducible genes include cytokines, adhesion proteins, and enzymes that produce low molecular weight inflammatory mediators. Together the products of these inducible genes upregulate host defense systems that participate in eliminating the bacterial infection (26). When purified from gram negative bacteria and injected into experimental animals, LPS induces an array of physiological responses. LPS can provoke many of the same pathophysiological symptoms that are characteristic of gram-negative infection (e.g., fever, vaso-constriction, hypoglycemia, systemic arterial hypotension, diarrhea, shock, and death). Host responsiveness to LPS is under genetic control and has been mapped to the "LPS gene" (27).

LPS induces the production of the pro-inflammatory cytokines, principally IL-1, TNF-α, and IL-6 by activated immune cells (28). There is a hierarchy of cytokine secretion, with TNF-α levels peaking and declining rapidly, followed by IL-1, then IL-6, which remains elevated. The LPS response is also characterized by stimulation of the hypothalamus–pituitary–adrenal axis (HPA) (8, 9, 29, 30), activation of the sympathetic nervous system (31–34) increases in peripheral prostaglandin levels (35, 36), and rapid increases in levels of the neurohypophyseal hormone arginine vasopressin (AVP) (36–41). LPS stimulates the expression of the inducible form of nitric oxide synthase (iNOS) and causes plasma and tissue levels of NO to increase (42, 43). Thus the systemic response to LPS results in the production of a host of inflammatory mediators and signals that are known effectors of Leydig cell steroidogenesis. In addition to soluble, blood borne messengers released in response to LPS, direct neuronal connections may deliver regulatory signals to Leydig cells (7, 9, 44–46), as has been shown in the ovary (47, 48). Indeed, LPS itself may exert a direct inhibitory effect on Leydig cells, as has been shown in the ovary (24, 49, 50).

Leydig Cells and Steroidogenesis

Leydig cells are the site of androgen production in the testis. The principal and most important androgen produced by Leydig cells is testosterone. Testosterone biosynthesis is primarily under the control of the pituitary gonadotropin luteinizing hormone (LH). LH stimulates the production of cAMP by binding to specific receptors on the surface of Leydig cells that are coupled to adenylate cyclase. Human chorionic gonadotropin (hCG) binds to LH receptors and is used to study LH action. Cyclic AMP is the intracellular second messenger for LH and mediates LH action in Leydig cells by activating the cAMP-dependent protein kinase, PKA (for a review see ref. 51). Cyclic AMP has two principal activities in the control of Leydig cell steroidogenesis. The first action of cAMP is the acute stimulation of testosterone biosynthesis via mobilization and transport of cholesterol into the steroidogenic pathway, an action that takes place within minutes. The second action of cAMP in Leydig cells is the chronic and prolonged stimulation of gene expression of the steroidogenic enzymes, a slower action that requires several hours (for a review see ref. 52).

Testosterone biosynthesis depends on the action of two cytochrome P450 enzymes and two flavoprotein dehydrogenase enzymes. The first and rate-limiting *enzymatic* step in testosterone synthesis is the conversion of cholesterol to pregnenolone that is catalyzed by cholesterol side-chain cleavage (P450scc), encoded by the *Cyp11A1* gene, located on the inner mitochondrial membrane. Pregnenolone diffuses out of the mitochondria to the smooth endoplasmic reticulum, where it is further metabolized via the action of 3ß-hydroxysteroid dehydrogenase Δ^4-Δ^5-isomerase (3ß-HSD) to progesterone. Progesterone in turn is converted by a two step process to androstenedione via the action of 17α-hydroxylase/C_{17-20} lyase (P450c17), encoded by the

Cyp17 gene. The conversion of androstenedione to testosterone is catalyzed by 17ß-hydroxysteroid dehydrogenase (17ß-HSD) (for reviews see refs. 53, 54).

Cholesterol is the precursor for all steroid hormones. Regardless of its source, its mobilization and transport into the inner mitochondrial membrane to P450scc is cAMP-dependent. Transfer of cholesterol across the inner mitochondrial space is regulated by, and dependent on, the action of steroidogenic acute regulatory protein (StAR). It has long been appreciated that acute production of steroids depends on a hormone stimulated, rapidly synthesized, and highly labile protein whose function is to mediate the transfer of cholesterol from the outer mitochondria to the inner mitochondrial membrane to P450scc. Although several candidate proteins have been considered, StAR is the only protein that has all of the necessary characteristics of the acute regulatory protein (52). The discovery that a deficiency in StAR accounts for the genetic defect associated with congenital adrenal lipoid hyperplasia was the essential proof of StAR's critical role in the acute regulation of steroidogenesis (55).

Testosterone is essential for the maintenance of spermatogenesis (56). Recent studies have demonstrated the importance of high local concentrations of androgens to the development of functional spermatozoa (57–62). Moreover, maintenance of accessory duct function depends on high concentrations of testosterone (63). One mechanism subserving inflammatory disease-associated decreases in male fertility is inhibition of testosterone production.

IMMUNE–ENDOCRINE CONTROL OF LEYDIG CELL FUNCTION

Although there is some controversy about the effect of cytokines on basal testosterone synthesis, the overwhelming consensus is that pro-inflammatory cytokines inhibit gonadotropin or cAMP-stimulated steroidogenesis in Leydig cells (for a review see ref. 10). Many factors have been implicated in mediating the pathological effects associated with endotoxemia and sepsis, cytokines are generally believed to be the decisive factors in determining the pathology (64–66). The cytokines most strongly associated with LPS endotoxemia and sepsis are TNF, IL-1, and IL-6. Considerable attention has been paid to the effects of TNF and IL-1 on Leydig cell function, but the effects of IL-6 have not been as extensively studied (9). Cytokines are released in a sequential manner following exposure to bacterial endotoxin resulting in a cytokine cascade (64). IFN-γ and IL-2 are also elevated in amounts that correlate with the severity of illness. With the exception of IL-6, each of these cytokines (TNF, IL-1, IFN-γ, and IL-2) has been shown to inhibit cAMP-stimulated steroidogenesis in Leydig cells at the level of steroidogenic enzyme gene expression (10). Recently, IL-6 was shown to have similar effects on Leydig cell steroidogenesis and inhibit cAMP-stimulated testosterone and P450c17 mRNA expression. IL-6 is unique in that it also inhibits the cAMP-induced expression of 17ß-HSD (type 3) in Leydig cells. It is noteworthy that the distal cytokine in the pro-inflammatory cascade inhibits the last enzyme in testosterone biosynthetic pathway (67). Testosterone production in Leydig cells is primarily under the control of LH acting via cAMP second messenger system. Cyclic AMP has two major roles in steroidogenesis: acute stimulation of cholesterol transfer to the inner mitochondria and chronic stimulation of steroidogenic enzyme gene expression. LPS endotoxemia results in a biphasic inhibition of steroidogenesis—acute inhibition at the level of cholesterol transport and chronic inhibition at the level of steroidogenic enzyme gene expression (23).

Leydig Cells and Macrophages

Leydig cells and macrophages in the interstitial tissue of the testis are closely associated. This close physical association suggests that testicular interstitial macrophages and Leydig cells are functionally related (10). Resident macrophages have specialized functions in addition to the classical macrophage activities. The structural, phagocytic, and immunological functions of resident testicular macrophages appear to be normal (68–70), and they express major histocompatibility complex class II (MHC II) molecules characteristic of normal antigen presenting cells (71, 72). Immune activated testicular macrophages have been shown to express mRNA for IL-1 α IL-6, TNF-α, and granulocyte macrophage colony stimulating factor (GM-CSF) (74–76) and secrete bioactive IL-1, IL-6, TNF-α, and GM-CSF protein (74, 76–78). Although testicular macrophages have numerous characteristics common to macrophages from other sources, they have unique and highly specialized properties, presumably important for their interaction with Leydig cells. Though testicular macrophages have been shown to secrete cytokines, as described above, it has been suggested that they have a blunted secretory response compared to peritoneal macrophages (76, 78). In addition, testicular macrophages demonstrate a pattern of protein secretion distinct from peritoneal macrophages (79) and express FSH receptors (80, 81).

Morphological examination of the adult rat testis indicated that there was a direct structural interaction between these cells (82). Cytoplasmic processes of Leydig cells were observed that extended to membrane invaginations of adjacent macrophages (68, 82). These specialized membrane associations have been termed "digitations" (69). During development, changes in Leydig cell and macrophage morphology are coordinated (83, 84). Macrophages are present in the rodent testis throughout postnatal prepubertal development (85). Macrophages also have been identified in the interstitial tissue of the human testis (86).

LPS injection stimulates the local expression of TNF-α by testicular interstitial macrophages (for a review see refs. 10, 69). TNF-α expression can be induced in isolated testicular macrophages in vitro (74, 77). In addition, testicular macrophages have been shown to produce IL-1 in vivo (73) and in vitro (76, 78). Thus testicular macrophages express and secrete TNF and IL-1 in the microenvironment of the Leydig cell. The local concentration of these cytokines is likely to be very high and will produce immediate and sustained inhibitory effects on Leydig cell function. In addition to testicular macrophages as paracrine sources of cytokines, many other testicular cells have been shown to produce cytokines in the microenvironment of the Leydig cell (for a review see ref. 54). In particular, Sertoli cells are known to secrete IL-1 and IL-6 (87–92). Thus there are several potential paracrine sources of cytokines, in addition to resident testicular macrophages. Furthermore, there is a large peripheral response to LPS (for reviews see refs. 28, 65, 93–97). LPS injection results in a rapid peripheral increase in TNF (75). Thus systemic increases in pro-inflammatory cytokines are of sufficient magnitude to contribute to the inhibition of Leydig cell function. Moreover, Leydig cells themselves are a potential source of pro-inflammatory cytokines. Leydig cells express and produce IL-1, TNF, and IL-6, suggesting a possible autocrine regulatory role of these cytokines on Leydig cell function (98–101). It is clear from these studies that Leydig cells are exposed to cytokines from the peripheral circulation, from adjacent testicular cells, and from Leydig cells themselves.

EFFECTS OF CYTOKINES ON LEYDIG CELL STEROIDOGENESIS

Interleukin-1

Interleukin-1 (IL-1) is a family of three distinct single-chain glycosylated 17 kDa proteins, IL-α, IL-1ß, and IL-1 receptor antagonist (IL-1a). IL-1α and ß share only 22% amino acid homology but bind to the same receptors and have similar biological activities. Both are important in the initiation of an inflammatory response, and coordinate the proliferation and activation of T lymphocytes, B lymphocytes, and monocytes. IL-1Ra is a naturally occurring antagonist that modulates the activity and toxicity of IL-1α and IL-1ß. IL-1α and ß are secreted by a host of differentiated cells, but most characteristicaly by activated macrophages and monocytes (for a review see ref. 102).

A review of the literature on the effects of IL-1 on basal testosterone production reveals that IL-1 is either stimulatory or has no effect (103–105). However, there is general agreement that IL-1 inhibits LH/hCG and/or cAMP stimulated testosterone production (73, 103, 104, 106–110). The major site of inhibition is at the level of the 17α-hydroxylase/C_{17-20} lyase enzyme. IL-1 causes a dose-dependent inhibition of cAMP-stimulated induction of P450c17 expression in macrophage depleted mouse Leydig cells in primary culture. IL-1 mediated inhibition of testosterone biosynthesis was primarily mediated by the inhibition of P450c17 (109). IL-1 inhibited cAMP-induction of P450c17, P450scc, and 3 ß-HSD, but did not inhibit the basal or constitutive expression of these enzymes (109, 111).

Tumor Necrosis Factor α

TNF-α is a 17 kDa glycosylated polypeptide secreted principally by activated monocytes and macrophages (65). It binds as a trimer to either of the two TNF receptors, which are found on most cells in the body, and plays a central role in the initiation of the inflammatory response (28). TNF-A stimulates the release of IL-1 and IL-6 from activated monocytes and macrophages, and its synthesis and release is enhanced by interferon- γ (IFN-γ) secreted from activated T lymphocytes (66). The sequelae following immune activation in vivo are complex but the network of cytokines that are produced depend on the secretion of TNF-α (28).

There are a number of reports in the literature describing the effects of TNF-α on Leydig cell steroidogenesis (75, 112–118). Although one group concludes that

TNF-α stimulates steroidogenesis (118), the majority of these reports describe inhibitory effects and a decrease in the production of testosterone. These studies have been performed in a variety of systems, including whole animal studies (114, 115), isolated primary cultures of Leydig cells (116, 117), and MA-10 tumor Leydig cells transfected with Cyp17-reporter constructs (113). TNF-α mediated inhibition of hCG binding has been reported (116), but the majority of these reports suggest that TNF-α inhibition occurs downstream of cAMP production, at the level of steroidogenic gene expression. In mouse Leydig cells in primary culture, TNF-α caused a decrease in P450scc, P450c17, and 3ßHSD expression (117). TNF-α has no effect on the basal expression of P450scc but does inhibit basal expression of 3ßHSD (111).

Other Cytokines

IL-2 is primarily a T cell growth factor that enhances the activity and formation of cytotoxic cells. IL-2 also stimulates TNF-α, IL-1, and IFN secretion. IL-2 inhibits gonadotropin-stimulated testosterone production by rat Leydig cells at the level of the P450c17 enzyme, similar to TNF-α, and IL-1 (119). Male patients treated with high doses of IL-2, as therapy for metastatic cancer, had significantly reduced serum testosterone levels (115). IL-2 causes a robust peripheral response resulting in elevation of numerous serum cytokines, in particular, TNF-α, IL-1, and IFN-γ (120, 121). The inhibitory effects of IL-2 could therefore be directly on Leydig cells, or indirectly mediated by activation of testicular macrophage TNF-α and IL-1 secretion. IL-2, similar to other cytokines, stimulates the hypothalamus–pituitary–adrenal axis, resulting in increased ACTH and corticosteroid levels. Glucocorticoids have direct inhibitory effects on Leydig cell steroidogenesis; thus elevated glucocorticoids could also contribute to the in vivo inhibitory effects of IL-2 (122).

Interferons (IFNs) are a group of structurally and functionally related polypeptides that comprise three main groups, IFN-α, IFN-ß, and IFN-γ. The best known effects of IFNs are their antiviral, antiproliferative, and immunomodulatory actions. The major cellular sources for the interferons are different: IFN-α is produced by monocyte/macrophages, IFN-ß is produced by fibroblasts and epithelial cells, and IFN-γ is produced by T-lymphocytes (for a review see ref. 123). IFNs have also been shown to have effects on the endocrine system. In particular, both IFN-α and IFN-γ have been shown to inhibit testosterone production in primary cultures of porcine Leydig cells (124, 125). IFN-γ exerts its inhibitory effect on testosterone production at the level of cholesterol transport into the mitochondria. IFN-γ inhibits the expression of both P450scc and P450c17 (126), similar to the effect of TNF-α on mouse Leydig cells (117). Normal healthy men who were treated with human leukocyte-derived IFN (IFN-α) had significantly decreased serum testosterone levels (127). The observed decrease in testosterone was most likely due to a direct inhibition of Leydig cell steroidogenesis because serum gonadotropin levels were unaffected by the treatment.

Transforming growth factor ß (TGF-ß) belongs to a family of at least five distinct dimeric proteins, of which three are expressed in mammals (ß1, ß2, ß3). These proteins are part of the superfamily of dimeric proteins that includes inhibin, activin, and anti-Mullerian hormone. TGF-ß proteins are multifunctional growth and differentiation factors involved in many aspects of tissue remodeling and repair as well as interacting with cytokines in the regulation of the immune system. Nearly all cells synthesize a form of TGF-ß and possess functional membrane receptors for this family of polypeptides. In vitro studies have shown that TGF-ß is a potent inhibitor of Leydig cell steroidogenesis. TGF-ß inhibits steroidogenesis at the level of LH receptor number and signaling as well as distal to cAMP production at the level of P450c17 expression (for a review see ref. 128).

PATHOLOGY AND TESTIS FUNCTION

The question arises, then, why is there a mechanism in place for the cytokine-mediated inhibition of testosterone production? It is widely recognized that in most species studied, males have weaker immune responses than females (129–131). The weaker immune response contributes to higher susceptibility to infection, and poorer survival of males compared to females. One consequence of the increased immune response in females, compared to males, is an increased incidence of autoimmune disease (13, 129). Studies in many experimental models have established that the underlying basis for this sex-related difference in susceptibility is due to differences in gonadal steroids. Indeed, androgens are immunosuppressive and often used for the treatment of autoimmune disorders such as rheumatoid arthritis (13). The effects of androgens on peripheral blood monocytes collected from patients with rheumatoid arthritis indicated that testosterone inhibited IL-1 secretion, which was interpreted to suggest that men with lower androgen levels are more susceptible to the disease (132). Moreover, dihydrotestosterone depresses the production of IL-4, IL-5, and IFN-γ by activated murine T lymphocytes, suggesting that androgens are important in the regulation of certain aspects of the immune response (133). Administration of testosterone decreases thymus weight and causes a depletion of cortical lymphocytes, whereas castration causes thymic hyperplasia due to withdrawal of androgenic steroids. The mechanism of androgen-induced thymolysis is unknown, but it has been suggested that nonlymphoid cells in the thymus are targets for androgens and that these nonlymphoid cells mediate the androgen-induced depletion of thymocytes (134). The testis has long been considered as immunologically privileged and it has been suggested that locally produced androgens are immunosuppressive and important to testicular immune privilege (71). These observations, together with the data that demonstrate that cytokines are elevated during conditions associated with decreased serum testosterone, provide the basis for the hypothesis: in order for the animal to wage the maximum possible immune response, products of the immune reaction (cytokines) inhibit the production of immunosuppresive androgens.

Nature provides an example that supports this hypothesis. The male marsupial mouse, *Antechinus stuartii*, is overtly preoccupied with copulation and dies abruptly at the conclusion of the mating season (135). In contrast, the female *A. stuartii* is longer lived and survives several mating seasons. To determine the mechanism behind the difference in longevity between males and females, autopsies of males revealed a variety of disease states, all associated with suppression of immune and inflammatory responses. It was observed that castrated males survived in the field well beyond the period of natural mortality. Males who were captured and raised in a pathogen-free environment lived up to 3 years, equivalent to the life-span of females (136). Thus these observations support the hypothesis that androgens are immunosuppressive. It follows, then, that inhibition (or removal) of androgens allows the animal to mount an effective immune response.

Autoimmune Disease of the Testis

When the immune system encounters testis-specific autoantigens, they are recognized as foreign despite their endogenous origin. Thus antibodies to sperm antigens are elicited in animal models of experimental autoimmune orchitis (EAO) when animals are immunized with autologous sperm or testicular cells. Animal models of EAO have provided important insights into human pathological incidence of autoimmune orchitis that results from testicular injury associated with biopsy, vasectomy, or an obstructed vas deferens (137). Indeed, there is a correlation between elevated anti-sperm antibodies and testicular lesions after vasectomy (138). Similar inflammatory changes have also been reported in the epididymis after vasectomy (139).

Historically, the sole mechanism believed to be necessary to protect autologous sperm antigens against immune destruction was their sequestration behind the blood–testis barrier. However, evidence has emerged suggesting testis autoantigens are exposed to circulating immune cells and that active immunoregulatory mechanisms are involved in preventing autoimmune responses to testis antigens (137). The blood–testis barrier is composed of tight junctions between adjacent Sertoli cells and the basal laminae of the seminiferous epithelium and separates germ cells in the basal compartment from those in the adluminal compartment. This barrier prevents antibody and lymphoid cells from reaching the adluminal compartment, and normally, lymphocytes and macrophages are not detected on the adluminal side of the tubule. Germ cell stages sequestered within the tubule include pachytene spermatozoa, spermatids, and testicular spermatozoa. All known orchitogenic antigens are present within the protected compartment (137). It is presumed that mechanisms subserving the pathogenesis of EAO are responsible for the etiology of autoimmune orchitis in humans. The progression of the disease is first accompanied by activation of testicular macrophages surrounding the tubules, demonstrated by a 20-fold increase in Ia+ immunoreactivity. Stimulation of macrophages and upregulation of Ia+ depends on circulating interferon (IFN-γ) and requires CD4+ lymphocytes. Evidence suggests sperm antigens are presented by IFN-γ stimulated MHC class II cells (Ia+ macrophages) to activated CD4+ lymphocytes which in turn initiate lesions in tubules and vas deferens (137). Once the blood–testis barrier is breached, immune complexes are formed outside the barrier on the peritubular basal lamina. The T cell response is then potentiated by the ensuing inflammatory response resulting from activation of macrophages that remove the exposed intratubular germ cells.

Orchitis is the most common complication of mumps in postpubertal men. Mumps orchitis is characterized by decreased serum testosterone and impaired Leydig cell responsiveness to gonadotropin (140). The etiology of orchitis in mumps has not been determined but it has been suggested that autoantigens from the salivary gland cross react with testicular antigens, resulting in autoimmune orchitis (Ken Tung, personal communication). Infection by the mumps virus results in elevated IFN-γ secretion, and IFN-γ activates a number of macrophage functions including upregulation of MHC class II antigens and cytokine secretion (123). Presumably the accompanying inflammatory response observed in autoimmune orchitis results in the elaboration of a cascade of pro-inflammatory cytokines. The resultant sequelae of cytokine secretion in the microenvironment of the testis likely affects Leydig cell function. Indeed, a characteristic consequence of vasectomy is marked depression of testicular androgen output with concomitant increase in LH secretion (141–144).

IMMUNE–ENDOCRINE INTERACTIONS IN THE TESTIS

In addition to macrophages, lymphocytes and other immune cells are found in the rodent (145) and human testis (72) and thus can also serve as potential sources for immune regulatory molecules such as lymphocyte derived cytokines (IFN-γ and IL-2). Leydig cells are also known to interact directly with lymphocytes, as well as with macrophages. In fact, Leydig cells are the only normal highly differentiated endocrine cells that spontaneously form rosettes with lymphocytes, macrophages, and eosinophils, consistent with specific receptors and recognition molecules encoded on the surface of Leydig cells (146). Following depletion of testicular Leydig cells by EDS injection (see below), precursor Leydig cells are recruited, proliferate, differentiate, and within a month repopulate the testis with normal adult Leydig cells. Mast cells proliferate and differentiate in parallel to Leydig cells and are subject to the same regulatory influences (147). It has been suggested that Leydig cells mediate local regulation of testicular leukocyte populations (148). Indeed, Leydig cells, macrophages, and Sertoli cells are all sources for immunoregulatory polypeptides (for a review see refs. 2 and 149).

The testis is considered to be an immunologically privileged site. Allografts and xenografts have been shown to survive in the testes of rodents (71). Despite the presence of normal components of the immune system (macrophages and lymphocytes) the regulation of these cells in the testis must be altered. Testicular macrophages constitute approximately 25% of the cells of the interstitium and have numerous characteristics of macrophages from other tissues, including structural, phagocytic, bactericidal functions, and express major histocompatibility complex class II (MHC II) molecules and Fc receptors (for a review see ref. 69). Macrophages participate in the initiation of the immune response by antigen presentation and co-stimulation of T lymphocytes, and by secreting pro-inflammatory cytokines, in particular, IL-1 (150). In addition to pro-inflammatory cytokines, macrophages also secrete anti-inflammatory cytokines such as TGF-ß and IL-1 receptor antagonist. Thus there exists a dynamic balance between immune activation and suppression. Androgens are also known to be immunosuppressive, in particular toward T lymphocyte mediated responses (133). It is possible that immunologic suppression of the testis is due, in part, to the high local concentration of testosterone in the interstitial tissue. Indeed, androgens have been shown to inhibit IL-1 secretion by blood mononuclear cells (132), and orchidectomy markedly increases the number of macrophages in the adrenal cortex, suggesting that androgens regulate macrophage numbers as well as secretory activities (151). Thus it is entirely plausible that macrophage activitation of T lymphocytes is inhibited in the androgen rich milieu of the testis. Leydig cells may also secrete other factors, in addition to steroid hormones, that regulate macrophages and/or affect the immune reactivity of the testis (148, 152, 153). Among these potential immune regulatory factors, pro-opiomelanocortin (POMC) and derived peptides (154), inhibin (155) and activin (156), have been shown to be produced by Leydig cells. Immunoreactive AVP is expressed in the testis and has been show to be secreted in vitro by Leydig cells (157). Other immunomodulatory factors shown to be secreted by Leydig cells include gonadotropin-releasing hormone (GnRH), growth hormone releasing hormone (GHRH), corticotrophin releasing hormone (CRH), oxytocin (OT), proenkephalin B, and dynorphin (54, 158–160). Recently Meinhardt et al., demonstrated that Leydig cells produce macrophage inhibitory factor (MIF) and presented evidence for its role in the regulation of testicular function (161). In addition to Leydig cell elaborated immune regulatory factors, the testis is a rich milieu of locally produced growth and differentiation fators (2). Immune–endocrine interactions in the testis are complex and the subject of much current research.

PHYSIOLOGICAL IMMUNE–ENDOCRINE INTERACTIONS

Macrophages–Leydig Cell Interactions during Development

Macrophages play important roles in the regeneration of many cell types after tissue injury. For example, macrophages secrete several growth factors and are central to the wound healing response, which requires proliferation of several regenerating cell types. Testicular macrophages are potential sources for several growth and differentiation factors and are closely associated, both physically and developmentally, to Leydig cells. Macrophages are therefore ideally located to provide some of the regulatory factors that govern Leydig cell proliferation and differentiation.

The cytotoxic drug ethane 1,2-dimethanesulfonate (EDS) causes the acute and selective destruction of Leydig cells and has been used extensively to study Leydig cell regeneration (for a review see ref. 162). After EDS treatment, there is extensive phagocytosis of dead Leydig cells by testicular macrophages. Following the destruction of the Leydig cells, there is a wave of proliferative activity and new Leydig cells repopulate the interstitium. During this time there is an increase in the number of resident macrophages and the first morphological signs of inflammation. These observations are consistent with the involvement of the inflammatory response in the stimulation of the proliferative activity of interstitial cells (163). It is probable that phagocytosis of atretic Leydig cells, and/or other signals, activates testicular macrophages to secrete growth factor (s) that stimulate the proliferative activity of the interstitial cells.

Macrophage-secreted factors such as IL-1 are known mitogens for lymphocytes. These same factors also have been shown to stimulate the proliferation of immature Leydig cells. Khan et al. reported that interleukin-1ß caused a dose-dependent stimulation of the incorporation of [³H]thymidine into the DNA in Leydig cells from 10 and 20 day old rats, but had no effect on DNA synthesis in Leydig cells from adult rats (164). They also reported that IL-1α and TNF-α stimulated DNA synthesis in immature Leydig cells, but that these cytokines were much less potent than IL-1ß. The close association of macrophages with Leydig cells, the invasion of the testicular interstitium by macrophages during prepubertal development, and the detection of IL-1-like activity in the testes from 20 days of age coincide with the development and differentiation of Leydig cells. Because IL-1 has been shown to stimulate proliferation of a variety of cells, these data are consistent with the role of IL-1, or other macrophage secreted cytokine-like growth factors, in signaling Leydig cell growth and differentiation both during normal development and during Leydig cell regeneration following EDS treatment. Another macrophage secreted cytokine-like factor, TGF-α, also stimulates DNA synthesis in immature, but not adult, Leydig cells (164).

Colony stimulating factor 1 (CSF-1) stimulates the survival, proliferation, and differentiation of mononuclear phagocytes and their precursors (for a review see ref. 165). Osteopetrotic (*op/op*) mice are characterized by an autosomal recessive mutation in the CSF-1 gene resulting in the absence of CSF-1. Consequently, *op/op* mice have impaired mononuclear phagocyte development, resulting in a deficiency of both macrophages and osteoclasts. Only bone marrow macrophages show some restoration with age. All other populations of macrophages, including those in the testis, do not recover with age. The importance of macrophages in the gonads is clearly demonstrated with *op/op* mice, which have markedly reduced fertility (for a review see ref. 166). Notably, *op/op* mice have severely reduced numbers of testicular interstitial macrophages (167). Serum testosterone levels in *op/op* mice are significantly reduced compared to op/+ mice. The Leydig cells in testes of *op/op* mice appear to be abnormal and may not be fully differentiated (168). Together these observations suggest that testicular macrophages secrete factor (s) necessary for the proliferation and differentiation of Leydig cells. The op/op mice have a phenotype similar to the IGF-1 null mutation, suggesting that one factor secreted by testicular macrophages may be IGF-1.

Other models of testicular macrophage depletion further demonstrate that in the absence of testicular macrophages, the development and normal functioning of Leydig cells is impaired. This suggests that the role of macrophage–Leydig cell associations during development and under noninflammatory conditions is to provide an appropriate microenvironment and extracellular milieu for the support of Leydig cell functions (10).

Cytokines and Spermatogenesis

Historically, much emphasis has been placed on understanding the roles of gonadotropins and androgens in the control of spermatogenesis (169). In recent years the emphasis has shifted to elucidating paracrine control mechanisms in the regulation of spermatogenesis (4). Mammalian spermatogenesis encompasses three phases: proliferation and renewal of spermatogonia by mitosis; meiosis; and metamorphosis of spermatids to mature spermatozoa by spermiogenesis. Spermatogonial proliferation, meiosis, and spermiogenesis occur continuously throughout the testis, thus spermatogonia, spermatocytes, and spermatids coexist in the seminiferous tubule. These cohorts form specific associations during their development resulting in defined stages of differentiation referred to as the wave of the seminiferous epithelium (169).

Paracrine control of spermatogenesis by peptide growth factors and cell–cell interactions has been reviewed (2, 4, 5). Cytokines have pleiotropic actions and act as growth and differentiation factors within the seminiferous tubule. An interleukin-1-like activity was observed in rat testis (170), and this activity was shown to be produced coincidentally with the initiation of active spermatogenesis (171). Gerard et al. demonstrated that an IL-1-like factor is IL-1α and that Sertoli cells are the site of its synthesis (87). They suggested that Sertoli cell-derived IL-1α is important in the paracrine regulation of germ cells by Sertoli cells. Subsequently, phagocytic activity of Sertoli cells has been shown to stimulate IL-1 production (90, 91). Sertoli cells are also known to produce IL-6 (88, 89, 91, 92). IL-6 was shown to be produced in the seminiferous epithelium in a stage-dependent manner, with highest levels at stages XIII–XIV–I–V. FSH stimulated IL-6 production at most stages, especially at stage VII. Exogenous IL-6 inhibited the onset of meiotic DNA synthesis of spermatocytes and to a lesser extent of spermatogonia. These results suggest that IL-6 is a stage-specific paracrine regulator of the seminiferous epithelium exerting specific inhibitory action on meiotic DNA synthesis (172).

Cytokines have been shown to modulate Sertoli cell transferrin release (173), supporting the hypothesis that there is a cytokine-mediated bidirectional communication between testicular cells. De et al. have shown that pachytene spermatocytes and round spermatids express TNF-α mRNA and that Sertoli cells, but not spermatogenic cells, express TNF-α receptors (174).

Interferon (IFN) α and γ expression was examined in the rat testis. IFNs are well known for their antiviral and immunoregulatory activities. Several studies have suggested an involvement of IFNs in the spermatogenic processes, but Dejucq et al. were the first to demonstrate that IFN-α/ß and γ mRNA and protein were produced by testicular cells. Sertoli cells produced the highest concentrations of IFN-α/ß, followed by peritubular cells. In contrast, IFN-γ was found only in early spermatids, but not in Sertoli cells, peritubular cells, or pachytene spermatocytes (175). However, studies on the effects of IFN-γ revealed that male mice treated chronically with IFN-γ had delayed sexual development, reduced testis and epididymal weights, reduced sperm counts, abnormal sperm morphology, and reduced mating performance and fertility (176).

Macrophage stimulating protein (MSP), a member of the hepatocyte growth factor (HGF) family, is a ligand for receptor tyrosine kinases in the HGF receptor family. In situ hybridization revealed that MSP mRNA was localized to spermatogonia and early spermatocytes in the testis and in the epithelial lining of the epididymis.

This localization suggests that MSP may be involved in germ cell–germ cell interactions during spermatogenesis (177).

These observations further support the role of cytokines as paracrine regulators of testicular function. Nonlymphoid cells secrete cytokines in a stage specific manner during spermatogenesis, presumably as growth and differentiation factors, whereas in the adult, macrophages and lymphocytes secrete cytokines under conditions causing immune activation, such as inflammation.

THE ROLE OF THE NEURAL–IMMUNE–ENDOCRINE AXIS IN THE CONTROL OF TESTICULAR STEROIDOGENESIS

A hallmark of immune–endocrine interactions is immune activation of the hypothalamus–pituitary–adrenal axis, resulting in the activation of the "stress response" (for a review see refs. 178, 179). The interaction between the stress and reproductive axes has been studied extensively. The reproductive axis can be suppressed by hormones from all levels of the stress axis (for a review see refs. 8, 180). Glucocorticoids have been shown to inhibit LH and FSH secretion. Such suppression takes days to become evident, suggesting a more chronic role for adrenal corticosteroids in the inhibition of gonadotropin secretion. Similarly, the direct inhibitory effects of glucocorticoids on Leydig cell steroidogenesis are manifested over a longer time course and act at the level of transcriptional repression (for a review see ref. 53). In contrast, the hypothalamic hormone CRH appears to repress the reproductive axis more acutely (for a review see ref. 8). Rivest et al. demonstrated that intracerebroventricular (icv) injection of IL-1ß into the rat inhibited GnRH release into the median eminence (180). Recently, Battaglia et al. have shown that injection of the bacterial endotoxin LPS into ovariectomized sheep inhibited pulsatile GnRH secretion into the hypothalamic–pituitary portal blood, further supporting the hypothesis that inflammatory stimuli inhibit the reproductive axis by acting centrally (181). Rivier and co-workers (182, 183), and subsequently Kalra and co-workers (184, 185), demonstrated that IL-1 inhibits LH secretion. Although perturbation of the LH secretion by central mechanisms would certainly result in a concomitant inhibition of gonadal steroidogenesis, evidence suggests that in addition there is a neural pathway through which icv IL-1 directly inhibits steroidogenesis. During stress conditions that lower LH levels, decreased testosterone levels are undoubtedly due at least in part to a pituitary mediated event. However, there are many stresses that lead to low testosterone levels in the absence of decreased LH secretion. These observations lead Rivier and co-workers to postulate that there may be a direct neuronal connection between the brain and testes that is activated by CNS cytokines (9). Recent support for this hypothesis comes from the demonstration that icv IL-1ß decreases testicular responsiveness to hCG in rats pretreated with a GnRH antagonist which therefore lack LH secretion (186). This inhibitory effect of centrally injected IL-1ß precedes elevation of peripheral cytokine levels or decreases in plasma LH. Recent studies support the existence of a direct neural link between the ventral medial hypothalamus and the testes that is influenced by IL-1, which regulates testicular responsiveness independently of the pituitary (187). The possible involvement of prolactin and opiods as mediators of the IL-1ß effect was ruled out; however, it appears that central catecholamine pathways may be involved. Of pharmacological interventions tested, propranolol effectively reversed the inhibitory effect of icv injected IL-1b (C. Rivier, personal communication).

In light of the large body of evidence demonstrating the existence of neuronal peptide signaling pathways that affect Leydig cell function (for reviews see refs. 2, 54, 128), it is tempting to speculate that these neuronal peptides are the efferent effectors of the direct brain-to-gonad signal produced in response to immune activation. In support of this hypothesis, surgical or pharmacological denervation of the testes blocks the effects of oxytocin on steroidogenesis. Oxytocin has been shown to stimulate steroidogenesis in immature rat testis. Serotonergic elements were destroyed by treatment with 5,6-dihydroxytryptamine, and the transection of the inferior testicular nerve by vasectomy produced similar results. These results support the concept that testicular innervation is involved in the control of local peptide effects (188).

The testis lacks somatic nerves and is supplied only with autonomic nerves, and the bulk of testicular nerves are sympathetic. The neurotransmitter associated with the sympathetic fibers innervating the testis appears to be norepinephrine. Other neuropeptides are co-expressed with norepinephrine in nerve fibers innervating the testis (for a review see ref. 7). Considerable evidence demonstrates the importance of catecholaminergic control of Leydig cell function and development, notably denervation by intratesticular injection of 6-hydroxydopamine inhibited LH responsiveness and testosterone production in the hamster (44). Surgical denervation of the rat testes induced a decline in gonadotropin responsiveness and resulted in a decrease in LH receptor numbers (189). However, high concentrations of catecholamines are correlated with decreased androgen production (44). These findings suggest that local intratesticular actions of catecholamines acting in concert with other central and peripheral mechanisms may be involved with suppression of testicular functions during times of acute stress and activation of the sympathetic nervous system (7).

Under normal physiological conditions, the pituitary gonadotropins, direct neural innervation, local neuroactive peptides, and catecholamines act in concert to control testicular function, especially Leydig cell androgen biosynthesis. During stress and inflammation perturbation of pituitary gonadotropin secretion, activation or suppression of direct neural connections, production of local inflammatory mediators, and inhibition or activation of local neuroactive peptide pathways act in concert to suppress testicular androgen production. The highly complex integration of the neural–immune–endocrine signals that control of testis function awaits elucidation.

PROSPECTS FOR FUTURE STUDIES

Our understanding of the neural circuitry that controls testicular function is in its infancy. The proposed direct neuronal control of Leydig cell steroidogenesis must be elucidated before we can fully understand the integration of neural–immune–endocrine regulatory mechanisms that control testicular function. Classic neurological approaches that identify nerve fibers involved in control of Leydig cells coupled with molecular biological techniques are being applied to the problem. The use of gene knockout mice and transgenic approaches will be invaluable when candidate regulatory genes have been identified.

The role of the testicular microcirculation in the control of steroidogenesis and spermatogenesis needs further evaluation. The recent demonstration that Leydig cells secrete angiogenic factors such as vascular endothelial growth factor (VEGF) is a compelling observation (190). Leydig cell stimulation of endothelial cell proliferation suggests that the testicular microvasculature is constantly being remodeled. Classic studies by Desjardins and colleagues have emphasized the importance of the testicular microcirculation in the local control of cells in the interstitial and tubular compartments of the testis (191). It will be important for our understanding of the integrative processes that control testis function to elucidate the role of vasoactive factors such as endothelin, nitric oxide, atrial natriuretic peptide, arginine vasopressin, oxytocin, and prostaglandins, all of which have been implicated as potential regulators of testicular function.

Much has been learned about paracrine and cell–cell interactions in the testis, yet our understanding of the integration of these processes into the control of testicular function is incomplete. Epithelial cell biology approaches, such as have recently been described by Jegou and colleagues (88), who examined the vectoral secretion of IL-1 and IL-6 from Sertoli cells in culture, provide important insights into control and integration of testicular processes.

In this era of the genome project, much emphasis has been placed on the use of homologous recombination, transgenic animal studies, gene knockout, and anti-sense knockout approaches. Clearly, these experimental approaches, which are in active use in the study of testicular function, are essential tools to further understanding. It is important, however, to continue to conduct more traditional, even descriptive studies, which are absolutely required to define all of the players involved in the control and integration of neuro–immune–endocrine regulation of testicular function.

ACKNOWLEDGMENTS

The author wishes to acknowledge the critical and insightful comments of Dr. Karen Held Hales, as well as funding from NIH HD27516.

REFERENCES

1. Bellanti JA, Kadlec JV, Escobar-Gutierrez A. Cytokines and the immune response. Clin Immunol 1994;41 (4):597–621.
2. Gnessi L, Fabri A, Spera G. Gondal peptides as mediators of development and functional control of the testis: an integrated system with hormones and local environment. Endocr Rev 1997;18 (4):541–609.
3. Skinner MK. Cell-cell interactions in the testis. Endocrine Rev 1991;12 (1):45–77.

4. Jegou B, Sharpe RM. Paracrine mechanisms in testicular control. In: de Krester D, ed. Molecular Biology of the Male Reproductive System. San Diego: Academic Press, 1993:271–310.

5. Robertson DM, Risbridger GP, Hedger M, et al. Growth factors in the control of testicular function. In: de Krester D, ed. Molecular Biology of the Male Reproductive System. San Diego: Academic Press, 1993:411–438.

6. Giordano G, Del Monte P, Minuto F. Growth factors and testis. J Endocrinol Inv 1991;15:67–75.

7. Mayerhofer A. Leydig cell regulation by catecholamines and neuroendocrine messengers. In: Payne AH, Hardy MP, Russell LD, eds. The Leydig Cell. Vienna, IL: Cache River Press, 1996:407–417.

8. Rivier C, Rivest S. Effect of stress on the activity of the hypothalamic-pituitary-gonadal axis: peripheral and central mechanisms. Biol Reprod 1991;45:523–532.

9. Turnbull A, Rivier C. Brain-periphery connections: do they play a role in mediating the effect of centrally injected interleukin-1b on gonadal function. Neuroimmuno-modulation 1995;2:224–235.

10. Hales DB. Leydig cell-macrophage interactions: an overview. In: Payne AH, Hardy MP, Russell LD, eds. The Leydig Cell. Vienna, IL: Cache River Press, 1996:451–466.

11. Christeff N, Auclair MC, Benassayag C, et al. Endotoxin-induced changes in sex steroid hormone levels in male rats. J Steroid Biochem 1987;26 (1):67–71.

12. Christeff N, Benassayag C, Carli-Vielle C, et al. Elevated oestrogen and reduced testosterone levels in the serum of male septic shock patients. J Steroid Biochem 1988; 29 (4):435–440.

13. Cutolo M, Balleari E, Giusti M, et al. Androgen replacement therapy in male patients with rheumatoid arthritis. Arthritis Rheum 1991;34 (1):1–5.

14. Fourrier F, Jallot A, Leclerc L, et al. Sex Steroid Hormones in Circulatory Shock, Sepsis Syndrome, and Septic Shock. Circ Shock 1994;43:171–178.

15. Handelsman DJ. Testicular dysfunction in systemic disease. Clin Androl 1994; 23 (4):839–856.

16. Lephart ED, Baxter CR, Parker CRJ. Effect of burn trauma on adrenal and testicular steroid hormone production. J Clin Endocrinol Metabol 1987;64:842–848.

17. Lindh A, Carlstrom K, Eklund J, et al. Serum steroid and prolactin during and after major surgical trauma. Acta Anesthesiol Scand 1992;36:119–121.

18. Martens HF, Sheets PK, Tenover JS, et al. Decreased testosterone levels in men with rheumatoid arthritis: Effects of low dose prednisone therapy. J Rheumatol 1994;21: 1427–1431.

19. Spector TD, Ollier W, Perry LA, et al. Free and serum testosterone levels in 276 males: A comparative study of rheumatoid arthritis, ankylosing spondylitis and healthy control. Clin Rheumatol 1989;8 (1):37–41.

20. Spratt DI, Bigos ST, Beitins I, et al. Both hyper- and hypogonadotropic hypogonadism occur transiently in acute illness: bio- and immunoactive gonadotropins. J Clin Endocrinol Metabol 1992;75 (4–6):1562–1570.

21. Spratt DJ, Cox P, Orav J, et al. Reproductive axis suppression in acute illness is related to disease severity. J Clin Endocrinol Metabol 1993;76:1548–1554.

22. Bruot BC, Clemens JW. Effect of adjuvant-induced arthritis on serum luteinizing hormone and testosterone concentrations in the male rat. Life Sciences 1987;41:1559–1565.

23. Bosmann HB, Hales KH, Li X, et al. Acute in vivo inhibition of testosterone by endotoxin parallels loss of steroidogenic acute regulatory (StAR) protein in Leydig cells. Endocrinology 1996;137 (10):4522–4525.

24. Sancho-Tello M, Tash JS, Roby KF, et al. Effects of lipopolysaccharide on ovarian function in the pregnant mare serum gonadotropin-treated immature rat. Endocrine J 1993;1 (6):503–511.

25. Sharma AC, Bosmann HB, Motew SJ, et al. Steroid hormone alterations following induction of chronic intraperitoneal sepsis in male rats. SHOCK 1996;6 (2):150.

26. Ulevitch RJ, Tobias PS. Receptor-dependent mechanisms of cell stimulation by bacterial endotoxin. Ann Rev Immunol 1995;13:437–457.

27. Vogel SN. The LPS gene: Insights into the genetic and molecular basis of LPS responsiveness and macrophage differentiation. In: Beutler B, ed. Tumor Necrosis Factors: The Molecules and Their Emerging Role in Medicine. New York: Raven Press, 1992:485–513.

28. Cerami A. Inflammatory Cytokines. Clin Immunol Immunopathol 1992;62 (1):S3–S10.

29. Spangelo BL, Judd AM, Call GB, et al. Role of cyotkines in the hypothalamic-pituitary-adrenal and gonadal axes. Neuroimmunomodulation 1995;2:299–312.

30. Munck A, Guyre PM, Holbrook NJ. Physiological functions of glucocorticoids in stress and their relation to pharmacological actions. Endocr Rev 1984;5 (1):25–44.

31. Delrue-Perollet C, Li K-S, Vitiello S, et al. Peripheral catecholamines are involved in the neuroendocrine and immune effects of LPS. Brain Behavior and Immunity 1995;9:149–162.

32. Jones SB, Romano FD. Plasma catecholamines in the conscious rat during endotoxicosis. Circ Shock 1984;14:189–201.

33. Jones SB, Yelich MR. Simultaneous elevation of plasma insulin and catecholamines in the conscious and anesthezied rat . Life Sci 1987;41 (13–18):1935–1943.

34. Jones SB, Westfall MV, Sayeed MM. Plasma catecholamines during E. coli bactermia in conscious rats. Am J Physiol 1988;254:R470–R477.

35. Garcia-Barreno P, Suarez A. Modification of catecholamine and prostaglandin tissue levels in E. coli endotoxin-treated rats. J Surg Res 1988;44.

36. Turnbull AV, Rivier C. Corticotropin-releasing factor, vasopressin, and prostaglandins mediate, and nitric oxide restrains, the hypothalamic-pituitary-adrenal response to acute local inflammation in the rat. Endocrinology 1996;137 (2):455–463.

37. Cronenwett JL, Baver-Neff BS, Grekin RJ, et al. The role of endorphins and vasopressin in canine endotoxin shock. J Surg Res 1986;41:609–619.

38. Egan JW, Jugus M, Kinter LB, et al. Effect of a selective V1 vasopressin receptor antagonist on the sequelae of endotoxemia in the conscious rat. Circ Shock 1989;29 (2):155–166.

39. Kasting NW, Mazurek MF, Martin JB. Endotoxin increases vasopressin release independently of known physiological stimuli. Am J Physiol 1985;248 (4):E420–424.

40. Kasting NW. Stimultaneous and independent release of vasopressin and oxytocin in the rat. Can J Physiol Pharm 1988;66 (1):22–26.

41. Schaller MD, Waeber B, Nussberger J, et al. Angiotension II, vasopressin, and sympathetic activity in conscious rats with endotoxemia. Am J Physiol 1985;249 (6):H1086–1092.

42. Thiemermann C, Wu C-C, Szabo C, et al. Role of tumor necrosis factor in the induction of nitric oxide synthase in a rat model of endotoxin shock. Br J Pharmacol 1993;110 (1–2):177–182.

43. Tracey WR, Tse J, Carter G. Lipopolysaccharide-Induced Changes in Plasma Nitrite and Nitrate Concentrations in Rats and Mice: Pharmacological Evaluation of Nitric Oxide Synthase Inhibitors. J Pharmacol Exp Ther 1995;272 (3):1011–1015.

44. Mayerhofer A, Amador AG, Steger RS, et al. Testicular function after local injection of 6-hydroxydopamine or norepinephrine in the golden hamster. J Androl 1990;11:301–311.

45. Mayerhofer A, Danilchik M, Pau K-YF, et al. Testis of prepubertal rhesus monkeys receives a dual catecholaminergic input provided by the extrinsic innervation and an intragondal source of catecholamines. Biol Reprod 1996;55:509–518.

46. Rauchenwald M, Steers WD, Desjardins C. Efferent innervation of the rat testis. Biol Reprod 1995;52:1136–1143.

47. Aguado LI, Ojeda SR. Prepubertal ovarian function is finely regulated by direct adrenergic influences. Role of noradrenergic innervation. Endocrinology 1984; 114:1845–4853.

48. Weiss G, Dail W, Ratner A. Evidence for direct neural control of ovarian steroidogenesis in rats. J Reprod Fert 1982;65:507–511.

49. Sancho-Tello M, Chen T-Y, Clinton TK, et al. Evidence for lipopolysaccharide binding in human granulosa-luteal cells. J Endocrinol 1992;135:571–578.

50. Taylor C, Terranova PF. Lipopolysaccharide inhibits in vitro luteinizing hormone-stimulated rat ovarian granulosa cell estradiol but not progesterone secretion. Biol Reprod 1996;54:1390–1396.

51. Cooke BA. Transduction of the luteinizing hormone signal within the Leydig cell. In: Payne AH, Hardy MP, Russell LD, eds. The Leydig Cell. Vienna, IL: Cache River Press, 1996:351–364.

52. Stocco DM, Clark BJ. Regulation of the acute production of steroids in steroidogenic cells. Endocr Rev 1996;17 (3):221–244.

53. Payne AH, O'Shaughnessy PJ. Structure, function and regulation of steroidogenic enzymes in the Leydig cell. In: Payne AH, Hardy MP, Russell LD, eds. The Leydig Cell. Vienna, IL: Cache River Press, 1996:259–285.

54. Saez JM. Leydig cells: Endocrine, paracrine, and autocrine regulation. Endocr Rev 1994;15 (5):574–626.

55. Lin D, Sugawara T, Strauss JFI, et al. Role of Steroidogenesis Acute Regulatory Protein in Adrenal and Gonadal Steroidogenesis. Science 1995;267:1828–1831.

56. Sharpe RM. Regulation of spermatogenesis. In: Knobil E, Neill JD, eds. The Physiology of Reproduction. 2 ed. New York: Raven Press, 1994:1363–1434. vol I).

57. Bremner WJ, Millar MR, Sharpe RM, et al. Immunohistochemical localization of androgen receptors in the rat testis: evidence for stage-dependent expression and regulation by androgens. Endocrinology 1994;135 (3):1227–1234.

58. Chen H, Chandrashekar V, Zirkin BR. Can spermatogenesis be maintained quantitatively in intact adult rats with exogenously administered dihydrotestosterone? J Androl 1994;15 (2):132–138.

59. McLachlan RI, Wreford NG, Meachem SJ, et al. Effects of testosterone on spermatogenic cell populations in the adult rat. Biol Reprod 1994;51 (5):945–955.

60. O'Donnell L, McLachlan RI, Wreford NG, et al. Testosterone promotes the conversion of round spermatids between stages VII and VIII of the rat spermatogenic cycle. Endocrinology 1994;135 (6):2608–2614.

61. Singh J, O'Neill C, Handelsman DJ. Induction of spermatogenesis by androgens in gonadotropin-deficient (hpg) mice. Endocrinology 1995;136 (12):5311–5321.

62. Troiano L, Faustini Fustini M, Lovato E, et al. Apoptosis and spermatogenesis: evidence from an in vivo model of testosterone withdrawal in the adult rat. Biochem Biophys Res Commun 1994;202 (3):1315–1321.

63. Luke MC, Coffey DS. The Male Sex Accessory Tissues: Structure, Androgen Action, and Physiology. In: Knobil E, Neill JD, eds. The Physiology of Reproduction. 2nd ed., Vol. 1. New York: Raven Press, 1994:1435–1487.

64. Blackwell TS, Christman JW. Sepsis and cytokines: current status. Br J Anaesth 1996;77:110–117.

65. Aggarwal BB, Pocsik E. Cytokines: From clone to clinic. Arch Biochem Biophys 1992;292 (2):335–359.

66. Spooner CE, Markowitz NP, Sarvolatz LD. The Role of Tumor Necrosis Factor in Sepsis. Clin Immunol Immunopathol 1992;62 (1):S11–S17.

67. Hales DB, Rivier C, Shankar B. Interleukin-6 (IL-6) inhibits cAMP-stimulated testosterone by blocking P450c17 expression in mouse Leydig cells. Endocrine Society Annual Meeting. Minneapolis, MN, 1997:209.

68. Miller SC, Bowman BM, Rowland HG. Structure,cytochemistry, endocytic activity, and immunoglobulin (Fc) receptors of rat testicular interstitial-tissue macrophages. Am J Anat 1983;168:1–13.

69. Hutson JC. Testicular macrophages. Int Rev Cytol 1994;149:99–143.

70. Yee JB, Hutson JC. Testicular macrophages: isolation, characterization and hormonal responsiveness. Biol Reprod 1983;29:1319–1326.

71. Head JR, Billingham RE. Immune priviledge in the testis. II: Evaluation of potential local factors. Transplantation 1985;40 (3):269–275.

72. Pollanen P, Niemi M. Immunohistochemical identification of macrophages, lymphoid cells and HLA antigens in the human testis. Int J Androl 1987;10:37–42.

73. Hales DB, Xiong Y, Tur-Kaspa I. The role of cytokines in the regulation of Leydig cell P450c17 gene expression. J Steroid Biochem Mol Biol 1992;43 (8):907–914.

74. Xiong Y, Hales DB. Expression, regulation, and production of tumor necrosis factor-a in mouse testicular interstitial macrophages in vitro. Endocrinology 1993;133 (6):2568–2573.

75. Xiong Y, Hales DB. Immune-endocrine interactions in the mouse testis: cytokine-mediated inhibition of Leydig cell steroidogenesis. Endocr J 1994;2:223–228.

76. Kern S, Robertson SA, Mau VJ, et al. Cytokine secretion by macrophages in the rat testis. Biol Reprod 1995;53:1407–1416.

77. Hutson JC. Secretion of tumor necrosis factor alpha by testicular macrophages. J Reprod Immunol 1993;23:63–72.

78. Hayes R, Chalmers SA, Nikolics Paterson DJ, et al. Secretion of bioactive interleukin-1 by rat testicular macrophages in vitro. J Androl 1996;17:41–49.

79. Hutson JC, Stocco DM. Comparison of celluar and secreted proteins of macrophages from the testis and peritoneum on two-dimensional polyacrylamide gels: Evidence of tissue specific function. Reg Immunol 1989;2:249–253.

80. Orth J, Christensen AK. Localization of 125I-labeled FSH in the testes of hypophysectomized rats by autoradiography at the light and electron microscope levels. Endocrinology 1977;101:262–278.

81. Yee JB, Hutson JC. Biochemical consequences of follicle-stimulating hormone binding to testicular macrophages in culture. Biol Reprod 1985;32:872–879.

82. Christensen AK, Gillman SW. The correlation of fine structure and function in steroid-secreting cells, with emphasis of those of the gonads. In: McKerns KW, ed. The Gonads. New York: Appleton-Century-Crofts, 1969:415–488.

83. Bergh A. Effect of cryptorchidism on the morphology of testicular macrophages: Evidence for a Leydig cell-macrophage interaction in the rat testis. Intl J Androl 1985; 8:86–96.

84. Bergh A. Treatment with hCG increases the size of Leydig cells and testicular macrophages in unilaterally cryptorchid rats. Intl J Androl 1987;10:765–772.

85. Niemi M, Sharpe RM, Brown WRA. Macrophages in the interstitial tissue of the rat testis. Cell Tissue Res 1986;243:337–344.

86. El-Demiry MI, Hargreave TB, Busuttil A, et al. Immunocompetent Cells in Human Testis in Health and Disease. Fertil Steril 1987;48 (3):470–479.

87. Gerard N, Syed V, Bardin W, et al. Sertoli cells are the Site of Interleukin-1a Synthesis in the Testis. Mol Cell Endocrinol 1991;82:R13–R16.

88. Cucicini C, Kercret H, Touzalin A-M, et al. Vectorial Production of Interleukin 1 and Interleukin 6 by Rat Sertoli Cells Cultured in a Dual Culture Compartment System. Endocrinology 1997;138 (7):2863–2870.

89. Syed V, Gerard N, Kaipia A, et al. Identification, ontogeny, and regulation of an interleukin-6-like factor in the rat seminiferous tuble. Endocrinology 1993;132:293–299.

90. Gerard N, Syed V, Jegou B. Lipopolysaccharide, latex beads and residual bodies are potent activators of Sertoli cell interleukin-1 production. Biochem Biophys Res Commun 1992;185:154–161.

91. Syed V, Stephan JP, Gerard N, et al. Residual bodies activate Sertoli cell IL-1 release which triggers IL-6 production by an autocrine mechanism, through the lipoxygenase pathway. Endocrinology 1995;136:3070–3078.

92. Okuda Y, Sun XR, Morris PL. Interleukin-6 (IL-6) mRNAs expressed in Leydig and Sertoli cells are regulated by cytokines, gonadotropins and neuropeptides. Endocrine 1994;2:617–624.

93. Tracey KJ, Cerami A. Tumor necrosis factor, other cytokines, and disease. Ann Rev Cell Biol 1993;9:317–343.

94. Dinarello CA. Biologic basis for interleukin-1 in disease. Blood 1996;87:2095–2147.

95. Kishimoto T. The biology of interleukin-6. Blood 1989;74 (1):1–10.

96. Koj A. Initiation of acute phase response and synthesis of cytokines. Biochim Biophys Acta 1996;1317:84–94.

97. Stewart RJ, Marsden PA. Biologic control of the tumor necrosis factor and interleukin-1 signaling cascade. Am J Kidney Dis 1995;25:954–966.

98. Xiong Y, Hales DB. Expression of tumor necrosis factor-a and interleukin-1b in mouse Leydig cells. Biol Reprod 1993;48 (Suppl. 1):376.

99. Boockfor FR, Wang D, Lin T, et al. Interleukin-6 secretion from rat Leydig cells in culture. Endocrinology 1994;134 (5):2150–2155.

100. Okuda Y, Bardin CW, Hodgskin LR, et al. Interleukins-1 alpha and -1 beta regulate interleukin-6 expression in Leydig and Sertoli cells. Recent Prog Horm Res 1995; 50:367–372.

101. Wang D, Nagpal ML, Calkins JH, et al. Interleukin-1b induces interleukin-1a messenger ribonucleic acid expression in primary cultures of Leydig cells. Endocrinology 1991;129 (6):2862–2866.

102. Dinarello CA. The Interleukin-1 family: 10 years of discovery. FASEB J 1994;8:1314–1325.

103. Moore C, Moger WH. Interleukin-1a-induced changes in androgen and cyclic adenosine 3′,5′-monophosphate release in adult rat Leydig cells in culture. J Endocrinol 1991;129:381–390.

104. Verhoeven G, Cailleau J, Damme JV, et al. Interleukin-1 stimulates steroidogenesis in cultured rat Leydig cells. Mol Cell Endocrinol 1988;57:51–60.

105. Watson ME, Newman RJ, Payne AM, et al. The effect of macrophage conditioned media on Leydig cell function. Ann Clin Lab Sci 1994;24 (1):84–95.

106. Calkins JH, Sigel MM, Nankin HR, et al. Interleukin-1 inhibits Leydig cell steroidogenesis in primary culture. Endocrinology 1988;123:1605–1610.

107. Calkins JH, Guo H, Sigel MM, et al. Differential effects of recombinant interleukin-1α and ß on Leydig cell function. Biochem Biophys Res Commun 1990;167:548–553.

108. Fauser BCJM, Galway AB, Hsueh AJW. Inhibitory actins of interleukin-1b on steroidogenesis in primary cultures of neonatal rat testicular cells. Acta Endocrinol 1989;120:401–409.

109. Hales DB. Interleukin-1 inhibits Leydig cell steroidogenesis primarily by decreasing 17α-hydroxylase/C17-20 lyase cytochrome P450 expression. Endocrinology 1992; 131 (5):2165–2172.

110. Mauduit C, Chauvin MA, Hartmann DJ, et al. Interleukin-1a as a potent inhibitor of gonadotropin actin in porcine Leydig cells: site (s) of action. Biol Reprod 1992;46:1119–1126.

111. Xiong Y, Hales DB. Differential effects of tumor necrosis factor-a and interleukin-1 on 3ß-hydroxysteroid dehydrogenase/Δ^5-Δ^4 isomerase expression in mouse Leydig cells. Endocrine 1997 7:295–301.

112. Calkins JH, Guo H, Sigel MM, et al. Tumor necrosis factor-a enhances inhibitory effects of intrleukin-1b on Leydig cell steroidogenesis. Biochem Biophys Res Commun 1990; 166 (3):1313–1318.

113. Li X, Youngblood GL, Payne AH, et al. Tumor necrosis factor-a inhibition of 17α-hydroxylase/C17-20 Lyase Gene (Cyp-17) Expression. Endocrinology 1995;136 (8): 3519–3526.

114. Mealy K, Robinson B, Millette CF, et al. The testicular effects of tumor necrosis factor. Ann Surg 1990;211:470–475.

115. Meikle AW, Cardoso De Sousa JC, Ward JH, et al. Reduction of testosterone synthesis after high dose interleukin-2 therapy of metastatic cancer. J Clin Endocrinol Metab 1991;73 (5):931–935.

116. Mauduit C, Hartmann DJ, Chauvin MA, et al. Tumor necrosis factor a inhibits gonadotropin action in cultured porcine Leydig cells: Site (s) of action. Endocrinology 1991;129 (6):2933–2940.

117. Xiong Y, Hales DB. The role of tumor necrosis factor-a in the regulation of mouse Leydig cell steroidogenesis. Endocrinology 1993;132 (6):2438–2444.

118. Warren DW, Pasupuleti V, Lu Y, et al. Tumor necrosis factor and interleukin-1 stimulate testosterone secretion in adult male rat Leydig cells in vitro. J Androl 1990;11 (4):353–360.

119. Guo H, Calkins JH, Sigel MM, et al. Interleukin-2 is a potent inhibitor of Leydig cell steroidogenesis. Endocrinology 1990;127:1234–1239.

120. Kasahara T, Hooks JJ, Dougherty SF, et al. Interleukin-2-mediated immune interferon (IFN-gamma) production by human T cells and T cell subsets. J Immunol 1983;130 (4):1784–1789.

121. Nedwin GE, Svedersky LP, Bringman TS, et al. Effect of interleukin-2, inteferon-gamma, and mitogens on the production of tumor necrosis factors α and ß. J Immunol 1985;135 (4):2492–2497.

122. Hales DB, Payne AH. Glucocorticoid-mediated repression of P450scc mRNA and de novo synthesis in cultured Leydig cells. Endocrinology 1989;124 (5):2099–2104.

123. Borden EC. Interferons: pleiotropic cellular modulators. Clin Immunol Immunopathol 1992;62 (1):S18–S24.

124. Orava M, Voutilainen R, Vihko R. Interferon-y inhibits steroidogenesis and accumulation of mRNA of the steoidogenic enzymes P450scc and P450c17 in cultured porcine Leydig cells. Mol Endocrinol 1989;3:887–894.

125. Orava M, Cantell K, Vihko R. Human leukocyte interferon inhibits human chorionic gonadotropin stimulated testosterone production by porcine Leydig cells in culture. Biochem Biophy Res Commun 1985;127 (3):809–815.

126. Orava M. Comparison of the inhibitory effects of interferons-a and -g on testosterone production in porcine Leydig cell culture. J Interferon Res 1989;9:135–141.

127. Orava M, Cantell K, Vihko R. Treatment with preparations of human leukocyte interferon decreases serum testosterone concentrations in men. Int J Cancer 1986;38:295–296.

128. Saez JM, Lejeune H. Regulation of Leydig cell functions by hormones and growth factors other than LH and IGF-1. In: Payne AH, Hardy MP, Russell LD, eds. The Leydig Cell. Vienna, IL: Cache River Press, 1996:383–406.

129. Ahmed SA, Penhale WJ, Talal N. Sex hormones, immune responses, and autoimmune diseases: Mechanisms of sex hormone action. Am J Pathol 1985;121:531–551.

130. Cohn DA. Sensitivity to Androgen: A possible factor in sex differences in the immune response. Clin Exp Immunol 1979;38:218–227.

131. Cohn DA. High sensitivity to androgen as a contributing factor in sex differences in the immune response. Arthritis Rheum 1979;22 (11):1218–1233.

132. Li ZG, Danis VA, Brooks PM. Effect of gonadal steroids on the production of IL-1 and IL-6 by blood mononuclear cells in vitro. Clin Exp Rheumatol 1993;11:157–162.

133. Araneo BA, Dowell T, Diegel M, et al. Dihydrotestosterone Exerts a Depressive Influence on the Production of Interleukin-4 (IL-4),IL-5, and y-Interferon, But Not IL-2 by Activated Murine T Cells. Blood 1991;78 (3):688–699.

134. Sasson S, Mayer M. Effect of androgenic steroids on rat thymus and thymocytes in suspension. J Steroid Biochem 1981;14:509–517.

135. Lee AK, Cockburn A. Antechinus as a paradigm in evolutionary ecology. In: Press CU, ed. Monographs on Marsupial Biology. Cambridge: Cambridge University Press, 1985:162–169.

136. Stein-Behrens BA, Sapolsky RM. Stress, glucocorticoids, and aging. Aging Clin Exp Res 1992;4:197–210.

137. Tung KSK. Regulation of testicular autoimmune disease. In: Desjardins C, Ewing LL, eds. Cell and Molecular Biology of the Testis. New York: Oxford University Press, 1993:474–490.

138. Herr JC, Flickinger CJ, Howards SS, et al. The relationship between antisperm antibodies and testicular alterations after vasectomy and vasovasotomy in Lewis rats. Biol Reprod 1987;37:1297–1305.

139. Flickinger CJ, Herr JC, Caloras D, et al. Inflammatory changes in the epididymis after vasectomy in the Lewis rat. Biol Reprod 1990;43:34–45.

140. Adamopoulos DA, Lawrence DM, Vassilopoulos P, et al. Pituitary-testicular interrelationships in mumps orchitis and other viral infections. Br Med J 1978;1:1177–1180.

141. Fisch H, Laor E, BarChama N, et al. Detection of testicular endocrine abnormalities and their correlation with serum antisperm antibodies in men following vasectomy. J Urol 1989;141 (5):1129–32.

142. Geierhaas B, Bornstein SR, Jarry H, et al. Morphological and hormonal changes following vasectomy in rats, suggesting a functional role for Leydig cell associated macrophages. Horm Metabol Res 1991;23:373–378.

143. Gerendai I, Nemeskeri A, Csernus V. The effect of neonatal vasectomy on testicular function. Andrologia 1986;18 (4):353–359.

144. Kessler DL, Smith WD, Hamilton MS, et al. Infertility in mice after unilateral vasectomy. Fertil Steril 1985;43 (2):308–312.

145. Pollanen P, Maddocks S. Macrophages, lymphocytes and MHCII antigen in the ram and rat testis. J Reprod Fertil 1988;82:437–445.

146. Rivenson A, Ohmori T, Hamazoki M, et al. Cell surface recognition: spontaneous identification of mouse Leydig cells by lymphocytes, macrophages and eosinophils. Cell Molec Biol 1981;27:49–56.

147. Gaytan F, Aceitero J, Lucena C, et al. Simultaneous proliferation and differentiation of Mast cells and Leydig cells in rat testis: Are common regulatory factors involved. J Androl 1992;13 (5):387–397.

148. Wang J, Wreford NGM, Lan HY, et al. Leukocyte Populations of the Adult Rat Testis Following Removal of the Leyding Cells by Treatment with Ethane Dimethane Sulfonate and SubcutaneousTestosterone Implants. Biol Reprod 1994;51:551–561.

149. Pollanen P, von Euler M, Soder O. Testicular immunoregulatory factors. J Reprod Immunol 1990;18:51–76.

150. Weaver CT, Unanue ER. The costimulatory function of antigen-presenting cells. Immunol Today 1990;11 (2):49–55.

151. Magalhaes MM, Magalhaes MC. Effects of ovariectomy and estradiol administration on the adrenal macrophage system of the rat. Cell Tissue Res 1984;238:559–564.

152. Hedger MP, Qin J, Robertson DM, et al. Intragonadal regulation of immune system functions. Reprod Fertil Dev 1990;2:263–280.

153. Raburn DJ, Coquelin A, Reinhart AJ, et al. Regulation of the macrophage population in postnatal rat testis. J Reprod Immunol 1993;24:139–151.

154. Bardin CW, Chen C-LC, Morris PL, et al. Proopiomelanocortin-derived peptides in testis, ovary, and tissues of reproduction. Rec Prog Horm Res 1987;43:1–28.

155. Risbridger GP, Clements JA, Robertson DM, et al. Immuno- and bioactive inhibin and inhibin a-subunit expression in rat Leydig cell cultures. Mol Cell Endocrinol 1989;66:119–122.

156. Lee W, Mason AJ, Schwall R, et al. Secretion of activin by interstitial cells in the testis. Science 1989;243:396–398.

157. Ivell R, Hunt N, Hardy M, et al. Vasopressin biosynthesis in rodent Leydig cells. Mol Cell Endocrinol 1992 (59–66).

158. Foo N-C, Carter D, Murphy D, et al. Vasopressin and oxytocin gene expression in rat testis. Endocrinology 1991;128:2118–2128.

159. Sharpe RM, Cooper I. Comparison of the effects on purified Leydig cells of four hormones (oxytocin, vasopressin, opiates and LHRH) with suggested paracrine roles in the testis. J Endocrinol 1987;113:89–96.

160. Fabri A, Knox G, Buczko E, et al. b-endorphin production by the fetal Leydig cell: regulation and implications for paracrine control of Sertoli cell function. Endocrinology 1988;122 (2):749–755.

161. Meinhardt A, Bacher M, McFarlane JR, et al. Macrophage migration inhibitory factor produciton by Leydig cells: evidence for a role in the regulation of testicular function. Endocrinology 1996;137 (11):5090–5095.

162. Teerds KJ. Regeneration of Leydig cells after depletion by EDS: a model for postnatal Leydig cell renewal. In: Payne AH, Hardy MP, Russell LD, eds. The Leydig Cell. Vienna, IL: Cache River Press, 1996.

163. Teerds KJ, De Rooij DG, Rommerts FFG, et al. Stimulation of the proliferation and differentiation of Leydig cell precursors after the destruction of existing Leydig cells with ethane dimethyl sulphonate (EDS) can take place in the absence of LH. J Androl 1989;10 (6):472–477.

164. Khan SA, Teerds K, Dorrington J. Growth factor requirements for DNA synthesis by Leydig cells from the immature rat. Biol Reprod 1992;46 (3):335–341.

165. Pollard JW, Role of colony-stimulating factor-1 in reproduction and development. Mol Reprod Dev 1997:46(1)54–61.

166. Cohen PE, Pollard JW. Use of osteopetrotic mouse for studying macrophages in the reproductive tract. In: Hunt JS, ed. Immunobiology of Reproduction. New York: Springer-Verlag, 1994:104–122.

167. Pollard JW, Dominguez MG, Mocci S, et al. Effect of the colony-stimulating factor-1 null mutation, osteopetrotic (csfmop), on the distribution of macrophages in the male mouse reproductive tract. Biol Reprod 1997;56:1290–1300.

168. Cohen PE, Chisholm O, Arceci RJ, et al. Absence of Colony-Stimulating Factor-1 in Osteopetrotic (csfmop /csfm op) Mice Results in Male Fertility Defects1. Biol Reprod 1996;55:310–317.

169. Zirkin BR. Regulation of spermatogenesis in the adult mammal: gonadotropins and androgens. In: Desjardins C, Ewing LL, eds. Cell and Molecular Biology of the Testis. New York: Oxford University Press, 1993:166–188.

170. Khan SA, Soder O, Syed V, et al. The rat testis produces large amounts of an interleukin-1-like factor. Intl J Androl 1987;10:495–503.

171. Syed V, Soder O, Arver S, et al. Ontogeny and cellular origin of an interleukin-1-like factor in the reproductive tract of the male rat. Intl J Androl 1988;11:437–447.

172. Hakovirta H, Syed V, Jegou B, et al. Function of interleukin-6 as an inhibitor of meiotic DNA synthesis in the rat seminiferous epithelium. Molec Cell Endocrinol 1995;108:193–198.

173. Boockfor FR, Schwarz LK. Effects of Interleukin-6, Interleukin-2, and Tumor Necrosis Factor-a on Transferrin Release from Sertoli Cells in Culture. Endocrinology 1991;129 (1):256–262.

174. De SK, Chen H, Pace JL, et al. Expression of Tumor Necrosis Factor-a in Mouse Spermatogenic Cells. Endocrinology 1993;133 (1):389–396.

175. Dejucq N, Dugast I, Ruffault A, et al. Interferon-α and -γ expression in the rat testis. Endocrinology 1995;136 (11):4925–4931.

176. Bussiere JL, Hardy LM, Hoberman AM, et al. Reproductive effects of chronic administration of murine interferon-gamma. Reproduc Toxicol 1996;10 (5):379–391.

177. Ohshiro K, Iwama A, Matsuno K, et al. Molecular cloning of rat macrophage-stimulating protein and its involvement in the male reproductive system. Biochem Biophys Res Commun 1996;227:273–280.

178. Bateman A, Singh A, Kral T, et al. The immune-hypothalamic-pituitary-adrenal axis. Endocr Rev 1989;10 (1):92–112.

179. Besedovsky HO, Del Rey A. Immune-neuro-endocrine interactions: facts and hypotheses. Endocr Rev 1996;17 (1):64–102.

180. Rivest S, Rivier C. Interleukin-1b inhibits the endogenous expression of the early gene c-fos located within the nucleus of LHRH neurons and interferes with hypothalamic LHRH release during proestrus in the rat. Brain Res 1993;613:132–142.

181. Battaglia DF, Bowen JM, Krasa HB, et al. Endotoxin inhibits the reproductive neuroendocrine axis while stimulating adrenal steroids: a simultaneous view from hypophyseal portal and peripheral blood. Endocrinology 1997;138 (10):4273–4281.

182. Rivier C, Vale W. In the rat, interleukin-1a acts at the level of the brain and the gonads to interfere with gonadotropin and sex steroid secretion. Endocrinology 1989;124 (5):2105–2109.

183. Rivier C, Vale W. Cytokines act within the brain to inhibit LH secretion and ovulation in the rat. Endocrinology 1990;127:849–856.

184. Bonavera JJ, Kalra SP, Kalra PS. Mode of action of interleukin-1 suppression of pituitary LH release in castrated male rats. Brain Res 1993;612:1–8.

185. Kalra PS, Fuentes M, Sahu A, et al. Endogenous opioid peptides mediate the interleukin-1-induced inhibition of the release of Luteinizing Hormone (LH)-Releasing Hormone and LH. Endocrinology 1990;127 (5):2381–2386.

186. Turnbull AV, Rivier C. Inhibition of gonadotropin-induced testosterone secretion by the intracerebroventricular injection of interleukin-1b in the male rat. Endocrinology 1997;138 (3):1008–1013.

187. Rivier C. The intracerebroventricular injection of interleukin-1b or corticotropin-releasing factor-like peptides decreases testicular responsiveness independently of altered LH secretion. Biol Reprod 1997;56(Suppl.):35.

188. Gerendai I, Csaba Z, Csernus V. Testicular injection of 5,6-dihydroxytryptamine or vasectomy interferes with local stimulatory effect of oxytocin on testicular steroidogenesis in immature rats. Neuroendocrinology 1996;63:284–289.

189. Campos MB, Vitale RS, Calandra RS, et al. Effect of bilateral denervation of the immature testis on testicular gonadotropin receptors and in vitro androgen production. Neuroendocrinology 1990;57:189–194.

190. Collin O, Bergh A. Leydig cells secrete factors which increase vascular permeability and endothelial cell proliferation. Int J Androl 1996;19:221–228.

191. Desjardins C. Design and function of the microcirculation. In: Desjardins C, Ewing LL, eds. Cell and Molecular Biology of the Testis. New York: Oxford University Press, 1993:126–136.

3

CYTOKINES IN OVARIAN FUNCTION

Craig L. Best and Joseph A. Hill

*Brigham and Women's Hospital, Harvard Medical School,
Boston, Massachusetts*

Cytokines are protein products of immune and nonimmune cells that exert autocrine, paracrine, juxtacrine and perhaps endocrine effects on target cells. Immunologic cytokines are those cytokines that are primarily derived from white blood cells. However, an expanded analysis of cells throughout the body has shown that most cytokines are synthesized by many different nonimmune cells. Cytokines may be growth promoting, growth inhibiting, or have no effect on the growth of adjacent cells. Likewise, proteins that are classically referred to as growth factors are often secreted by both immune cells and nonimmune cells. The distinction between cytokines and growth factors is rather arbitrary. The involvement of cytokines/growth factors in ovarian function is becoming increasingly apparent.

The ovary conducts an orchestra of biologic events culminating in sexual maturation, ovulation, and pregnancy maintenance. In the past, ovarian follicular development was explained solely through the two cell, two gonadotropin theory of estradiol production. Recently, it has become clear that cytokines (Table 3.1) and other peptides affect regulatory events within the ovary. An anatomic basis for immunologic cytokine involvement has recently been provided using techniques to determine the

Cytokines in Human Reproduction, Edited by Joseph A. Hill
ISBN 0-471-35242-X   Copyright © 2000 Wiley-Liss, Inc.

Table 3.1. Cytokine and growth factor localization and function in the ovary

Cytokine	GC	TL	CL	S	P^4 Synthesis	E^2 Synthesis	A Synthesis	GFC Proliferative	Oocyte Maturation
	Location/Source				Function				
TNF-α	+	+	+	+	↑↓	↓	↓	↑→	?
IL-1	+	+	?	+	↑↓	↓	↓	→	↑?
IFN-γ	−	?	+	+	↓	↓	↓?	→	?
IL-6	+	?	?	+	↓?	?	?	?	?
IGF-I	−	+	−?	?	↑	↑	↑	↑	?
IGF-II	+	+	+	?	↑	↑	?	↑	↑
TGF-γ	+	+	+	?	?	?	?	↑	↑?
EGF	?	?	?	?	↑?	↓	?	↑	↑
TFG-ß	+	+	+	?	↑↓	↑	↓→	↑	↑
GM-CSF	+?	+?	+	+?	?	?	?	?	?

GC = Granulosa cells; TL = Theca Luteal Cells; CL = Corpus Luteal; S = Stroma; +, − = presence (+) or absence (−) of cytokine or cytokine mRNA; ? = unknown; ↑ = stimulating; ↓ = inhibiting.

immune cells and cytokines present within the ovary. Recombinant cytokines have been used in in vitro experiments to analyze their specific effects on ovarian function. Utilization of molecular techniques has revealed sources of cytokine biosynthesis within the ovary. Thus a clearer understanding of the actions and relationships of the various ovarian cytokines and growth factors is emerging.

WHITE BLOOD CELL SUBPOPULATIONS IN THE OVARY

Leukocyte subpopulations within the ovary have been studied in both animals (1–5) and humans (6–8). The presence of white blood cells in the ovary provides an anatomic basis for immunologic cytokine involvement in ovarian function.

Macrophages

Resident macrophages are present in almost every tissue of the body. These cells are involved in antigen recognition and presentation. Macrophages are also directly involved in local cellular immune defense through the secretion of cytotoxic cytokines and through phagocytosis. Macrophages are known to secrete a number of cytokines and growth factors including IL-1, IL-6, IL-8, TNF-α, TNF-ß, G-CSF, M-CSF, GM-CSF, and bFGF (9).

Macrophages are associated with many of the anatomic structures within the ovary and their numbers fluctuate depending on the menstrual cycle phase. Compartments of the ovary that contain macrophages include the hilum, stroma, follicles, and corpora lutea (8). Important differences in the concentration of macrophages exist during different stages of follicle and corpus luteum development and regression.

Furthermore, macrophage concentrations in the various ovarian compartments may be different between pathological and normal ovaries (10, 11).

Relatively few macrophages are observed in the theca of the developing follicle, whereas macrophage numbers have been found to increase around the time of ovulation (7). Atretic follicles, in contrast, contain moderate numbers of macrophages in the granulosa and theca interstitial compartments (8) (Fig. 3.1A). Macrophages in atretic follicles express HLA-DR, indicating that they are activated and capable of cytokine secretion (8) (Fig. 3.1B).

Studies in animals have demonstrated the presence of macrophages in the corpus luteum (1, 2). The primary function of these resident ovarian macrophages was presumed to be phagocytosis of regressing luteal cells (1, 2). Marked differences in the concentrations of macrophages have been observed in the early corpus luteum compared to the late or regressing corpus luteum. Early corpora lutea contain very few macrophages, whereas regressing corpora lutea contain abundant numbers of these cells (8, 12) (Figs. 3.2A and B). As in atretic follicles, macrophages in regressing corpora lutea are activated as evidenced by their expression of cell surface HLA-DR antigens (8). Lei and co-workers also found that the number of macrophages in the human corpus luteum increased from early to mid luteal phase and then increased again from mid to late lutea phase (13). These data are consistent with data from rat (1), guinea pig (2), and bovine corpora lutea (13), which have all shown macrophage numbers to increase with the duration of the lutea phase.

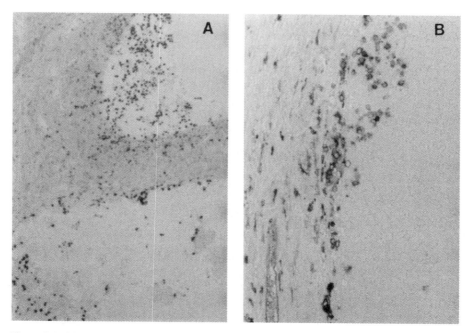

Figure 3.1. Macrophages numbers are increased in the atretic follicle (A) and they express MHC class II antigens (B).

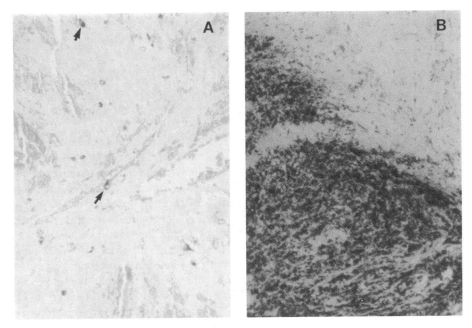

Figure 3.2. Macrophages in early (A) versus late (B) corpus luteum.

Macrophages in and around atretic follicles and in regressing corpora lutea are speculated to play a role in the process of apoptosis (programmed cell death) but it is unclear whether macrophages contribute to the initiation of apoptosis or arrive after the process of apoptosis has been established. Because macrophages participate in the process of tissue repair throughout the body, they may provide a similar function in the ovary. Macrophages in regressing corpora lutea are larger and are lipid laden (8), which supports the hypothesis that they are involved in tissue cleanup and repair within the ovary. However, the macrophage secretory products TNF-α and IFN-γ have been shown to facilitate cellular apoptosis (14). Follicular atresia could therefore be enhanced by activated macrophages providing a central role for macrophages in the cellular events of the ovarian cycle. However, more research is needed to determine whether macrophages initiate apoptosis and thus atresia within the ovary.

Macrophage numbers within benign pathological conditions of the ovaries such as in endometriomas and in polycystic ovarian syndrome have been determined. Endometriotic ovaries contain significantly greater numbers of macrophages in the stroma at the sites of endometriotic implants than does normal ovarian stroma (10) (Fig. 3.3A). Macrophage numbers also appear to be higher in the atretic follicles of endometriotic ovaries when compared with normal ovaries (10). Developing follicles

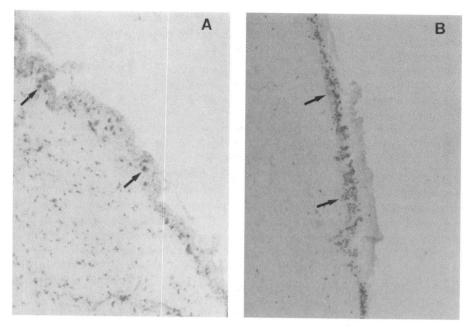

Figure 3.3. Macrophages (A) and granulocytes (B) are present in high numbers at sites of ovarian endometriosis.

and the early corpus luteum (1 day 19 CL) in endometriotic ovaries contain mild to moderate numbers of macrophages, which represent a substantial increase in macrophage concentration compared within these same structures in normal ovaries (10). The greater macrophage content within the endometriotic ovary may influence intraovarian strereoidogenesis and potentially ovum quality, thereby contributing to reproductive difficulty in these women. Fewer numbers of developing follicles and corpora lutea in endometriotic ovaries have been observed (10), lending further support to the hypothesis that macrophages may facilitate the atretic process in the endometriotic ovary.

Macrophage numbers have not been observed to be different in atretic follicles from polycystic ovaries compared to normal ovaries (11). However, greater numbers of atretic follicles are present in the polycystic ovary compared with the normal ovary. The number of macrophages in the stroma, hilum, and corpora lutea of the polycystic ovary compared to the normal ovary is also not different (11).

Lymphocytes

Antigens, along with class II MHC molecules, are presented to the CD4+ T-helper/inducer lymphocyte by antigen presenting cells, which include macrophages, dendritic cells, Langerhans cells, Kupffers cells, microglial cells and B lymphocytes. Following activation, CD4+ T lymphocytes produce predominantly one of two distinctive cytokine profiles termed T-helper1 (TH1) and T-helper2 (TH2). TH1 cells induce cellular immunity through the secretion of interferon-gamma (IFN-γ), interleukin-2 (IL-2), and tumor necrosis factor beta (TNF-ß, lymphotoxin). Th2 cells downregulate cellular immunity while facilitating antibody production and thus humoral immunity through the secretion of primarily, interleukin-4, but also interleukin-5, 6, and 10.

The distribution of T lymphocytes in the ovary is similar to the distribution of ovarian macrophages, which have not been found in great numbers in the developing follicle (7). Developing follicles have been observed to contain focal small numbers of T lymphocytes in the blood vessels of the theca. In contrast, atretic follicles contained few T lymphocytes in the granulosa but moderate numbers in the theca (8). In another report, no difference was reported in T lymphocyte numbers in follicles throughout the human menstrual cycle (7). The function of T lymphocytes in the human ovarian follicle is unknown, but they have been shown to possess memory (8). T lymphocytes in atretic follicles are activated and express the activation marker HLA-DR (8). The T lymphocyte cytokine IFN-γ has been found in human ovarian follicles (15, 16) and has been shown to inhibit estradiol biosynthesis (17–19) and to facilitate the process of apoptosis (14). The inhibitory effect of IFN-γ on ovarian estradiol secretion can be enhanced by TNF-α (18). Therefore T lymphocytes may facilitate follicular atresia though the biosynthesis and secretion of the cytokine IFN-γ acting synergistically with TNF-α.

Controversy also exists regarding the status of T lymphocytes in human corpora lutea. Some reports agree with animal data in showing few T lymphocytes in the early corpora lutea, whereas regressing corpora lutea contained moderate to abundant numbers of T lymphocytes (8, 13). However, another report did not detect differences in the concentration of T lymphocytes between the early and late luteal phases of the cycle (7). The ratio of CD4 (T helper/inducer) to CD8 (T suppresser/cytotoxic) T lymphocytes in the early corpora lutea favored the CD4 T cells, but in regressing corpora lutea, the ratio was 1:1. T lymphocytes that were found to be increased in the regressing corpora lutea were activated (6, 8) and may be secreting IFN-γ, which has been shown to inhibit progesterone biosynthesis. IFN-γ may also act synergistically with the macrophage cytokines TNF-α and IL-1 to limit the production of progesterone and facilitate the regression of the corpus luteum through the apoptotic process.

Natural killer cells have been detected in the ovary but are relatively few and do not vary with phases of the ovarian cycle (7). B lymphocytes are not present in the ovary and therefore any immunoglobulins found in the ovary are likely the result of serum transudation (7, 8).

Endometriotic ovaries have been reported to contain T lymphocytes in the stroma in areas of endometriotic implants, but roughly similar numbers of T lymphocytes in other ovarian compartments (10). Natural killer cells and B lymphocytes have not been observed in the endometriotic ovary (10).

Polycystic ovaries are reported to contain T lymphocytes in essentially the same numbers as in normal ovaries in all structures observed, follicles, corpora lutea, hilum, and stroma (11). Neither natural killer cells nor B lymphocytes have been observed in the polycystic ovary (11).

Other Immune Cells

Neutrophils and granulocytes are present in the human ovary and their concentrations may vary with the location and timing of the ovarian cycle. Two human studies differ in their assessment of the number of neutrophils at different sites within the ovary (7, 8). In the first report, high numbers of neutrophilic granulocytes were detected in the theca of the preovulatory follicle and high numbers were detected in the corpora lutea (7). No increase in neutrophil numbers were detected with regression of the corpora lutea. In another report, low numbers of neutrophils and granulocytes in both follicles and corpora lutea were detected without a difference in cell numbers between phases of the ovarian cycle (8).

Endometriotic ovaries contained moderate numbers of granulocytes (CD15+ cells) in the regressing corpora lutea and in other sites of endometriosis within the ovary (10) (Fig. 3.3). Neutrophil numbers were not observed to be increased in the endometriotic ovary (10). Granulocyte and neutrophil numbers were similar in both polycystic ovaries and in normal ovaries (11).

White Blood Cell Influence on Ovarian Steroid Production

White blood cells and their secreted proteins have been demonstrated to influence ovarian steroid biosynthesis. Peritoneal macrophages may modulate granulosa cell progesterone production directly or through the secretion of cytokines and other factors. The effects of macrophages on human granulosa cell progesterone production have been studied (20). Peritoneal macrophages were reported to increase basal progesterone production of human granulosa cells cultured in vitro (20). When conditioned medium derived from cultured human peritoneal macrophages was added to porcine granulosa cells in vitro, progesterone biosynthesis was increased whereas LH receptor content was attenuated (21). Progesterone production of hCG primed granulosa cells was not affected significantly. Thus it appears that peritoneal macrophages may increase basal progesterone, while attenuating the effect of hCG stimulation on granulosa cells.

To determine whether white blood cells specifically affect granulosa cells, progesterone production co-culture experiments using granulosa cells cultured with associated ovarian white blood cells have been compared to granulosa cells cultured free of white blood cells (Fig. 3.4). These experiments revealed that granulosa cells co-cultured with white blood cells do not respond normally to hCG stimulation. hCG stimulation of leukocyte-free granulosa cells resulted in a three- to fourfold increase in progesterone production compared to granulosa cells cultured with associated white blood cells (19). Thus white blood cells may exert a tonic inhibitory influence on granulosa cell progesterone synthesis in response to hCG, suggesting that these cells may regulate hormone production during the luteal phase of the menstrual cycle and potentially during early pregnancy.

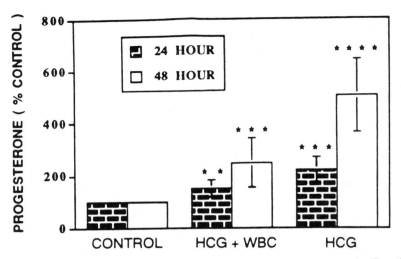

Figure 3.4. Luteinized human granulosa cells stimulated with hCG produced significantly less progesterone in the presence of white cells (WBC) at both 24 and 48 h of culture.

CYTOKINE LOCALIZATION AND FUNCTION IN THE OVARY

Tumor Necrosis Factor α

Tumor necrosis factor α (TNF-α) is a 17kDa cytokine secreted by activated macrophages and other cell types (22). TNF-α has been found to be present in the rabbit (23) and human (24) corpus luteum. Roby and co-workers (24) found cells that stained positive for TNF-α in human corpus luteum and cultured granulosa cells. Follicular fluid and granulosa cell culture supernatants contain immunoreactive TNF-α as measured by ELISA in levels of 100–170 pg/mL and 145–806 pg TNF-α/500,000 cells, respectively. The possibility that immune cells in the corpus luteum and in granulosa cell cultures were the source of TNF-α was not ruled out but subsequent investigations in our laboratory using RT-PCR on purified cells have confirmed that human granulosa cells are a source of TNF-α in the ovary (unpublished observations). In murine tissues, TNF-α was detected by immunohistological staining in the corpus luteum and in atretic and antral follicles (25). TNF-a has also been found in the corpora lutea of sheep (26), cows (25, 27), and rabbits (28, 29).

TNF-α has been reported to be present in the sera (30) (concentration ranging from 84 to 920 pg/mL) and follicular fluid (22, 31) (concentration ranging from 20 to 700 pg/mL) of women having in vitro fertilization (IVF). Punnanen et al. (31) reported that women with detectable levels of TNF-α in follicular fluid had lower follicular fluid estradiol and progesterone levels. Furthermore, it has been demonstrated, utilizing in vitro granulosa cell cultures, that TNF-α directly and specifically inhibits luteinized granulosa cell progesterone and estradiol biosynthesis (32–35) (Figs. 3.5 and 3.6). However, some investigators have reported that TNF-α increases proges-

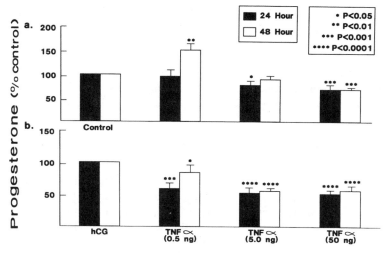

Figure 3.5. TNF-α elicited a biphasic modulation of progesterone production in basal granulosa cells (a) whereas all concentrations of TNF-α significantly decreased progesterone production in hCG-stimulated granulosa cells (b).

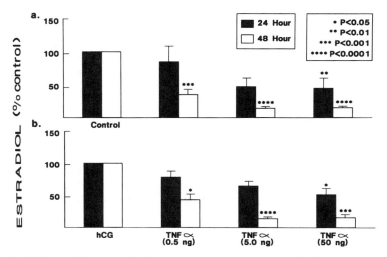

Figure 3.6. TNF-α inhibited estradiol biosynthesis in both basal (a) and hCG-stimulated (b) granulosa cells.

terone biosynthesis under certain in vitro culture conditions (36, 37). The discrepant results regarding the effect of TNF-α on basal and hCG primed progesterone production in the human may be explained by differences in the differentiation of the granulosa cells, species differences, and also the association of white blood cells in granulosa cell cultures. This is an important confounding variable that has not been addressed by all investigators because up to 50% of cells in human granulosa cell suspensions prepared using traditional techniques are white blood cells, but these cells can be reduced to less than 4% (<1% macrophages) by using anti-CD45 magnetic immunobeads (35). Thus relatively pure human granulosa cells have been studied in culture and comparisons made with white blood cell associated granulosa cells (35). TNF-α is likely to be an important regulator of the corpus luteum. However, the timing of synthesis and secretion, cell receptor location, and regulation in humans is presently unknown.

Interleukin-1

Interleukin-1 (IL-1α and IL-1ß) circulates as 17kDa polypeptides. The two cytokines originate from distinct loci on chromosome 2; however, they possess 25% homology and bind to the same two receptor types (38). Cellular sources of IL-1 production have been ascribed to a broad range of cell types including macrophages, T and B lymphocytes, neutrophils, fibroblasts, dendritic cells, and endothelial cells (39, 40). Evidence suggests that IL-1 plays an important role in male and female reproductive function. IL-1 has been reported to modulate human testicular steroidogenesis (41, 42) and spermatogenesis (43). Many female reproductive events may also be influenced by IL-1α and IL-1ß including embryo development (44, 45), blastocyst implantation (46–48), and trophoblast outgrowth (49).

The relative amounts of IL-1α and IL-1ß mRNA transcripts have been determined in whole human ovary, granulosa cultures, and cell suspensions using solution hybridization/RNAse protection assays (24). This study also determined the level of type I, IL-1 receptor (IL-1R) gene expression and mRNA for the IL-1 receptor antagonist (IL-1RA). Associated macrophages in granulosa cell cultures were removed using anti-CD68-coupled magnetic immunobeads. However, associated T lymphocytes were not removed from the granulosa cells harvested from follicular fluid aspirates. IL-1 mRNA was not found in whole ovarian tissue on cycle days 4 and 12 of natural cycles. Preovulatory follicular fluid containing granulosa cells and T lymphocytes did contain IL-1α and Il-1ß, but IL-α mRNA was in greater abundance than IL-1ß. Granulosa cell suspensions essentially free of macrophages but containing T lymphocytes exhibited IL-1ß gene transcripts. IL1R was found in whole ovary, and in macrophage depleted granulosa cell suspensions, whereas IL-1RA mRNA was expressed only in macrophage-free follicular aspirates.

Although this excellent work represents the best knowledge of human ovarian IL-1 localization and quantification, many questions still remain. First is the concern that IL-1 message may have been attributed to T lymphocytes (T lymphocytes were not removed from the suspensions) and not macrophages within the granulosa cell suspensions. Although macrophages are generally thought of as the predominant immunologic source of IL-1, T and B lymphocytes may also secrete IL-1 (40, 50, 51). Significant lymphocyte numbers (40% to 52% of cells) are present in follicular fluid aspirates of women undergoing IVF (35, 52–54). IL-1α and IL-1ß mRNA was detected only in cell suspensions and not in whole ovary at cycle day 4 and 12, suggesting that lymphocytes that are known to exist in follicular cell suspensions may have accounted for the detection of IL-1 mRNA. Another possibility was that whole human ovaries are sufficiently replete with cells not containing IL-1 transcripts, thus making it difficult to determine quantitatively the levels of IL-1 mRNA in these tissues. IL-1ß was not detected in granulosa cells after 48 h of culture, a process that would effectively reduce total white blood cell numbers, supporting the contention that lymphocyte contamination in ovarian granulosa cell culture harvested from women having IVF may explain the detection of IL-1ß mRNA in macrophage-free follicular aspirates. Peripheral blood monocytes that were negative for IL-1α and ß mRNA were used as a further control in this study of IL-1 in the human ovary, but these cells were not activated, and therefore it may not be surprising to find that they did not express IL-1 mRNA transcripts. However, data from the rat indicate that IL-1ß is synthesized by theca interstitial cells with synthesis regulated by both gonadotropins and IL-1ß (55).

IL-1 has been proposed to be involved in the process of ovulation with serum levels of IL-1 peaking following ovulation (56). IL-1 has also been detected in whole sections of rat ovary in association with developing follicles and corpora lutea (57), suggesting that IL-1 may have a role in ovarian physiological events.

The importance of IL-1α and IL-1β as intraovarian regulators is becoming increasingly apparent. IL-1 has been found to affect in vitro human luteinized granulosa cell estradiol but not progesterone production at concentrations of 1–50 ng/mL in some, but not all studies (36, 58–62). One report studying the effects of IL-1α and IL-1ß in luteinized human granulosa cells cultured with and without associated white blood cells concluded that IL-1α but not IL-1ß inhibited estradiol biosynthesis, but neither influenced progesterone biosynthesis by granulosa cells cultured free of white blood cells (62). IL-1 has also been reported to inhibit gonadotropin-induced androgen biosynthesis in human theca cells (63). Animal data in both porcine (64–66) and murine (67–69) in vitro models have consistently demonstrated inhibition of estradiol and progesterone secretion. It is not clear why animal data are more consistent but two possibilities are that (1) animals provide a more homogeneous sample whereas human granulosa cells are derived from women with many different fertility problems and thus different ovarian pathologies, or (2) the association of white blood cells with granulosa cells may not be as great in animals as in humans. The presence of IL-1 in the human corpus luteum has not been previously demonstrated nor has the cellular origin and regulation of IL-1 been clearly defined.

Interferon-gamma

Interferon-gamma (IFN-γ), is a heterogeneous 15–25 kDa polypeptide secreted by many cell types including lymphocytes (69, 70). General immunologic effects of IFN-γ include induction of class I and class II (DR) major histocompatability antigens on several cell types; macrophages and endothelial cell activation; stimulation or inhibition of lymphokine activities; enhancement of natural killer cell activity; and antiviral activity (69–71). IFN-γ has also been reported to inhibit hormone production in a variety of endocrine cells including Sertoli and Leydig cells (72–74), thyroid cells (75, 76), and pancreatic beta cells (77, 78). Adrenal steroidogenesis has been reported to be enhanced by IFN-γ (79).

IFN-γ has been demonstrated immunohistochemically in the normal human ovary using a polyclonal sheep anti-human IFN-γ (16). IFN-γ has also been demonstrated in follicular fluid (80) of women during IVF cycles at concentrations ranging from 5 to 35 IU/mL (0.25–1.75 ng/mL). Cell-specific staining of IFN-γ was demonstrated in new corpora lutea, while regressing corpora lutea contained moderate amounts of IFN-γ. Atretic follicles but not developing follicles contained cells that specifically stained for IFN-γ. Double immunofluorescent labeling experiments revealed co-localization of IFN-γ with macrophages and T lymphocytes in both atretic follicles and regressing corpora lutea. RT-PCR analysis of ovarian granulosa cells confirmed that granulosa cells do not synthesize IFN-γ but that stimulated ovarian and peripheral white blood cells do (16). Thus ovarian immune cells are implicated as the one potential source of IFN-γ in the ovary.

Ovarian steroid production in the rat (81) and human (17–19, 82, 83) has been reported to be inhibited by IFN-γ. Rat granulosa cell progesterone, 20α-hydroxypregn-4-en-3-one, and estrogen production were inhibited in a dose dependent manner by IFN-γ through LH and hCG receptor regulation (81). In women, administration of IFN-γ resulted in decreased serum estrogen and progesterone concentrations without affecting the concentrations of serum FSH and LH, suggesting that it acts directly on the granulosa and theca cells within the ovary (82). Reports concerning the in vitro effects of IFN-γ on human granulosa cell steroid production are controversial. Fukuoka et al. (17) reported that IFN-γ decreased both progesterone and estradiol production, whereas Wang and associates (18), using similar IFN-γ concentrations, demonstrated decreased progesterone production but no effect on estradiol biosynthesis. In another report, the effects of IFN-γ were determined on human luteinized granulosa cell progesterone and estrogen production with and without associated white blood cells in co-culture (19). In these experiments IFN-γ alone, and with associated leukocytes, inhibited granulosa cell progesterone, estrone, and estradiol biosynthesis. These effects were abrogated with a neutralizing antibody to IFN-γ, indicating specificity for IFN-γ action. IFN-γ was not cytotoxic to granulosa cells but specifically inhibited gonadal steroidogenesis (19). Thus INF-γ may participate in the processes of follicular atresia and corpus luteum regression by influencing ovarian steroid biosynthesis.

Recent evidence indicates that elevated levels of INF-γ in the range of 1.25 to 125 × 10^5 ng/mL may play a role in premature ovarian failure and perhaps corpus luteum regression through the induction of HLA class II antigens on granulosa cells (71). Varying degrees of immune activation and ovarian sensitivity to secreted immunologic cytokines may result in a continuum of luteal-phase insufficiency, anovulation, and in susceptible women premature ovarian failure.

Interleukin-6

Interleukin-6 (IL-6) is a multifunctional cytokine that has been reported in human follicular fluid in significant concentrations (84). IL-6 levels in human follicular fluid have not been found to be different between women with tubal factor (155 ± 0.53 pg/mL), endometriosis (1.15 ± 0.53 pg/mL), and antisperm antibodies (1.58 ± 0.46

pg/mL). Studies in the rat indicate that granulosa cells are the most likely source of IL-6 in the ovary and that IL-6 production appears to be regulated by FSH, IL-1α, and IL-1ß, but not by TNF-α (85). Although IL-6 levels appear to be constant throughout the menstrual cycle (86), there is evidence that this cytokine may be involved in follicular angiogenesis (87). IL-6 in the follicular fluid at the time of ovulation may also be important to the neovascularization of the developing corpus luteum. IL-6 has also been shown to influence FSH-stimulated progesterone production in the rat (88). However, the potential contribution of IL-6 to corpus luteum development requires further study.

GROWTH FACTOR LOCALIZATION AND FUNCTION IN THE OVARY

Insulin-like Growth Factor I

Insulin-like growth factor (IGF-I), like IGF-II, is a mitogenic, low molecular weight protein that is structurally related to proinsulin. The main source of circulating IGF-I is the liver and its synthesis is regulated by growth hormone (GH). IGF-I is also synthesized by many other somatic cells including immune and ovarian cells. The role of IGF-I as a putative intraovarian regulator has been established over the past two decades. The existence of an intraovarian IGF system complete with ligands (IGF-I and IGF-II), receptors (I and II), and binding proteins (IGFBPs 1-4) has been established. Each component of the IGF system plays a unique and important role in the autocrine and paracrine regulation of steroid producing granulosa and theca lutean cells, thereby contributing to the fate of the ovarian follicle (and ultimately the oocyte) as well as the corpus luteum.

IGF-I was first discovered in porcine follicular fluid, where it was found to be in greater concentrations than in serum (89). Ovulation induction with gonadotropins elevated the follicular fluid concentrations of IGF-I in parallel with the follicular fluid levels of progesterone and estradiol (90). Production of IGF-I by porcine granulosa cells in vitro was found to be gonadotropin dependent (91). Estradiol was synergistic with FSH in stimulating IGF-I biosynthesis in the pig (91). Growth hormone was also found to stimulate IGF-I production alone and in synergy with FSH and E_2 (92). Epidermal growth factor (EGF) and transforming growth factor-α (TGF-α) stimulated immunoreactive IGF-I secretion but platelet derived growth factor (PDGF) and fibroblast growth factor (FGF) alone had no effect. However, PDGF can enhance EGF's ability to stimulate IGF-I secretion (93).

In porcine and in murine models, IGF-I mRNA expression has been detected in granulosa cells (94–97). IGF-I gene expression is also found in the rat corpus luteum (98). There are important species differences in the location of IGF-I ligands. In humans, IGF-I gene expression is found in the theca of small antral follicles but not in granulosa cells or in dominant follicles (99). Therefore, in the human, the origin of IGF-I secretion is likely to be theca lutea cells of antral follicles with an added contribution provided through serum transudation.

In the human, IGF-I stimulates basal and FSH-primed biosynthesis of P and E_2 (100–107), as was found in porcine (108–111) and murine systems (112–115). The effect of IGF-I on granulosa cell P production in healthy follicles is small, but in the presence of FSH, IGF-I acts as a profound stimulator of granulosa cell P synthesis (106). Thus it appears that IGF-I acts to amplify the gonadotropin effect on granulosa cells rather than as a primary stimulus to the ovary. Both granulosa cells and theca cells contain IGF-I receptors and IGF-I stimulates androgen biosynthesis (116). IGF-I may facilitate providing androgen substrate for E_2 biosynthesis, although this potential role for IGF-I is not fully understood.

IGF-I has also been shown to stimulate mitotic division of granulosa cells in pigs and humans (117–123). This function may be important in the growth and development of the dominant ovarian follicle where granulosa cell proliferation is essential.

IGFBPs are believed to be important in the regulation of IGF action and in extending the half-life of IGF. IGFBPs-1 to 4 are produced by human granulosa cells and are central to IGF-I regulation in the ovary. IGFBP-3 is also produced in the CL and may be important for the regulation of IGF action in the CL (124). IGFBPs are capable of binding and thereby sequestering IGF-I so that it is not free to bind its receptor and exert its gonadotropin enhancing actions. IGFBP-1 has been shown to inhibit the synergistic action of FSH and IGF-I on rat granulosa cell P biosynthesis (125, 126). FSH may in turn accelerate the availability of IGF-I through its ability to inhibit the constitutive release of IGFBP by granulosa cells (126, 127). Remarkably, FSH produces a biphasic effect of IGFBPs secretion depending on the concentration of FSH (128). IGFBPs appear to continue their IGF regulation at low concentrations of FSH. With higher FSH concentrations and thus lower concentrations of IGFBPs, IGF-I levels are increased, and this may promote granulosa cell proliferation and steroid biosynthesis necessary for further maturation of the dominant follicle. This pattern of IGFBP regulation by FSH may be necessary for follicle recruitment to occur and development of the dominant follicle.

Although it is not clear whether IGF-I plays a critical role in oocyte maturation, it does stimulate maturation of cumulus–oocyte complexes in both rats and humans (129, 130). Furthermore, IGF-I receptor mRNA is present in human oocytes (131). Higher levels of IGF-I have been found in the follicular fluid from follicles containing mature cumulus–oocyte complexes (132). These data suggest that IGF-I may be important in oocyte maturation.

Insulin-like Growth Factor II

In contrast to IGF-I, IGF-II mRNA is expressed in theca cells in the rat but in the granulosa of dominant follicles and the theca of small antral follicles in the human (99, 133). Luteinized human granulosa cells also secrete IGF-II (134–136) which may be important in corpus luteum development. IGF-II acts via both type I and type II IGF receptors in contrast to IGF-I, which acts primarily through the type I receptor (137–139). Also in contrast to IGF-I, IGF-II synthesis is minimally influenced by GH (137, 140).

The in vivo ovarian actions of IGF-II are less well understood that those of IGF-I. In vitro, IGF-II has been shown to stimulate human granulosa cell proliferation (123). In the in vitro porcine model, IGF-II stimulated FSH-induced E_2 biosynthesis (108).

In the human, IGF-II was also able to increase the synthesis of E_2 from granulosa cells in the absence of FSH (141). In porcine (111) and human (141) in vitro culture models, IGF-II stimulated basal P biosynthesis. In the pig, IGF-II also stimulated an increase in LDL induced P production (111). Thus, IGF-II may be an important stimulator of follicular growth and corpus luteum development. Like IGF-I, IGF-II stimulates the maturation of the cumulus–oocyte complexes (129) and therefore may also be important in oocyte maturation. IGF-II is also regulated by IGFBPs through the influence of FSH.

Transforming Growth Factor α

Transforming growth factor α (TGF-α) is a polypeptide that possesses 20% structural homology with epidermal growth factor (EGF), which interacts with the same receptor (142) and exerts similar biologic effects as EGF (143). TGF-α has been found in numerous sites in the ovary. Immunohistochemically, TGF-α has been detected in the theca lutea (144, 145), granulosa (145), corpus lutea (145), and oocytes (145) in the human (145) as well as bovine (144) species. TGF-α gene expression is detected in the theca lutea (144), granulosa (146), and corpus luteum (147), indicating that sites of TGF-α production are not isolated to a single cell type within the ovary. However, the primary site of TGF-α production in the ovary is thought to be theca lutean cells (148, 149), and the in vitro accumulation of TGF-α mRNA is increased by FSH (148). The TGF-α/EGF shared receptor is under the regulatory control of gonadotropins, which may stimulate (150, 151) or inhibit (152) receptor function.

TGF-α is growth promoting to granulosa cells in bovine species (144) but not in the rat (153, 154). Because EGF is mitogenic to granulosa cells in a number of species including humans (155, 156) but not rats, and it utilizes the same receptor as TGF-α, it is likely that TGF-α is also mitogenic to human granulosa cells. TGF-ß, on the other hand, appears to inhibit the ability of TGF-α/EGF to promote granulosa cell growth (157, 158). In the rat, TGF-α inhibits FSH receptor gene expression and FSH receptor binding (159). TGF-α is also inhibitory to rat granulosa cell E_2 biosynthesis (153, 154) but stimulates E_2 production in the porcine species (160). TGF-α does stimulate FSH-primed P and 20α-hydroxyprogesterone biosynthesis in the rat (146). In summary, TGF-α appears primarily to stimulate granulosa cell proliferation but also to have a role in the modulation of ovarian steroid biosynthesis. Its actions are attenuated by TGF-ß and regulated by gonadotropins. The overall importance of TGF-α to the development of the dominant follicle and to corpus luteum development deserves further investigation.

Epidermal Growth Factor

Epidermal growth factor (EGF), as previously mentioned, is a polypeptide possessing some structural homology with TGF-α and sharing the same receptor. The actions of EGF within the ovary are similar to TGF-α, providing functional diversity of more than one molecular source to ensure that their shared actions on ovarian function occurs. The source of EGF differs from TGF-α in that it does not appear to be produced locally in the ovary, but EGF activity has been detected in follicular fluid (161). EGF may function as a tropic regulator of ovarian granulosa cell differentiation rather than as an autocrine/paracrine intraovarian regulator. EGF receptor regulation is gondotropin-dependent and the type and degree of gonadotropin control depends on the stage of granulosa cell differentiation (150–152).

EGF stimulates granulosa cell growth in a number of species but not the rat (155, 156). In contrast to its promotion of granulosa cell growth, EGF inhibits LH receptor induction and FSH stimulated aromatase activity (162, 163). Therefore, E_2 production by ovarian granulosa cells is reduced in the presence of EGF. EGF also inhibits the basal and gonadotropin stimulated androgen production of cultured theca cells but does not influence theca cell prostaglandin production (164). EGF may have a positive influence on oocyte development for it has been shown to induce oocyte maturation in rat follicles (165).

Transforming Growth Factor ß

Transforming growth factor ß (TGF-ß) is a homodimer composed of two identical amino acid chains and exists in three different forms (TGF-ß 1, 2, 3). The three forms of TGF-ß have similar actions and are thought to be separated primarily by theca cells in murine, bovine, porcine, and human ovaries, allowing for a paracrine action on granulosa cells (145, 166–170). TGF-ß is also synthesized to a limited extent by granulosa cells as demonstrated by the presence of TGF-ß2 mRNA expression in rat (171) and TGF-ß 1 and 2 mRNA in human (145, 170, 172) granulosa cells, where it may exert autocrine action on granulosa cells. TGF-ß has also been detected using immunohistology in corpus lutea and oocytes of animals (173–175) and humans (145, 170) where they may exert paracrine effects.

Studies on the effects of TGF-ß on specific ovarian cells in animal models have reported conflicting results most likely due to species and cell differentiation differences. TGF-ß enhances FSH induced responses in granulosa cells while countering the actions of TGF-α and EGF. TGF-ß may inhibit EGF induced granulosa cell proliferation in the cow (157) and pig (176), and it has been shown to enhance the proliferation of rat granulosa cells in some (177–179) but not all (153, 180) studies. FSH has been shown to stimulate the proliferation of granulosa cells synergistically with TGF-ß (177, 178). TGF-ß does appear to increase FSH receptors on granulosa cells but has variable effects on FSH receptor binding (159, 181). In the rat, LH receptor induction stimulated by FSH was further enhanced by TGF-ß at low FSH concentrations, but was inhibited by TGF-ß at high FSH concentrations (182). This biphasic action regarding LH receptor induction may have physiological relevance in the selection of the dominant follicle. Likewise TGF-ß enhanced FSH stimulated cAMP production by granulosa cells at low FSH concentrations but inhibited FSH induced cAMP production at high FSH levels (182). In vitro granulosa cell P production responded variably to TGF-ß with both stimulatory (180) and inhibitory (176) responses, which may be partially explained by species differences. FSH induced inhibin production was stimulated by TGF-ß and FSH induced EGF receptor gene expression was also enhanced by TGF-ß (183).

TGF-ß also affects theca interstitial compartment of the follicle. TGF-ß inhibits TGF-α induced stimulation of theca cell proliferation (184). Reports on the effects of TGF-ß on theca cell steroid production are conflicting. Basal androgen production has been reported to be both inhibited (185) and unaffected (181, 186) by TGF-ß. LH and forskolin stimulated androgen production are reported to be inhibited by TGF-ß in several different species (186). Basal and hCG stimulated E_2 production may be enhanced with TGF-ß, but effects on P production have been reported to be variable (185, 186).

TGF-ß may have specific effects on the ovarian follicle. For example, in the hamster, TGF-ß stimulates follicular DNA synthesis but inhibits EGF-induced DNA synthesis (187).

The maturation of follicular oocytes is enhanced by TGF-ß as are cumulus–oocyte complexes (129). Oocytes that are denuded of the follicle or cumulus, however, are not affected by TGF-ß, suggesting that TGF-ß acts through stimulation of granulosa cell derived growth factors to enhance oocyte maturation (129). However, TGF-ß inhibited EGF induced oocyte maturation (129).

OVULATION

Immune Cells

Macrophages may be involved in the process of ovulation through the actions of IL-1ß, TNF-α, and GM-CSF. Macrophage induced synthesis of prostaglandins and proteases may facilitate follicular rupture. Because TNF-α is produced by a number of nonimmune cells in the ovary, such as endothelial cells, fibroblasts, and granulosa cells (188), it is unclear whether immune cell or nonimmune cell derived TNF-α and IL-1ß are involved in the process of ovulation. Further studies are necessary before concluding that immune cells contribute to the process of ovulation. Macrophages have been associated with ovulation by virtue of their increased numbers in the theca of rat ovarian follicles just prior to and after ovulation (5). Furthermore, ovulation is an inflammatory process and macrophages, which are present at the time of ovulation, secrete pro-inflammatory cytokines such as IL-1, TNF-α, and GM-CSF. Although TNF-α, IL-1ß, and GM-CSF have been found in the preovulatory follicular fluid of human (22, 24) and bovine (189) females, it has not been determined whether the source of these cytokines is primarily immune or nonimmune cells.

Cytokines

Interleukin-1ß.   Interleukin-1ß (IL-1ß), a macrophage secretory product and possibly also derived by ovarian cells, has been associated with several events in the ovulatory process. IL-1ß increases vascular permeability, collagenase activation, prostaglandin biosynthesis, plasminogen activator production, proteoglycan synthesis, and hyluronic acid secretion (190, 191).

In experiments using rat ovarian tissue, IL-1β transcripts, as assessed by hybridization/RNase protection assays, were increased by treatment of the ovarian cells

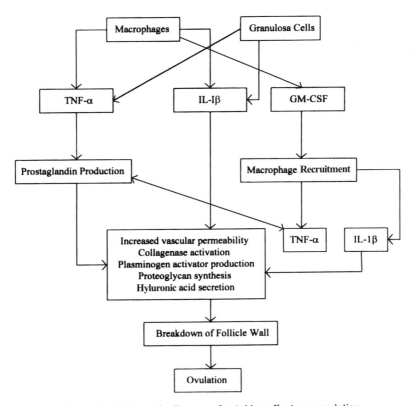

Figure 3.7. Schematic diagram of cytokine effects on ovulation.

with pregnant mare's serum gonadotropin (PMSG) followed by hCG. After 6h of hCG exposure a dramatic increase (four- to fivefold) was seen in the IL-1ß message (190). In separate experiments, exposure of rat ovarian cells to recombinant IL-1ß increased ovarian IL-1ß biosynthesis, indicating an autocrine regulatory role for IL-1ß in its own production.

The effect of IL-1β on ovulation was also studied in in vivo perfused rat ovaries (192). In these experiments, cannulation of the rat's aorta and vena cava was performed and the connecting vessels except the ovarian artery and vein were ligated so that the IL-1ß and LH could be selectively delivered to the ovary. In these experiments unstimulated ovaries did not ovulate, but the administration of 100 ng/mL of LH resulted in ovulations (3.4 ± 0.6). IL-1ß (4 ng/mL) alone caused ovulations (1.6 ± 0.4) in each of the ovaries studied. When IL-1ß was added with LH there was a threefold increase in the number of ovulations compared to when LH was added alone. IL-2 did not induce ovulations in this animal model. The presence of indomethacin in the medium reduced the number of ovulations when LH or LH plus IL-1ß was used to stimulate ovulation. Indomethacin did not alter the number of ovulations when IL-1ß was used alone to stimulate ovulation. These data support the hypothesis that IL-1ß plays a supportive rather than a primary role in the process of ovulation. This hypothesis was further supported by experiments in IL-1 knockout mice where no difficulty with ovulation was observed.

In the human, IL-1 like activity has been detected in peripheral blood immediately prior to ovulation (56) but there are no data in humans linking IL-1 directly with the ovulatory process.

Tumor Necrosis Factor α. Tumor necrosis factor α (TNF-α), which is secreted by both macrophages and granulosa cells, promotes ovulation in the in vitro perfused rat ovary (6). TNF-α enhanced prostaglandin production but not plasminogen activator activity in the rat perfused ovary and did not act synergistically with LH (193). TNF-α has also been reported to increase prostaglandin production by human luteinized granulosa cells (194, 195). The presence of TNF-α in bovine and human preovulatory follicular fluid lends further support to the concept that TNF-a may be a factor in the ovulatory process. Because prostaglandins are believed to be involved in the process of ovulation, TNF-α may be an important stimulus for the production of periovulatory prostaglandins.

Granulocyte Macrophage Colony Stimulating Factor. Granulocyte macrophage colony stimulating factor (GM-CSF) is another macrophage product that may be involved in ovulation. It is present in human follicular fluid in significant concentrations and is synthesized in elevated concentrations just prior to ovulation in the rat (196). In the rat, the preovulatory rise in GM-CSF may be facilitated by TNF-α and IL-1ß in conjunction with LH (196). GM-CSF, known for its ability to recruit and activate macrophages and granulocytes, may be involved in establishing the periovulatory increase in inflammatory cells at the time of ovulation. However, it is not likely that GM-CSF plays a major role in the process of ovulation, for GM-CSF mutant mice have no difficulty with ovulating (197, 198).

CYTOKINES, GROWTH FACTORS, AND FOLLICULAR FATE

Follicular development, as described by the two cell theory, depends on the production of androstenedione substrate by follicular theca interstitial cells and a conversion of androstenedione to estradiol by follicular granulosa cells. LH promotes the synthesis of androstenedione in the theca whereas FSH stimulates the conversion of androstenedione to estradiol via the aromatase enzyme in granulosa cells.

Growth factors including IGF-I, IGF-II, EGF, TGF-α, and TGF-ß promote granulosa cell proliferation as well as E_2 biosynthesis, which are important to follicle and oocyte development. Although it is not likely that any one growth factor is critical for follicular development, collectively growth factors appear to be essential for normal ovarian function. The number of growth factors involved in the processes leading to oocyte maturation—and possibly more will be discovered—provide numerous cooperative pathways contributing to the successful development of the dominant follicle and ultimately the release of a mature oocyte. Each growth factor has its own set of regulators. In most cases, ovarian growth factors are regulated by gonadotropins, in particular FSH. IGF-I and IGF-II are regulated by FSH through the intermediary IGF-BPs. FSH inhibits IGFBP production in the ovary, which in turn allows unbound IGF-I and IGF-II to exert their actions. IGF-I appear to enhance the action of FSH with regard to steroid biosynthesis (100–115) but is a less important modulator in the absence of FSH. IGF-I thus appears to serve as an amplifier of FSH action at the ovarian tissue level despite relatively low serum concentrations of FSH during the follicular phase. IGF-II, on the other hand, stimulates basal granulosa cell biosynthesis of P and E_2 and thus acts independently of FSH (111, 141). TGF-ß is another growth factor that acts primarily in conjunction with FSH in stimulating granulosa cell proliferation (177, 178). TGF-ß also enhances FSH induced inhibin and EGF production (183). Furthermore, TGF-ß increases the FSH receptor content of granulosa cells allowing for further amplification of FSH action (159).

Cytokines, particularly TNF-α, IL-1, and INF-γ, are present in the ovary in significant concentrations and likely play important regulatory roles. Like growth factors, these cytokines appear to act collectively to assure normal ovarian function but during disease processes may contribute to ovarian dysfunction. Cytokines may contribute to follicular development as well as follicular atresia. TNF-α, for example, may enhance granulosa cell proliferation and P biosynthesis in early granulosa cell differentiation (36, 37) but appears to have no effect on granulosa cell proliferation and inhibits P biosynthesis in luteinized human granulosa cells. Furthermore, TNF-α may act synergistically with INF-γ to inhibit P production (18). Estrogen production of human granulosa cells is inhibited by TNF-α (35). Perhaps low levels of TNF-α enhance early follicle maturation whereas increasing concentrations present before ovulation in association with the increased numbers of immune cells and subsequent prostaglandin presence are important for follicular rupture and the decline in E_2 that occurs after ovulation.

INF-γ is a cytokine that has consistently been reported to inhibit both P and E_2 production (17–19). IFN-γ has been detected in the atretic follicle in greater concentrations than in the developing follicle (16). IFN-γ has also been shown to induce apoptosis in granulosa cells (14). Thus it is possible that IFN-γ is involved in the process of follicular atresia. IFN-γ induced expression of HLA class II antigens on granulosa cells may further contribute to the cytotoxic T cell induced destruction of the follicle (71). Although plasma cells and B lymphocytes are not generally present in the ovary, induction of MHC class II antigens by IFN-γ may also lead to humoral immune responses within the ovary, contributing to premature ovarian failure. Varying degrees of immune cell activation and ovarian sensitivity to IFN-γ may result in a continuum of luteal phase insufficiency, anovulation, and in susceptible women, premature ovarian failure. Human granulosa cells have been ruled out as a source of INF-γ but INF-γ mRNA expression has been detected in ovarian white blood cells (16). Therefore, activated resident ovarian T lymphocytes that are present in high concentrations in the atretic follicle appear to contribute to the process of follicular atresia through the secretion of INF-γ (8, 16).

Because a complete IL-1 system (receptors, ligands, and receptor antagonist) has been detected in the ovary, it is likely that IL-1 plays a significant role in ovarian physiology. Although IL-1 has consistently inhibited P and E_2 biosynthesis in murine and porcine models, IL-1 has variable effects on the steroid production of human granulosa cells. In some studies using luteinized human granulosa cells, IL-1 at concentrations of 1–50 ng/mL has been shown to inhibit estradiol but not progesterone production (36, 58–62). Reasons for the discrepant results may again be due to differences in the differentiation of the granulosa cells and to contamination of the granulosa cell cultures with associated white blood cells. In an attempt to clarify the white blood cell contamination issue, experiments were done with the associated leukocytes removed from culture (62). In these studies, IL-1α but not IL-1ß inhibited estradiol biosynthesis (62). Neither IL-1α or IL-1ß inhibited progesterone production (62). However, in the same report, hCG stimulated granulosa cells cultured with associated white blood cells produced less progesterone than the same granulosa cells cultured in the absence of white blood cells. Therefore, although IL-1α may inhibit estradiol production in luteinized granulosa cells, white blood cells appear to suppress progesterone production (62). The role of IL-1α or ß in the maturation of the dominant follicle has not been determined. It is difficult to speculate from experiments using luteinized granulosa cells whether an effect on granulosa cells early in the differentiation process exists. On the other hand, more solid data are available to substantiate a role for IL-1ß in the process of ovulation. IL-1ß, which increases at the time of ovulation, has been shown to enhance many ovulation associated phenomena, including but not limited to an increase in the production of prostaglandins, collagenase, hyaluronic acid, and proteoglycans.

CYTOKINES AND CORPUS LUTEUM REGRESSION

Following ovulation the corpus luteum forms from the transformation of theca lutea cells and granulosa cells, which become luteinized. Progesterone secretion by the corpus luteum is essential for endometrial development allowing implantation and pregnancy maintenance. In the absence of pregnancy, corpus luteum regression must occur to allow for new follicular recruitment. Immune cells and their secreted cytokines appear to facilitate the process of corpus lutea regression by downregulating progesterone production (fig. 3.8). Because granulosa cells are also a source of TNF-α and IL-1, they may also contribute to the process of luteal regression through the secretion of these cytokines.

Macrophages, activated T lymphocytes, and granulocytes are present in the corpus luteum and have been shown to increase markedly in numbers as the corpus luteum regresses (8, 13). Cytokines such as TNF-α and IFN-γ also are present in the corpus luteum and IFN-γ has been show to increase in the regressing corpus luteum (16). Macrophages may be involved in corpus luteum regression through phagocytosis of dying luteal cells and therefore play an active role in this tissue remodeling process (1, 2, 8). Macrophages may also contribute to luteolysis directly through the secretion of the cytokines TNF-α and IL-1. T lymphocyte secretion of IFN-γ may also be contribute to luteolysis. In the rabbit, T lymphocytes are present in the corpus luteum and precede the appearance of macrophages (199). These T lymphocytes may secrete

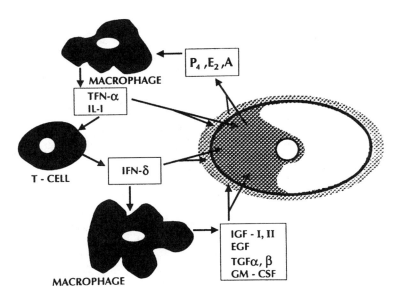

Figure 3.8. Diagram of cytokine interaction with granulosa and theca cells.

chemotactic factors, attracting macrophages to participate in corpus luteum regression. Granulocytes are increased in the regressing corpus luteum and may directly contribute to the destruction of luteal cells through peroxide secretion (200, 201).

TNF-α and IFN-γ inhibit luteinized granulosa cell P production in both animals (32, 34, 74, 81) and humans (18, 31, 35). TNF-α has also been reported to act synergistically with IFN-γ in the inhibition of P biosynthesis (18). TNF-α, in some human experiments, has not been shown to inhibit granulosa cell P production alone and therefore may only act to enhance the inhibitor effect of IFN-γ (18, 36, 37). These cytokines acting in concert may cause a significant reduction in the P levels before complete regression of the corpus luteum. This inhibition of gonadal steroid production within luteal cells is independent of granulosa cell death and likely precedes cell death, which may not be immediate (35). IL-1 inhibits P biosynthesis in animals but has not been shown to inhibit P production in humans consistently (62, 64–69). However, IL-1 may indirectly contribute to corpus luteum regression by causing further immune cell activation, leading to enhanced secretion of both TNF-α and IFN-γ. IL-6 has also been reported to inhibit FSH stimulated P biosynthesis in the rat (88).

The cytokines TNF-α and IFN-γ have been found to enhance the apoptotic (programmed cell death) process of granulosa and other cells. Specifically, IFN-γ may facilitate apoptosis through regulation of anti-apo-1 (14). It is unclear to what extent these cytokines induce apoptosis within the corpus luteum, but this may be another mechanism contributing to corpus luteum regression.

The expression of MHC class I antigens are increased under the influence of TNF-α (202). TNF-α also enhances the production of prostaglandin $F_{2\alpha}$ in bovine luteal cells, which may contribute to luteal regression (202). IFN-γ enhances the expression of MHC class II antigens on bovine luteal cells (203). LH attenuates IFN-γ induced expression of MHC class II antigens in the bovine corpus luteum, which appears to provide initial protection to the early corpus luteum and may continue to protect the corpus luteum during early pregnancy (203). MHC class II antigen expression on luteinized human granulosa cells is also induced by IFN-γ (71). The immunohisto-logical presence of MHC class II antigens has been demonstrated in the human cor-pus luteum and expression increases as the corpus luteum regresses (8). These antigens are also present on luteal cells and vascular epithelial cells (8). MHC class I and class II antigens are important activators of immunologic responses by facilitat-ing antigen presentation to CD8 (cytotoxic/inducer) T lymphocytes and macrophage activation.

In summary, immune and nonimmune cells within the corpus luteum may con-tribute to the demise of the corpus luteum through secretion of the cytokines IFN-γ, TNF-α, and to a lesser extent, IL-1. The T lymphocyte cytokine IFN-γ may be the first and most important cytokine secreted in this cascade because T lymphocytes are pres-ent early in luteal regression and IFN-γ may facilitate chemotaxis of macrophages and granulocytes to the corpus luteum. In response to these cytokines, P biosynthesis is im-paired, apoptosis is induced, and MHC class I and II antigens are expressed on granu-losa/luteal cells. Through these immune mediated mechanisms the corpus luteum undergoes orderly regression remodeling and replacement by the corpus albicans.

CONCLUSION

Cytokines and growth factors are present in the ovary and appear to play important roles in the ovarian cycle. Specifically, cytokines and growth factors appear to be im-portant in folliculogenesis and ovulation and in the processes of follicular atresia and corpus luteum regression through immune cell activation. In the pathological ovary, such as in polycystic ovarian disease and in endometriosis, normal ovarian functions may be disturbed through immune cell and cytokine perturbations. Our understand-ing of the role cytokines and growth factors play in ovarian function is still rudimen-tary. More work is needed to determine specifically the factors regulating cytokine synthesis and cytokine receptor location and regulation within the ovary and their in-volvement in ovarian health and disease.

REFERENCES

1. Bulmer D. The histochemistry of ovarian macrophages in the rat. J Anat Lond 965; 98:13–319.
2. Paavola LG. The corpus luteum of the guinea pig. Fine structure at the time of maximum progesterone secretion and during regression. Am J Anat 1977;150:565–604.
3. Kirsch TM, Friedman AC, Vogel RL, Flickinger GL. Macrophages in the corpora lutea of mice: characterization and effect on steroid seretion. Biol Reprod 1981;25:629–638.

4. Bagavandoss P, Kunkel SL, Wiggins RC, Keyes PL. Tumor necrosis factor-α (TNF-α) production and localization of macrophages and T lymphoytes in the rabbit corpus luteum. Endocrinology 1988;122:1185–1187.

5. Brannstrom M, Mayrhofer G, Robertson SA. Localization of leukocyte subsets in the rat ovary during the periovulatory period. Biol Reprod 1993a;48:277–286.

6. Brannstrom M, Norman RJ. Involvement of leukocytes and cytokines in the ovary process and corpus luteum function. Human Reprod 1993;8:1762–1775.

7. Brannstrom M, Pascoe V, Norman RJ, McClure N. Localization of leukocyte subsets in the follicle wall and in the corpus luteum throughout the human menstrual cycle. Fertil Steril 1994;61:488–495.

8. Best CL, Pudney J, Welch WR, Burger N, Hill JA. Localization and characterization of white blood cell populations within the human ovary throughout the menstrual cycle and menopause. Human Reprod 1996;11;790–797.

9. Cohen PE, Polland JW. Cytokines and growth factors in reproduction. In Bronson RA, ed., Reproductive Immunology. Cambridge, MA: V Blackwell Science, 1996:52–102.

10. Best CL, McKinley D, Hill JA. White blood cell subpopulations in the human endometriotic ovary. J Soc Gynecol Invest 1996;3(Suppl.):202A.

11. Best CL, Berger NZ, Hill, JA. White blood cell subpopulations in the polycystic oary. Presented at the Society for Gynecologic Investigation Meeting, 1995.

12. Wang LJ, Pascoe V, Petrucco OM, Norman RJ. Distribution of leukocyte subpopulations in the human corpus luteum. Human Reprod 1992b;7:197–202.

13. Lei ZM, Chegini N, Roa Ch V. Quantitative cell composition of human and bovine corpora lutea from various reproductive states. Biol Reprod 1991;44:1148–1156.

14. Cataldo NA, Jaffe RB. Human luteinizing granulosa cells express Apo-1/FAS, and interferon gamma (IFN-γ) increases their susceptibility to anti-Apo-1-mediated apoptosis. Abstract No. P25. Presented at the Meeting of the Society for Gynecologic Investigation, Philadelphia, PA, 1996.

15. Grasso G, Asano A, Tanaka T, Fujimoto S, Muscettola M. Immuohistochemical localization of interferon-γ in normal human ovary. Gynecol Endocrinol 1994;8:161–168.

16. Best CL, McKinney, Hill JA. Immunohistochemical localization of interferon-gamma and activated T-lymphocytes in the normal human ovary. Am Soc Reprod Med, 1995 (Abstract).

17. Fukoaka M, Yasuda K, Emi N, Fujiwara H, Iwai M, Takakura K, Kanzaki H, Mori T. Cytokine modulation of progesterone and estradiol secretion in cultures of luteinized human granulosa cells. J Clin Endocrinol Metab 1992;75:254–258.

18. Wang HZ, Lu SH, Han XJ, Zhou W, Sheng WX, Sun ZD, Gong YT. Inhibitory effect of interferon and tumor necrosis factor on human luteal funtion in vitro. Fertil Steril 1992;58:941–945.

19. Best CL, Griffin PM, Hill JA. Interferon gamma inhibits luteinized human granulosa cell steroid production in vitro. Am J Obstet Gynecol 1995;172:1505–1510.

20. Halme J, Hammond MG, Syrop CH, Talbert LM. Peritoneal macrophages modulate human granulosa-luteal cell progestreone prodution. J Clin Endocrinol Metab 1985;61:912–916.

21. Chen TT, Lane TA, Doody MC, Caudle MR. The effect of peritoneal macrophage-derived factor(s) on ovarian progesterone secretion and LH receptors. The role of calcium. Am J Reprod Immunol 1992;28:43–50.

22. Wang LJ, Brannstromm M, Robertson SA, Norman RJ. Tumor necrosis factor-α in the human ovary: Presence in follicular fluid and effects on cell proliferation and prostaglandin production. Fertil Steril 1992;58:934–940.

23. Bagavandoss P, Kunkel SL, Wiggins RC, Keyes PL. Tumor necrosis factor-α (TNF-α) production and localization of macrophages and T-lymphocytes in the rabbit corpus luteum. Endocrinology 1988;122:1185–1187.

24. Roby KF, Weed J, Lyles R, Terranova PF. Immunological evidence for a human ovarian tumor necrosis factor-α. J Cin Endocrinol Metab 1990;71:1096–1102.

25. Roby KF, Terranova PF. Localization of tumor necrosis factor (TNF) in rat and bovine ovary using immunocytochemistry and cell blot: evidence for granulosal production. In: Hirshfield AN, ed. Growth Factors and the Ovary. New York: Plenum Press, 1989:1096–1102.

26. Ji I, Slaughter RG, Ellis JA, Ji TH, Murdoch WJ. Analyses of oine corpora lutea for tumor necrosis factor mRNA and bioactivity during prostaglandin-induced luteolysis. Mol Cell Endocrinol 1991;81:77–80.

27. Zolti M, Meiron R, Shemesh M, et al. Granulosa cells as a source and target organ for tumor necrosis factor-α. FEBS Lett 1990;261:253–255.

28. Bagavandoss P, Kunkel SL, Wiggins RC, Keyes PL. Tumor necrosis factor α (TNF α) production and localization of macrophages and T lymphocytes in the rabbit corpus luteum. Endocrinology 1988;122:1185–1187.

29. Bagavandoss P, Wiggins RC, Kunkel SL, Remick DG, Keyes PL. Tumor necrossi factor production and accumulation of inflammatory cells in the corpus luteum of pseudopregnancy and pregnancy in rabbits. Biol Reprod 1990;42:367–376.

30. Witkin SS, Kiu HC, David OK, Rosenwaks S. Tumor necrosis factor is present in maternal sera and embryo culture fluids during in vitro fertilization. J Reprod Immunol 1991;19:85–93.

31. Punnanen J, Heinonen PK, Teisala K, Kujansuu E, Jansen CT, Punnanen R. Demonstration of tumor necrosis factor-α in preovulatory follicular fluid: Its association with serum 17ß-estradiol and progesterone. Gynecol Obstet Invest 1992;33:80–4.

32. Darbon JM, Oury F, Laredo J, Bayard F. Tumor necrosis factor-α inhibits follicle-stimulating hormone-induced differentiation in cultured rat granulosa cells. Biochem Biophys Res Commun 1989;1038–46.

33. Adashi EY, Resnick CE, Croft CS, Payne DW. Tumor necrosis factor-α inhibits gonadotropin hormonal action in nontransformed ovarian granulosa cells. J Biol Chem 1989;264:1591–1596.

34. Adashi EY, Resnick CE, Packman JN, Hurwitz A, Payne DW. Cytokine-mediated regulation of ovarian function: Tumor necrosis factor-α inhibits gonadotropin-supported progesterone accumulation by differentiating and luteinizing murine granulosa cells. Am J Obstet Gynecol 1990;162:889–99.

35. Best CL, Pudney J, Anderson DJ, Hill JA. Modulation of human granulosa cell steroid production in vitro by tumor necrosis factor alpha: implications of white blood cells in culture. Obstet Gynecol 1994;84:121–127.

36. Fukoka M, Yasuda K, Emi N, Fujjiwara H, Iwai M, Takakura K, Kanzaki H, Mori T. Cytokine modulation of progesterone and estradiol secretion in cultures of luteinized human granulosa cells. J Clin Endocrinol Metab 1992;75:254–258.

37. Yan Z, Hunter V, Weed J, Hutchinson S, Lytes R, Terranova P. Tumor necrosis factor-α alters steroidogenesis and stimulates proliferation of human ovarian granulosa cells in vitro. Fertil Steril 1993;59:332–338.

38. Dower SK, Kronheim SR, Hopp TP, Centrell M, Deeley M, Gillis S, Henney CS, Urdal DR. The cell surface receptors for interleukin-1 and interleukin-1 are identical. Nature 1986;324:266–268.

39. Oppenheim JJ, Kovacs EJ, Matsushima K, Durum SK. There is more than one interleukin-1. Immunol Today 1986;7:45–56.

40. Dinarello CA. Interleukin-1 and its biologically related cytokines. Adv Immunol 1989;44:153–205.

41. Vorhoeven G, Caillenu J, Van Damme J, Billiau A. Interleukin-1 stimulates steroidogenesis in cultured rat leydig cells. Mol Cell Endocrinol 1988;57:51–60.

42. Calkins JH, Sigel MM, Nonkin HR. Interleukin-1 inhibits leydig cell steroidogenesis in primary culture. Endocrinology 1988;123:1605–1610.

43. Pollanen P, Soder D, Parvinen M. Interleukin-1 stimulation of spermatogonial proliferation in vitro. Reprod Fertil Develop 1989;1:85–87.

44. Fakih H, Baggett B, Holtz G, Tsong KY, Lee JC, Williamson HO. Interleukin-1 possible role in the infertility associated with endometriosis. Fertil Steril 1987;47:213–217.

45. Hill JA, Haimovici F, Anderson DJ. Productions of activated T-lymphocytes and macrophages inhibit mouse development in vitro. J Immunol 1987;139:2250–2254.

46. Haimovici F, Hill JA, Anderson DJ. The effects of soluble products of activated lymphocytes and macrophages on blastocyst implantation events in vitro. Biol Reprod 1991;44:69–75.

47. Simón C, Frances A, Piquette G, et al. Interleukin-1 system in the materno-trophoblast unit in human implantation: Immunohistochemical evidence for autocrine/paracrine function. J Clin Endocrinol Metab 1994;78:847–854.

48. Simon C, Frances A, Piquette GN, et al. Embryonic implantation in mice is blocked by interleukin-1 receptor antagonist. Endocrinology 1994;134:521–528.

49. Berkowitz RS, Hill JA, Kurtz CB, Anderson DJ. Effects of products of activated leukocytes (lymphokines and monokines) on the growth of malignant trophoblast cells invitro. Am J Obstet Gynecol 1988;158:199–203.

50. Sander DN. Interleukin-1. Arch Dermatol 1989;125:679–682.

51. Dinarello CA. Interleukin-1 and interleukin-1 antagonism. Blood 1991;77:1627–1646.

52. Hill JA, Barbieri RL, Anderson DJ. Detection of T8 (suppressor/cytotoxic) lymphocytes in human ovarian follicular fluid. Fertil Steril 1987;47:114–117.

53. Hill JA, Anderson DJ. Distribution of T-cell subsets in follicular fluid. Fertil Steril 1989;51:736–737.

54. Beckmann MW, Polacek D, Saung L, Schreiber JR. Human ovarian granulosa cell culture: Determination of blood cell contamination and evaluation of possible culture purification steps. Fertil Steril 1991;10:299–304.

55. Hurwitz A, Ricciarelli E, BoteroL, et al. Endocrine- and autocrine-mediated regulation of rat ovarian (theca-interstitial) interleukin-1ß gene expression: gonadotropin-dependent preovulation acquisition. Endocrinology 1991;129:3427–3429.

56. Cannon JG, Dinarello CS. Increased plasma interleukin-1 activity in women after ovulation. Science 1985;227:1247-1249. Kokia E, Adashi EY. Potential role of cytokines in ovarian physiology: the case for interleukin-I. In: Adashi EY, Leung PCK, eds. The Ovary. New York: Raven Press, 1993;383–394.

57. Simon C, Frances A, Piquette G, Polan ML. Immunohistochemical localization of the interleukin-1 system in the mouse ovary during follicular growth, ovulation, and luteinization. Biol Reprod 1994;50:449–457.

58. Barak V, Yanai P, Treves AJ, Roisman I, Simon A, Laufer N. Interleukin-1: Local production and modulation of human granulosa luteal cell steroidogenesis. Fertil Steril 1992;58:219–225.

59. Polan ML, Daniele A, Kuo A. Gonadal steroids modulate human monocyte interleukin-1 IL-1) activity. Fertil Steril 1988;49:964–968.

60. Wang L, Robertson S, Seamark RF, Norman FJ. Lymphokines, including interleukin-2, after gonadotropin-stimulating progesterone production and proliferation of human granulosa-luteal cells in vitro. J Clin Endocrinol Metab 1991;72:824–831.

61. Sjogren A, Holmes RV, Hillensjo T. Interleukin-1 modulates luteinizing hormone stimulated cyclic AMP and progesterone release from human granulosa cells in vitro. Human Reprod 1992; 6:910–913.

62. Best CL, Hill JA. Interleukin-1 alpha and beta modulation of luteinized human granulosa cell estrogen and progesterone biosynthesis. Human Reprod 1996; 3206–3210.

63. Hurwitz A, Hernandez ER, Andreal CL, Resnick CE, Payne DW, Adashi EY. Cytokine-mediated regulation of ovarian function: interleukin-1 inhibits gonadotropin-induced androgen biosynthesis. Endocrinology 1991;1250–1257.

64. Fukuoka M, Mari T, Taii S, Yasuda K. Interleukin-1 inhibits luteinization of porcine granulosa cells in culture. Endocrinology 1988;122:367–369.

65. Fukuoka M, Yasuda K. Taii S, Takakuro K, Mori T. Interleukin-1 stimulates growth and inhibits progesterone secretion in cultures of porcine granulosa cells. Endocrinology 1989;124:884–890.

66. Yasuda K, Fukuoka M, Tali S, Takakura K, Mori T. Interleukin effects of interleukin-1 on follicle stimulating hormone induction of aromatase activity, progesterone secretion, and functional luteinizing hormone receptors in cultures of porcine granulosa cells. Biol Reprod 1990;43:90–96.

67. Gotschall PE, Uehara A, Hoffmann ST, Arimura A. Interleukin-1 inhibits follicle stimulating hormone-induced differentiation in rat granulosa cells in vitro. Biochem Biophys Res Comm 1987;149:502–509.

68. Gotschall PE, Katsuura G, Dahl RR, Hoffmann ST, Arimura A. Discordance in the effecf of IL-1 on rat granulosa cell differentiation induced by follicle-stimulating hormone or activators of adenylate cyclase. Biol Reprod 1988;39:1074–1085.

69. Pestka S, Langer JA, Zoon KC, Samuel CE. Interferons and their actions. Ann Rev Biochem 1987;56:727–777.

70. Dinarella CA, Mier JW. Lymphokines. New Engl J Med 1987;317:940–945.

71. Hill JA, Welch WR, Faris HM, Anderson DJ. Induction of class II major histocompatibility complex antigen expression in human granulosa cells by interferon gamma: a potential mechanism contributing to autoimmue ovarian failure. Am J Obstet Gynecol 1990:162:534–540.

72. Orava M, Cantell K, Vihko, R. Human leukocyte interferon inhibits human chorionic gonadotropin stimulated testosterone production by porcine leydig cells in culture. Biochem Biophys Res Commun 1985;127:809–815.

73. Branca AA, Franke MA, Sluss PM, Reichert LE. Interferon inhibits FSH-stimulated estradiol production in rat Sertoli cell cultures. Med Sci Res 1987;15:739.

74. Orava M, Voutilainen R, Vihko R. Interferon-gamma inhibits steroidogenesis and accumulation of mRNA of the steroidogenic enzymes P450scc and P450c 17 in cultured porcine leydig cells. Mol Endocrinol 1989;3:887–894.

75. Fentiman IS, Thomas BS, Galkwill FR, Rubens RD, Haywood JL. Primary hypothyroidism associated with interferon therapy of breast cancer. Lancet 1985;1:1166.

76. Nagayama Y, Izumi M, Ashizawa K, Kiriyama T, Yokoyama N, Morita S, Ohtakara S, Fukuda T, Equchi K, Morimoto I, Okamoto S, Ishikawa N, Ito K, Nagataki S. Inhibitory effect of interferon-gamma on the response to TSH and the expression of Dr antigen. J Clin Endocrinol Metab 1987;64:949–953.

77. Shimuzi F, Shimizu M, Kamaiyma K. Inhibitory effect of interferon on the production of insulin. Endocrinology 1985;117:2081–2084.

78. Campbell IL, Oxbrow L, Harrison L. Interferon-gamma pleiotropic effects on a rat pancreatic beta cell line. Mol Cell Endocrinol 1987;52:161–167.

79. Goldstein D, Cockerman J, Krishnan R, Ritchie J, Tso CY, Hood LE, Ellinwood E, Laszlo J. Effects of gamma-interferon on the endocrine system: results from a phase I study. Cancer Res 1987;47:6397–6401.

80. Grasso G, Muscettola M, Traina V, Causio F, Fanizza G, Cognazzo G. Presence of interferons in human follicular fluid after ovarian hyperstimulation for in vitro fertilization. Med Sci Res 1988;16:167–168.

81. Gorospe WC, Tuchel T, Kasson BG. Gamma-interferon inhibits rat granulosa cell differentiation in culture. Biochem Biophys Res Commun 1988;157:891–897.

82. Kauppila A, Cantell K, Janne O, Kokko E, Vihko R. Serum sex steroid and peptide hormone concentrations, and endometrial estrogen and progestin receptor levels during administration of human leukocyte interferon. Int J Cancer 1982;29:291–294.

83. Wang LJ, Brannatrom M, Robertson SA, Norman RJ. Tumor necrosis factor α in the human ovary: presence in follicular fluid and effects on cell proliferation and prostaglandin production. Fertil Steril 1992;58:934–940.

84. Buyaios RP, Watson JM, Martinez-Maza O. Detection of interleukin-6 in human follicular fluid. Fertil Steril 1992;1230–1234.

85. Gorospe WC, Spangelo BL. Interleukin-6 production by rat granulosa cells in vitro: effects of cytokines, follicle-stimulating hormone, and cyclic 3´5´-adenosine monophosphate. Biol Reprod 1993;48:538–543.

86. Mori T, Takakura K, Fujiwara H, Hayashi K. Immunology of ovarian function. In Bronson, ed. Reproductive Immunology. Cambridge, MA: Blackwell Science, 1996:240–274.

87. Motro B, Itin A, Sachs L, Keshet E. Pattern of interleukin-6 gene expression in vivo suggests a role for this cytokine in angiogenesis. Proc Natl Acad Sci USA 1990;87:3092–3096.

88. Gorospe WC, Hughes PM Jr, Spangelo BL. Interleukin-6: effects on and production by rat granulosa cells in vitro. Endocrinology 1992;130:1750–1752.

89. Hammond JM. Peptide regulators in the ovarian follicle. Aust J Biol Sci 1981;34:491.

90. Hammond JM, Hsu C-J, Klindt J, Tsang BK, Downey BR. Gonadotropin increase concentrations of immunoreactive insulin-like growth factor-I in porcine follicular fluid in vivo. Biol Reprod 1988;38:304.

91. Hsu CJ, Hammond JM. Gonadotropin and estradiol immunoreactive insulin-like growth factor-1 production by porcine granulosa cells in vitro. Endocrinology 1985;117–253.

92. Hsu CJ, Hammond JM. Concomitant effects of growth hormone secretion of insulin-like growth factor-I and progesterone by cultured porcine granulosa cells. Endocrinology 1987;121:1343.

93. Mondschein JS, Hammond JM. Growth factors regulate immunoreactive insulin-like growth factor-I by cultured porcine granulosa cells. Endocrinology 1988;123:463.

94. Oliver JE, Aitman TJ, Powell JF, et al. Insulin-like growth factor I gene expression in rat ovary is confined to the granulosa cells of developing follicles. Endocrinology 1989:124:2671–2679.

95. Hernandez ER, Roberts CT Jr, LeRoith D, Adashi EY. Rat ovarian insulin-like growth factor I (IGF-I) gene expression is granulosa cell-selective: 5'-untranslated mRNA variant representation and hormonal regulation. Endocrinology 1989;125:572–574.

96. Zhou J, Chin E, Bondy C. Cellular pattern of insulin-like growth factor-I (IGF-I)and IGF-receptor gene expression in the developing and mature ovarian follicle. Endocrinology 1991;129:3281–3288.

97. Hatey F, Langlois I, Mulsant P, et al. Gonadotropins induce accumulation of insulin-like growth factor I mRNA in pig granulosa cells in vitro. Mol Cell Endocrinol 1992;86:205–211.

98. Parmer TG, Roberts CT Jr, LeRoith D, et al. Expression, action, and steroidal regulation of insulin-like growth factor-I (IGF-I) and IGF-I receptor in the rat corpus luteum: their differential role in the two cell populations forming corpus luteum. Endocrinology 1993;133:2395–2398.

99. El-Roeiy A, Chen X, Roberts VJ, et al. Expression of insulin-like growth factor-I (IGF-I) and IGF-II and IGF-I, IGF-II, and insulin receptor genes and localization of the gene product in the human ovary. J Clin Endocrinol Metab 1993:77:1411–1418.

100. Mason H, Margara R, Winston R, et al. Insulin-like growth factor-I (IGF-I) inhibits production of IGF-binding protein-1 while stimulating estradiol secretion in granulosa cells from normal and polycystic human ovaries. J Clin Endocrinol Metab 1993;76:1275–1279.

101. Bergh C, Olsson J-H, Hillensjö T. Effect of insulin-like growth factor I on steroidogenesis in cultured human granulosa cells. Acta Endocrinol (Copenh) 1991;125:177–185.

102. Bergh C, Olsson J-H, Hillensjö T. Insulin-like growth factor I on steroidogenesis in cultured human granulosa cells. Acta Endocrinol (Copenh) 1991;125:177–186.

103. Erickson GF, Garzo VG, Magoffin DA. Insulin-like growth factor-1 regulates aromatase activity in human granulosa and granulosa-luteal cells. J Clin Endocrinol Metab 1989;89:716–724.

104. Erickson GF, Magoffin DA, Gragun JR, Change RJ. The effects of insulin and insulin-like growth factor-I and -II on estradiol production by granulosa cells of polycystic ovaries. J Clin Endocrinol Metab 1990;70:894–902.

105. Dor J Costritsci N, Pariente C, et al. Insulin-like growth factor-I and follicle-stimulating hormone suppress insulin-like growth factor binding protein-1 secretion by human granulosa-luteal cells. J Clin Endocrinol Metab 1992;75:969–971.

106. Erickson GF, Garzo VG, Magoffin DA. Progesterone production by human granulosa cells cultured in serum free medium: effects of gonadotrophins and insulin-like growth factor-I (IGF-I). Human Reprod 1991;6:1074–1081.

107. Christman GM, Rancolph JG, Peegel H, Menon KM. Differential responsiveness of luteinized human granulosa cells to gonadotropins and insulin-like growth factor-I for induction of aromatase activity. Fertil Steril 1991;55:1099–1106.

108. Veldhuis JD, Furlanetto RW, Jucther D, et al. Tropic actions of human somatomedin C/insulin-like growth factor I on ovarian cells: in vitro studies with swine granulos cells. Endocrinology 1985;116:1235–1242.

109. Veldhuis JD, Rogers RJ. Mechanisms subserving the steroidogenic synergism between follicle-stimulating hormone and insulin-like growth factor (somatomedin-C). J Biol Chem 1987;126: 7658–7664.

110. Veldhuis JD, Rodgers RJ, Furlanetto RW, et al. Synergistic actions of estradiol and the insulin-like growth factor somatomedin-C on swine ovarian (granulosa) cells. Endocrinology 1986;119:530–538.

111. Garmey JC, Day RN, Day KH, et al. Mechanisms of regulation of ovarian sterol metabolism by insulin-like growth factor type II: in vitro studies with swine granulosa cells. Endocrinology 1993;133:800–808.

112. Adashi EY, Resnick CE, Svoboda ME, Van Wyk JJ. Somatomedin-C synergizes with follicle-stimulating hormone in the acquisition of progestin biosynthetic capacity by cultured rat granulosa cells. Endocrinology 1985;116:2135–2142.

113. Adashi EY, Resnick CE, Brodie AMH, et al. Somatomedin-C-mediated potentiation of follicle-stimulating hormone-induced aromatase activity of cultured rat granulosa cells. Endocrinology 1985;117:2313–2320.

114. Adashi EY, Resnick CE, Svoboda ME, Van Wyk JJ. A novel role for somatomedin-C in the cytodifferentiation of the ovarian granulosa cell. Endocrinology 1984;115:1227–1229.

115. Rohan RM, Ricciarelli E, Kiefer MC, et al. Rat ovarian insulin-like growth factor-binding protein-6: a hormonally regulated theca-interstitial-selective species with limited antigonadotropic activity. Endocrinology 1993;132:2507–2512.

116. Hernandez ER, Resnick CE, Svoboda ME, et al. Somatomdein-C/insulin-like growth factor 1 (Sm-C/IGF-I) as an enhancer of androgen biosynthesis by cultured rat ovarian cells. Endocrinology 1988;122:1603.

117. Baranao JLS, Hammond JM. Comparative effects of insulin and insulin-like growth factors on DNA synthesis and differentiation of porcine granulosa cells. Biochem Biophys Res Commun 1984;124:484–490.

118. Maruo T, Hayashi M, Matsuo H, et al. Comparison of the facilitative roles of insulin and insulin-like growth factor I in the functional differentiation of granulosa cells. Acta Endocrinol (Copenh) 1988;117:230–240.

119. May JV, Frost JP, Schomberg DW. Differential effects of epidermal growth factor, somatomedin-C/insulin-like growth factor I, and transforming growth factor-ß on porcine granulosa cell deoxyrobonucleic acid synthesis and cell proliferation. Endocrinology 1988;123:168–179.

120. Olsson JH, Carlsson B, Hillensjö T. Effect of insulin-like growth factor I on deoxyribonucleic acid synthesis in cultured human granulosa cells. Fertil Steril 1990;54:1052–1057.

121. Angervo M, Koistinen R, Suikkari A-M, Seppälä M. Insulin-like growth factor binding protein-1 inhibits the DNA amplification induced by insulin-like growth factor 1 in human granulosa-luteal cells. Human Reprod 1991;6:770-773.

122. Yong EL, Baird DT, Yates R, et al. Hormonal regulation of the growth and steroidogenic function of human granulosa cells. J Clin Endocrinol Metab 1992;74:842–849.

123. Di Blasio QM, Viganó P, Ferrari A. Insulin-like growth factor-II stimulates human granulosa cell proliferation in vitro. Fertil Steril 1994;61:483–487.

124. Nakatani A, Shimasaki S, Erickson GF, Ling N. Tissue-specific expression of four insulin-like growth factor-I actions in the bovine luteal cells regulation of receptor tyrosine kinase activity, phosphatidylinosirol-3-kinase, and deoxyribonucleic acid synthesis. Endocrinology 1993;133:1331–1340.

125. Adashi EY, Resnick CE, Ricciarelli E, Hurwitz A, Hernandez ER. Insulin-like growth factor (IGF) binding protein-1 is an anti-gonadotropin: evidence that optimal FSH action is

contingent upon amplification by endogenously-derived IGFs. Thirty-eighth Annual Meeting, Society for Gynecologic Investigation, San Antonio, March 1991, Abstract No. 429.

126. Adashi EY, Resnick CE, Hurwitz A, Hernandez ER. Granulosa-derived insulin-like growth factor (IGF) binding proteins are inhibitory to IGF-I hormonal action: evidence derived from the use of a truncated IGF-I analogue. Seventy-third Annual Meeting, The Endocrine Society, Washington, DC, June 1991, Abstract No. 882.

127. Adashi EY, Resnick CE, Hernandez ER, et al. Follicle-stimulating hormone inhibits the constitutive release of insulin-like growth factor binding proteins by cultured rat ovarian granulosa cells. Endocrinology 1990;126:1305–1307.

128. Adashi EY, Resnick CE, Hurwitz A, Riciarelli E, Hernandez ER, Rosenfeld RG. Ovarian granulosa cell-derived insulin-like growth factor binding proteins: modulatory role of follicle-stimulating hormone. Endocrinology 1991;128:754.

129. Feng P, Catt KJ, Knecht M. Transforming growth factor-ß stimulates meiotic maturation of the rat oocyte. Endocrinology 1988;122:181–186.

130. Gómez E, Tarin JJ, Pellicer A. Oocyte maturation in humans: the role of gonadotropins and growth factors. Fertil Steril 1993;60:40–46.

131. Zhou J, Bondy C. Anatomy of the human ovarian insulin-like growth factor system. Biol Reprod 1993;48:467–482.

132. Roussie M, Royere D, Guillonueau M, Lansac J, Muth JP. Human antral fluid IGF-1 and oocyte maturity: effect of stimulation therapy. Acta Endocrinol (Copenh) 1989;121:90.

133. Hernandez ER, Roberts CT Jr, Hurwitz A, et al. Rat ovarian insulin-like growth factor II (IGF-II) gene expression is theca-interstitial cell-exclusive: hormonal regulation and receptor distribution. Endocrinology 1990;127:3249–3251.

134. Voutilainen R, Miller WL. Coordinate trophic hormone regulation of mRNAs for insulin-like growth factor II and the cholesterol side-chain cleavage enzyme, P450cc, in human steroidogenic tissues. Proc Natl Acad Sci USA 1987;84:1590–1594.

135. Geisthovel F, Moretti-Rojas I, Asch RH, Rojas FJ. Expression of insulin-like growth factor-II (IGF-II) messenger ribonucleic acid (mRNA), but not IGF-I mRNA in human pre-ovulatory granulosa cells. Proc Natl Acad Sci USA 1987;84:2643–2647.

136. Ramasharma K, Li CH. Human pituitary and placental hormones control human insulin-like growth factor II secretion in human granulosa cells. Proc Natl Acad Sci USA 1987;84:2643–2647.

137. Rechler MM, Nissley SP. Insulin-like growth factors. In: Sporn MB, Roberts AB (eds). Handbook of Experimental Pharmacology: Peptide Growth Factors and Their Receptors I. Berlin: Springer-Verlag, 1990;95:263.

138. Rotwein P. Structure, evolution, expression, and regulation of insulin-like growth factors I and II. Growth Factors 1991;5:3.

139. Rosenfeld RG. Receptors for insulin-like growth factors I and II. In: Miller EE, Cocchi D, Locatelli Y (eds). Advances in Growth Hormone and Growth Factor Research. Rome: Pythagora Press, 1989:133.

140. Daughaday WH, Rotwein P. Insulin-like growth factors I and II. Peptide, messenger ribonucleic acid and gene structures, serum, and tissue concentrations. Endocr Rev 1989;10:68.

141. Kubota T, Kamada S, Ohara M, et al. Insulin-like growth factor II in follicular fluid of the patients with in vitro fertilization and embryo transfer. Fertil Steril 1993;844–849.

142. Todato GJ, Fryling C, De Larco JE. Transforming growth factors produced by certain human tumor cells: polypeptides that interact with epidermal growth factor receptors. Proc Natl Acad Sci USA 1980;77:5258–5262.

143. Lee DC, Rose TM, Webb NR, Todaro GJ. Cloning and sequence analysis of cNA for rat transforming growth factor-alpha. Nature 1985;313:489.

144. Skinher MK, Coffey RJ Jr. Regulation of ovarian cell growth through the local production of transforming growth factor-α by theca cells. Endocrinology 1988;123:2632–2638.

145. Chegini N, Williams RS. Immunocytochemical localization of transforming growth factors (TGFs) TGF-α and TGF-ß in human ovarian tissues. J Clin Endocrinol Metab 1992;74:973–980.

146. Yeh J, Lee GY, Anderson E. Presence of transforming growth factor-alpha messenger ribonucleic acid (mRNA) and absence of epidermal growth factor mRNA in rat ovarian granulosa cells, and the effects of these factors on steroidogenesis in vitro. Biol Reprod 1993;48:1071–1081.

147. Kennedy TG, Brown KD, Vaughan TJ. Expression of the genes for the epidermal growth factor receptor and its ligands in porcine corpora lutea. Endocrinology 1993; 132:1857–1859.

148. Kudlow JE, Kobrin MS, Purchio AF, Twardzik Dr. Hernandez ER, Asa SL, Adashi EY. Ovarian transforming growth factor-alpha gene expression: immunohistochemical localization to the theca-interstitial cells. Endocrinology 121:1577, 1987.

149. Lobb DK, Kobrin MS, Kudlow JE, Dorrington JH. Transforming growth factor-alpha in the adult bovine ovary: identification in growing ovarian follicles. Biol Reprod 1989;40:1087–1093.

150. St. Arnaud R, Walker P, Kelly PA, Labrie F. Rat ovarian epidermal growth factor receptors: characterization and hormonal regulation. Mol Cell Endocrinol 1983;31:43.

151. Feng P, Knecht M, Catt K. Hormonal control of epidermal growth factor receptors by gonadotropins during granulosa cell differentiation. Endocrinology 1987; 120:1121.

152. Buck PA, Schmberg DW. [125]iodo-epidermal growth factor binding and mitotic responsiveness of porcine granulosa cells and modulating by differentiation and follicle-stimulating hormone. Endocrinology 1988;122:28.

153. Adashi EY, Resnick CE. Antagonistic interactions of transforming growth factors in the regulation of granulosa cell differentiation. Endocrinology 1986;119:1879–1881.

154. Adashi EY, Resnick CE, Twardzik DR. Transforming growth factor-α attenuates the acquisition of aromatase activity by cultured rat granulosa cells. J Cell Biochem 1987;33:1–13.

155. Gospodarowicz D, Mescher AL, Birdwell CR. Control of cellular proliferation by the fibroblast and epidermal growth factors. Natl Cancer Inst Monogr 1978;48:109.

156. Gospodarowicz D, Bialecki H. Fibroblast and epidermal growth factors are mitogenic agents for cultured granulosa cells of rodent, porcine and human origin. Endocrinology 1979;104:757.

157. Skinner MK, Keski-Oja J, Osteen KG, Moses HL. Ovarian theca cells produce transforming growth factor-ß which can regulate granulosa cell growth. Endocrinology 1987;121:1577–1579.

158. Kudlow JE, Kobrin MS, Purchio AF, et al. Ovarian transforming growth factor-alpha gene expression: immunohistochemical localization to the theca-interstitial cells. Endocrinology 1987;121:786–792.

159. Dunkel L, Tilly JL, Shikone T, et al. Follicle-stimulating hormone receptor expression in the rat ovary: increases during prepubertal development and regulation by the opposing actions of transforming growth factors ß and α. Biol Reprod 1994;50:940–948.

160. Gangrade BK, Davis JS, May JV. A novel mechanism for the induction of aromatase in ovarian cells in vitro role of transforming growth factor alpha-induced protein tyrosine kinase. Endocrinology 1991;129:2790–2792.

161. Hsu C, Holmes SD, Hammond JM. Ovarian epidermal growth factor-like activity. Concentrations in porcine follicular fluid during follicular development. Biochem Biophys Res Commun 1987;147:242–247.

162. Mondshein JS, Shomberg DW. Growth factors modulate gonadotropin receptor induction in granulosa cell cultures. Science 1981;211:1179.

163. Hsueh AJW, Welsh TH, Jones PBC. Inhibition of ovarian and testicular steroidogenesis by epidermal growth factor. Endocrinology 1981;108:2002.

164. Caubo B, Devinna RS, Tonetta SA. Regulation of sterodogenesis in cultured porcine theca cells by growth factors. Endocrinology 1989; 125:321.

165. Dekel N, Sherizl I. Epidermal growth factor induces maturation of rat follicle-enclosed oocytes. Endocrinology 1985;116;406.

166. Bendell JJ, Dorrington J. Rat thecal/interstitial cells secrete a transforming growth factor-ß-like factor that promotes growth and differentiation in rat granulosa cells. Endocrinology 1988;123:941.

167. Thompson NL, Flanders KC, Smith JM, Ellingsworth LR, Roberts AB, Sporn MB. Expression of transforming growth factor-ß 1 in specific cells and tissues of adult and neonatal mice. J Cell Biol 1989;108:661.

168. Skinner MK, Keski-Oja J, Oskeen KG, Moses HL. Ovarian thecal cells produce transforming growth factor ß gene expression. Biol Reprod 1987;36:58A.

169. Gangrade BK, May JV. The production of transforming growth factor-ß and their selective cellular localization in human ovarian tissue of various reproductive stages. Endocrinology 1992;130:1707–1715.

170. Chegini N, Flanders KC. Presence of transforming growth factor-ß and their selective cellular localization in human ovarian tissue of various reproductive stages. Endocrinology 1992;130:1707–1715.

171. Hernandez ER, Twardzik DR, Purchio A, Adashi EY. Gonadotropin-dependent ovarian transforming growth factor-ß gene expression. Biol Reprod 1987;36:58A.

172. Mulheron GW, Bossert NL, Lapp JA, et al. Human granulosa-luteal and cumulus cells express transforming growth factors-ß type 1 and type 2 mRNA. J Clin Endocrinol Metab 1992;74:458–460.

173. Teerds KJ, Dorrington JH. Immunohistochemical localization of transforming growth factor-ß1 and -ß2 during follicular development I the adult rat ovary. Mol Cell Endocrinol 1992;84:R7–R13.

174. Gangrade BK, Gotcher ED, David JS, May JV. The secretion of transforming factor-ß by bovine luteal cells in vitro. Mol Cell Endocrinol 1993;93:117–123.

175. Roy SK, Ogren C, Roy C, Lu B. Cell-type-specific localization of transforming growth factor-ß1 in the hamster ovary: differential regulation by follicle-stiumulating hormone and luteinizing hormone. Biol Reprod 1992;127:2372–2380.

176. Mondschein JS, Canning SF, Hammond JH. Effects of transforming growth factor-ß on the production of immunoreactive insulin-like growth factor I and progesterone

and the [3H]thymidine incorporation in porcine granulosa cell cultures. Endocrinology 1988;123:1970–1976.

177. Bendell JJ, Dorrington J. Rat thecal/interstitial cells secrete a transforming growth factor-ß-like factor that promotes growth and differentiation in rat granulosa cells. Endocrinology 1988;123:941–948.

178. Dorrington J, Chuma AV, Bendell JJ. Transforming growth factor ß and follicle-stimulating hormone promote rat granulosa cell proliferation. Endocrinology 1988;123:353–359.

179. Dorrington JH, Bendell JJ, Khan SA. Interactions between FSH, estradiol-17 beta and transforming growth factor-beta regulate growth and differentiation in the rat gonad. J Steroid Biochem Mol Biol 1993;44:441–447.

180. Dodson WC, Schomberg DW. The effect of transforming growth factor-ß on follicle-stimulating hormone-induced differentiation of cultured rat granulosa cells. Endocrinology 1987;120:512–516.

181. Adashi EY, Resnick CE, Hemandez ER, et al. Ovarian transforming growth factor-ß (TGF-ß): cellular site(s), and mechanism(s) of action. Mol Cell Endocrinol 1989;61:247–256.

182. Knecht M, Feng P, Catt K. Bifunctional role of transforming growth factor-ß during granulosa cell development. Endocrinology 1987;120:1243–1249.

183. Zhiwen Z, Findlay JK, Carson RS, et al. Transforming growth factor ß enhances basal and FSH-stimulated inhibin production by rat granulosa cells in vitro. Mol Cell Endocrinol 1988;58:161–166.

184. Roberts AJ, Skinner MK. Transforming growth factor-α and-ß differentially regulate growth and steroidogenesis of bovine thecal cells during antral follicle development. Endocrinology 1991;129:2041–2048.

185. Caubo B, DeVinna RS, Tonetta SA. Regulation of steroidogenesis in cultured porcine thecal cells by growth factors. Endocrinology 1989;125:321–326.

186. Magotfin DA, Gancedo B, Erickson GF. Transforming growth factor-ß promotes differentiation of ovarian thecal-interstitial cells but inhibits androgen production. Endocrinology 1989;125:1951–1958.

187. Roy SK. Epidermal growth factor and transforming growth factor-ß modulation of follicle-stimulating hormone-induced deoxyribonucleic acid synthesis in hamster preantral and early antral follicles. Biol Reprod 1993;48:552–557.

188. Vassalli P. The pathophysiology of tumor necrosis factors. Ann Rev Immunol 1992;10:411–452.

189. Zolti M, Meirom R, Shemesh M, Wollach D, Mashiach S, Shore I, Rafael ZB. Granulosa cells as a source and target organ for tumor necrosis factor-α. FEBS Lett 1990;261:253–255.

190. Kokia E, Adashi EY. Potential role of cytokines in ovarian physiology: The care for interleukin-1. In: Adashi EY and Leung PCK. The Ovary. New York: Raven Press;1993:383–394.

191. Dayer JM, Rochenonteix BD, Burrus S, et al. hrIL-1 stimulates collagenase and PGE_2 production by human synovial cells. J Clin Invest 1986;77:645–648.

192. Brännström M, Norman RJ, Seamark RF, Robertson SA. Ovulatory effect of interleukin-1ß on the perfused rat ovary. Endocrinology 1993;132:399–404.

193. Brännström M, Bonello N, Wang LJ, Norman RJ. Effects of tumor necrosis factor-α (TNFα) on ovulation in the rat ovary. 1995;7:67–73.

194. Wang LJ, Brännström M, Robertson A, Norman RJ. Tumor necrosis factor α in the human ovary: presence in follicular fluid and effects on cell proliferation and prostaglandin production. Fertil Steril 1992;58:934–940.

195. Brännström M, Wang L, Norman RUJ. Effects of cytokines on prostaglandin production and steroidogenesis of incubated preovulatory follicles of the rat. Biol Reprod 1993;48:165–171.

196. Brännström M, Normal RJ, Seamark RF, Robertson SA. Rat ovary produces cytokines during ovulatin. Biol Reprod 1994;50:88–94.

197. Stanley E, Lieschke GJ, Grail D, et al. Granulocyte/macrophage colony-stimulating factor-deficient mice show no major pertubation of hematopoiesis but develop a characteristic pulmonary pathology. Proc Natl Acad Sci USA 1994;91:5592–5596.

198. Dranoff G, Crawford AD, Sadelain M, et al. Involvement of granulocyte-macrophage colony-stimulating factor in pulmonary homeostasis. Science 1994;26:713–716.

199. Bagavandoss P, Kunkel SL, Wiggins RC, Keys PL. Tumor necrosis factor-α (TNF-α) production and localization of macrophages and T lymphocytes in the rabbit corpus luteum. Endocrinology 1988;122:1185–1187.

200. Wang LJ, Pascoe V, Petrucco OM, Normal RJ. Distribution of leukocyte subpopulations in the human corpus lutreum. Human Reprod 1992;7:197–202.

201. Pepperell JR, Wolcott K, Behrman HR. Effects of neutrophils on rat luteal cells. Endocrinology 1992;130:1001–1008.

202. Benyo DF, Pate JL. Tumor necrosis factor-alpha alters bovine luteal cell synthetic capacity and viability. Endocrinology 1992;130:854–860.

203. Fairchild DL, Pate JL. Interferon-γ induction of major histocompatibility complex antigens on cultured bovine luteal cells. Biol Reprod 1989;40:453–457.

4

CYTOKINES IN THE CERVICAL VAGINAL ENVIRONMENT

Raina N. Fichorova and Deborah J. Anderson

*Brigham and Women's Hospital, Harvard Medical School,
Boston, Massachusetts*

The lower female genital tract comprises a dynamic and complex biosystem that is influenced by hormonal changes associated with the menstrual cycle, pregnancy, lactation, contraception, and menopause; by blood and tissue products introduced during menses and parturition; by a diverse population of microorganisms including endogenous flora and pathogens that can reside in the cervicovaginal compartment; by semen and other secretions introduced with sexual intercourse; and by vaginal products, used for a variety of reasons including hygiene, lubrication, medication, and contraception. The primary function of the lower female genital tract is to provide a barrier against foreign materials including infectious organisms while serving as a conduit for delivery of spermatozoa to the upper genital tract, elimination of menstrual effluent, and passage of the fetus at parturition. Not surprisingly, epithelial cells, lymphocytes, macrophages, and dendritic cells residing in this region have been shown to have some unique characteristics. A selected population of lymphocytes, macrophages and dendritic cells populate the cervicovaginal epithelium [reviewed by

Cytokines in Human Reproduction, Edited by Joseph A. Hill
ISBN 0-471-35242-X   Copyright © 2000 Wiley-Liss, Inc.

Anderson, 1996 (1)] and are capable of producing a large array of cytokines and chemokines, depending on their differentiation and activation status and the nature of the activating stimulus. Cervical and vaginal epithelial cells can also be a primary source of many cytokines and chemokines, such as IL-1α, IL-1ß, IL-6, IL-8, M-CSF, TGF-ß, MIP1α, MIP1ß, and RANTES (2–5). Cytokines in the lower genital tract are thought to have important roles in intercellular communication underlying immune defense, epithelial cell growth and wound repair, and reproductive processes. This chapter presents an overview of the literature on cytokines in the lower human female genital tract, their significance, and prospects of future studies.

MEASUREMENT OF CYTOKINES IN CERVICOVAGINAL SECRETIONS

Studies on cytokines in the lower female genital tract have been driven by the need to understand and facilitate clinical management of genital tract infections, infertility, and pregnancy failure. Because cytokine profiles in cervicovaginal secretions are affected by hormonal status as well as other factors, it is important to establish age- and menstrual cycle-specific normal reference values for cytokine concentration ranges in cervicovaginal fluids. These should be established for women before puberty, during adolescence, at various stages of the menstrual cycle and pregnancy, and during the perimenopausal and postmenopausal stages of life. It is also important to determine the effects of intercourse, vaginal hygiene, and medication on cytokine levels in normal cervicovaginal secretions. The establishment of such reference values has been initiated in several laboratories and should include the following considerations: (1) detailed clinical information including patient age, reproductive history (parity status, sexual activity, use of contraceptives and vaginal products), hormonal profiles, vaginal microflora, vaginosis or vaginitis/cervicitis, medication, and symptoms of diabetes or other systemic autoimmune diseases; (2) documentation of recent intercourse with confirmatory testing (6). Because intercourse affects cytokine levels in the female genital tract, reference values should be obtained from women following a period of at least 72 h of abstinence; (3) use of a minimally invasive method of sample collection to avoid inflammation and bleeding. Collection techniques should be standardized and the location of collection and type of secretion noted; (4) collection, processing, and storage conditions that minimize cytokine entrapment, degradation, or inappropriate cytokine release from cells; (5) use of well established and controlled quantitative assay systems. The measurement of cytokines in biological fluids is now greatly facilitated by the large number of immunoassay kits available through various companies. Quantitative molecular (that is, reverse transcriptase polymerase chain reaction) and bioassay techniques have also been utilized.

Investigators studying cytokine expression in the lower human female genital tract have used various sample collection methods including cervicovaginal lavage (7–13), swab (14–16), and cervical brush (17). Cervicovaginal lavages (CVLs) have been performed in various volumes (i.e., 3, 5, or 10 mL) of isotonic or phosphate buffered saline. The swab technique usually entails saturating various sized cotton gauze or polyester fiber swabs with cervical or vaginal secretions by placing the swab for 10 s to 20 min into the cervix or vaginal fornix and subsequently eluting the secretions in 0.5 to 2 mL of saline or PBS with or without centrifugation. Cervical mucus collection for cytokine measurements has also been performed with an endocervical brush (17) or by direct aspiration (10, 18, 19). Each of these collection techniques has advantages and drawbacks.

Collection of cervical cells and mucus by endocervical brush provides a large amount of material for study, but is highly invasive (often associated with bleeding) and could stimulate the release of cytokines such as IL-1 by damaged epithelial cells. Swab and wick techniques are less invasive and are site specific, but usually yield a small amount of material for study. Furthermore, it needs to be determined in advance whether the material matrix of the swab or wick absorbs the cytokines being studied. The dilution factor of cervicovaginal secretions following elution from swabs and wicks can be accurately determined by weighing the swab/wick before and after sample collection. The lavage technique is minimally invasive and recovers a large amount of material for study, but assessing the dilution factor of secretions in cervicovaginal lavage specimens is problematic. Some investigators have presented cytokine concentrations per milligram of protein in diluted lavage samples (18, 19). However, the protein concentration in cervical and vaginal secretions is another independent variable, influenced by concentrations of mucins, antibodies, and so on, which are not necessarily regulated by the same factors that affect cytokine abundance. Belec et al. have assessed the dilution factor in cervicovaginal lavages by introducing 10 mM lithium chloride in 3 mL of washing buffer and measuring its concentration before and after washing by a spectrophotometer (20). This procedure resulted in a mean dilution factor of 12% ± 3.2% (range 5.6% to 18.8%), indicating that approximately 300 µL of cervicovaginal secretions are recovered by a single 3 mL wash. Belec noted that the mean volume of collected cervicovaginal secretions was significantly increased in the luteal phase in comparison with the follicular phase of the menstrual cycle (mean values 423 µL vs. 300 µL). Some investigators have used Belec's mean measure of 300 µL of recoverable cervicovaginal secretions by the lavage method to estimate a dilution factor; others have calculated the total amount of cytokine (s) recovered per CVL, and compared these total amounts in different groups.

CYTOKINES IN CERVICOVAGINAL SECRETIONS AND PRETERM LABOR

The earliest studies of cytokines in the human lower genital tract secretions were driven by growing evidence that certain cytokines (i.e., IL-1ß, IL-6, and TNF-α) play a role in the initiation of parturition, particularly in preterm labor (14–17, 21). Expression of cytokines at the fetal–maternal interface and their role in parturition is discussed elsewhere in this text. These early investigations, however, included small groups of healthy nonpregnant women and thus were the first published reports on "normal" cytokine levels in the cervicovaginal compartment. Cox et al. (21) published interesting data concerning IL-1ß. They found that 100% of their nonpregnant control group consisting of six premenopausal women and two postmenopausal women exhibited detectable but highly variable levels of IL-1ß in CVLs. Pregnant women during labor ($n = 17$) had significantly more (5–100 times) IL-1ß in CVL than term pregnant and nonpregnant women, most of it coming from vaginal rather than cervical secretions. Three pregnant women with long-standing vaginitis were also tested at multiple 7-day intervals. Their IL-1ß levels were consistently greater than those of pregnant women not in labor. Interestingly, antibiotic treatment led to decreased IL-1ß levels in CVLs from one of the women with vaginitis, whereas in another, IL-1ß levels were dramatically increased until antimycotic treatment was applied. Intercourse 4 h before CVL collection did not appear to influence IL-1ß levels in these patients. Interleukin-6 was detected in CVLs from only a few of the pregnant and none of the nonpregnant women, and levels were not affected by labor. In another study, genital tract concentrations of IL-6, recovered from swabs between 24 and 36 weeks of gestation, were significantly increased (3–4×) in women with preterm versus term delivery (15). According to other authors (16), increased levels of IL-6 in cervicovaginal secretions were predictive of preterm delivery in women whose cervical examination revealed dilatation or effacement; however, a stronger association was noted between preterm delivery and CVL TNFα levels in this study. Recently, increased IL-6 levels were also found in cervical secretions of women with intra-amniotic infection and premature rupture of membranes (22).

CYTOKINES IN CERVICOVAGINAL SECRETIONS AND FERTILITY

Studies in several laboratories have sought associations between elevated levels of cytokines in various reproductive tract fluids and infertility. It has been demonstrated that certain cytokines such as IFN-γ and TNF-α adversely affect sperm function, fertilization, and endocrine functions of the ovary and placenta [reviewed by Hill et al., 1993 (23)]. Naz et al. (18, 19) measured concentrations of IL-6, IL-8, TNF-α, and IFN-γ in cervical secretions aspirated from fertile, idiopathic infertile and infertile women with sperm antibodies in serum and/or cervical mucus to test the hypothesis that these cytokines are associated with infertility. All four cytokines were found at elevated concentrations in cervical mucus of women who remained infertile after at least 1 year of unprotected sexual intercourse; the increase in INF-γ and TNF-α concentrations were more pronounced in patients with sperm antibodies detectable by sperm agglutination, sperm immobilization, or indirect immunobead techniques.

Our research suggests that cytokines in CVLs of healthy ovulating women can be divided into four groups: cytokines detectable at menses only (LIF, RANTES, MIP-1α); cytokines detectable throughout the cycle but at highest levels at menses (IL-8, IL-6, TGF-ß and IL-1ß); cytokines detectable throughout the cycle but peaking during the late proliferative phase (M-CSF and EGF); and cytokines such as INF-γ and TNF-α, which are detectable in a subpopulation of women during nonmenses stages of the cycle and may be associated with inflammatory or immunologic events (24). Studies performed in our laboratory have also revealed that cytokines implicated in local modulation of endometrial receptivity to blastocyst implantation such as CSF-1, IL-1ß, TGF-ß1, TGF-ß2, and EGF are detectable in CVLs of fertile ovulatory reproductive-aged women throughout the menstrual cycle, with levels of CSF-1 and EGF higher in the late preovulatory proliferative phase of the cycle (11, 12). These findings encourage further use of cervicovaginal washings as a minimally invasive technique to monitor cytokine secretory patterns related to implantation and maintenance of normal pregnancy.

Following intercourse, cervicovaginal secretions contain cytokines originating from semen. A number of cytokines, chemokines, and growth factors can be constantly (IL-8, IL-6, TGF-ß, HGF, RANTES, MIP-1ß), or intermittently (IFN-γ, TNF-α, MIP-1α, IL-1ß) detected in seminal fluid of healthy fertile individuals (13, 25, 26). The presence of high levels of IL-8, TGF-ß, HGF, and RANTES in the majority of semen samples from healthy men suggests that these cytokines may have a beneficial role in human reproduction and that reduced rather than increased levels may have pathological consequences. On the other hand, increased semen levels of IL-6, TNF-α, IL-1α, IL-1ß, GROα, or IL-10 have been found by some investigators in patients with infertility, leukocytospermia, and various andrological diseases including genital infections (26–34). The immunomodulatory cytokine IL-2 was found at increased concentrations in seminal fluids of infertile patients (35, 36), but was significantly decreased in semen samples from men with genital tract infections or with antisperm antibodies (37, 38). Soluble cytokine receptors including sIL-2R, sIL-1R, sIL-6R, and sTNF-RI have also been detected in semen and may play a role in regulating the bioactivity of cytokines in semen and the cervicovaginal environment (25, 29, 39–41). Factors in semen can also affect cytokine responses by cells residing in the cervicovaginal epithelium. Kelly et al. (42) reported that prostaglandins of the E series, which are abundant in seminal fluid, enhance IL-10 production by activated T-cells and can bias the local immune response to a TH-2 (humoral) type response. Animal studies (43) have shown a dramatic increase in GM-CSF synthesis in the female reproductive tract following intercourse, and it has been hypothesized that this cytokine response enhances uterine receptivity to pregnancy. More studies are needed in this area to elucidate fully the role of cytokines in fertility and infertility.

CYTOKINES AND BACTERIAL INFECTIONS OF THE GENITAL TRACT

Cytokines in the lower female genital tract may play a role in maintaining the normal vaginal microflora while modulating potentially pathogenic host–microbial interactions. Normal vaginal fluid contains 10^5 to 10^7 microorganisms per milliliter with lactobacilli accounting for more than 90% of the bacteria. Numbers of bacteria in the vagina increase up to 1000-fold above normal in patients with vaginosis, a condition without apparent signs of inflammation (i.e., elevated number of polymorphonuclear leukocytes) (44). Studies on the relationship between vaginosis and cytokines in CVLs have focused on pregnant women with conflicting results. Platz-Christensen and colleagues (17) reported that IL-1α levels were significantly higher in vaginal fluid and lower in cervical mucus of 10 patients with bacterial vaginosis as compared to 17 pregnant women without vaginosis. Rizzo et al. (45) found no relationship between the presence of bacterial vaginosis and cervical levels of IL-1ß, IL-1ra, TNF-α, and IL-6, whereas Imseis et al. (46) found significantly elevated IL-1ß, but not

IL-1α, TNF-α, and IL-6 in nonlaboring pregnant women. Increased levels of IL-1ß were detected in cervicovaginal secretions of first trimester pregnant women with bacterial vaginosis, and BV-associated endotoxins were found to induce cytokine production by monocytic cells in vitro (47). Further information concerning the features of the inflammatory response associated with bacterial vaginosis, including cytokine levels, may provide important clues for the development of rational preventive and therapeutic strategies for this disease condition, which has been difficult to treat with conventional antibiotics.

It is important to elucidate further the role of vaginal and cervical epithelial cells as amplifiers of mucosal immune responses in cases of active bacterial, viral, and protozoan infections. In vitro models have been established to study constitutive and infection-induced expression of cytokines by epithelial cells originating from various mucosal sites. It is known that cytokines/chemokines with well defined roles in acute inflammation, such as IL-8, TNF-α, MCP-1, and GM-CSF, are upregulated in cultured human urogenital and gastrointestinal tract epithelial cells by adhesion and entry of invasive gram-positive and gram-negative bacteria including *E. coli* (48–50). Less work has been done with epithelial cell lines originating from the lower female genital tract. HPV-16/E6E7 immortalized normal human endocervical, ectocervical, and vaginal epithelial cell lines established in our laboratory all constitutively express IL-8, TGF-ß1, IL-1ß, M-CSF, and MIP-1ß, but not IFNγ, TNF-α and LIF (2). We recently showed that the endocervical cell line (columnar epithelial cells) constitutively expressed more cytokines than the ectocervical and vaginal cell lines (stratified squamous epithelial cells); the endocervical cell line expressed IL-6, IL-7, RANTES, and MIP-1α in addition to the five cytokines listed above, and the three cell lines produced higher concentrations of several of these cytokines following stimulation with IFN-γ and TNF-α. Woodworth and Simpson (3) demonstrated that primary cultures of normal human endocervical cells secrete significantly more IL-8, IL-1ß, IL-6, and TNF-α than primary human ectocervical cells, and that HPV-16 infection decreased IL-8 and totally inhibited TNF-α and IL-6 secretion. Rasmussen et al. (5) showed that chlamydial infection leads to expression of IL-1α by primary endocervical epithelial cultures and cell lines, leading to increased secretion of pro-inflammatory cytokines including IL-8, GROα, GM-CSF, and IL-6.

CYTOKINES AND VIRAL INFECTIONS OF THE GENITAL TRACT

Research on mechanisms of sexual transmission of HIV-1 has focused attention on cytokines in cervicovaginal secretions. It is well established that HIV-1 transmission is enhanced in individuals with concurrent genital tract infections (52). Demonstration that certain of the pro-inflammatory cytokines are strong promoters of HIV-1 replication has led to speculation that the presence of such cytokines in genital tract secretions of individuals with genital tract infections could play an important role in HIV-1 transmission.

It is now well established that TNF-α and TNF-ß are strong promoters of HIV-1 replication in cells of both monocytic and T lymphocytic lineages. The effect of several other cytokines on HIV-1 replication appears to be more restricted. HIV-1 replication in macrophages depends on the activation and differentiation state of the cell. Virus expression in primary macrophages is enhanced in the presence of IL-1, IL-3, low dose IL-4, GM-CSF, and M-CSF, but is inhibited by exposure to TGF-ß, IL-13, IFN-γ, IL-10, and high dose IL-4. IL-2, IL-7, and IL-12 stimulate HIV-1 replication specifically in T cells (reviewed by Meyaard et al., 1997) (53). The mechanism of action by which these cytokines regulate HIV-1 expression is not fully elucidated, but evidence suggests that the effect may be mediated through activation of the nuclear factor Kappa B (NF-KB), an intracellular regulatory factor that promotes transcription of HIV-1 proviral DNA through an interaction with the long terminal repeat region.

Recent studies have shown that dendritic and epithelial cells can also be infected by primary HIV strains (54–56) and thus may be other primary target cells in the heterosexual transmission of HIV. Little is known concerning cytokine effects on HIV-1 infection of cervicovaginal dendritic or epithelial cells.

Only a few studies have been published to date on cytokine concentrations in CVLs of HIV infected women (7, 9, 13, 57, 58). Belec et al. (7) showed that both the prevalence and levels of TNF-α, IL-1ß, and IL-6 are increased in CVLs of CDC stage IV patients as compared to earlier stages of AIDS or to healthy HIV negative women. The viral infection itself was not enough to stimulate continuously increased levels of these cytokines as shown also by a later study on IL-6 expression in CVLs of 17 women infected by human T cell leukemia/lymphotropic virus type I, another primarily sexually transmitted virus (8). We also detected significantly increased concentrations of IL-1ß in CVLs of HIV-1 infected women (13). We also found detectable levels of ß-chemokines RANTES, MIP-1α, and MIP1-ß in cervicovaginal secretions of HIV-1 infected women, whereas they are rarely detectable in nonmenstrual CVLs of HIV-1 negative women. Another recent study reported a significant correlation between cervical shedding of HIV-1 infected cells and the concentration of MIP-1ß in cervicovaginal secretions obtained from 40 women by cervical swab and/or cytobrush technique (57). Sha et al. (9) reported a trend toward higher IFN-γ levels in CVLs of HIV-1 infected women, with significantly higher levels of IFN-γ in women with vaginal infections or cervicovaginal dysplasia than in those without vaginal symptoms.

Recent studies have elucidated an important role of CXC and CC chemokines and their receptors in HIV transmission. HIV-1 uses the chemokine receptors CCR4, CCR5, and CCR3 as co-receptors for entry into target cells. The chemokines that normally bind to these receptors (i.e., RANTES, MIP1α, and MIP1ß) compete with HIV-1 for these receptors and can inhibit HIV-1 infection (59). Cells positive for chemokine receptors are especially abundant in the transformation zone of the cervix and at sites of inflammation (60). Chemokines have been detected in genital tract secretions at concentrations that inhibit HIV-1 infection in vitro (13, 24) and could play a significant role in regulating the sexual and vertical transmission of HIV-1 in the genital tract compartment.

Cytokines in cervicovaginal secretions may also affect HPV infection and pathogenesis. A study done on peripheral blood mononuclear cells suggested that interferons, particularly IFN-α ↑, may be a prognostic marker for HPV infection of human cervical epithelium (61). Another study also demonstrated that women with cervical intraepithelial neoplasia (CIN) had lost their ability to mount a cellular immune response (62). TNF and IL-1 have antiviral effects in HPV infection through downregulation of its gene transcription (63). Pao et al. (64) found that the transcription of IFN-γ was significantly reduced in both CIN and cervical cancer tissue as compared to normal cervix. Increased levels of IL-8 were also found in cervicovaginal lavages of HIV infected women with cervical dysplasia and HPV infection (58).

Larger studies of well defined cervicovaginal samples will be needed to further define the interrelationship between pro-inflammatory and anti-inflammatory cytokines and HIV, HPV, and other viral infections in the lower genital tract.

CONCLUSIONS AND PROSPECTS FOR FUTURE STUDIES

A variety of cytokines are detectable in cervical and vaginal secretions. Research in this area is clinically important because cytokines have been hypothesized to play a role in mucosal immune defense of the lower female genital tract, fertility, parturition, and the transmission and pathogenesis of genital tract infections including HIV-1 and HPV (Table 4.1). Further research is needed to define the role of genital tract cy-

Table 4.1. Cytokines detectable in human cervicovaginal secretions

Cytokine	Presence During the Menstrual Cycle in Healthy Women (24)	Putative Clinical Significance
IL-1ß	Throughout the cycle	↑ in labor (21), ↑ AIDS (CDC IV) (7, 13), ↑ in vaginosis (46)
IL-6	Throughout the cycle	↑ in preterm delivery (15, 16), ↑ in bacterial infection of epithelia (5), ↑ HIV expression (65), ↑ AIDS (CDC IV) (7), ↑ in primary infertility (19), ↑ HPV infection (4)
IL-8	Throughout the cycle	↑ in primary infertility (19), ↑ in bacterial infection of epithelia (5, 48–51)
IFN-γ	Rarely found	↑ in immunologic infertility (18), ↓ HIV expression (65), ↑ cervical dysplasia/HPV infection (61)
TNF-α	Rarely found	↑ in preterm delivery (16), ↑ in idiopathic and immunologic infertility (18), ↑ in bacterial infection of epithelia (48–51) ↑ HIV expression (65), ↑ AIDS (CDC IV) (7)
TGF-ß	Throughout the cycle	↑↓ HIV expression (65)
CSF-1	Throughout the cycle	↑ HIV expression (65)
LIF	At menses	↑ HIV expression (65)
RANTES	At menses	↓ HIV infection (59, 66)
MIP-1α	At menses	↓ HIV infection (59, 66)
MIP-1ß	Rarely found	↓ HIV infection (59, 66)

tokines in normal reproductive physiology and reproductive failure, and mucosal immune defense against infectious organisms and cancer.

ACKNOWLEDGEMENTS

Research described in this report was funded by grants from the National Institute of Health (AI35564, HD33276, and HD33205) and by contracts CSA-96-186, CSA-97-202, and CSA-88-020 from the Contraceptive Research and Development (CONRAD) Program of the U.S. Agency for International Development, which receives funds for AIDS research from an interagency agreement with NICHD.

REFERENCES

1. Anderson DJ. The importance of mucosal immunology to problems in human reproduction. J Reprod Immunol 1996;31:3–19.

2. Fichorova R, Rheinwald J, Anderson D. Differential expression of immunobiological mediators by immortalized human cervical and vaginal epithelial cells. Biol Reprod 1999;60:508–514.

3. Woodworth CD, Simpson S. Comparative lymphokine secretion by cultured normal human cervical keratinocytes, papillomavirus-immortalized, and carcinoma cell lines. Am J Pathol 1993;142:1544–1555.

4. Inglesias M, Plowman GD, Woodworth CD. Interleukin-6 and interleukin-6 soluble receptor regulate proliferation of normal human papillomavirus-immortalized, and carcinoma-derived cervical cells in vitro. Am J Pathol 1995;146:944–952.

5. Rasmussen SJ, Eckman L, Quayle AJ, Shen L, Zhang Y-X, Anderson DJ, Flere J, Stephens RS, Kagnoff MF. Secretion of proinflammatory cytokines by epithelial cells in response to Chlamidia infection suggests a central role for epithelial cells in chlamidial pathogenesis. J Clin Invest 1997;99:77–87.

6. Haimovici F, Anderson D. Detection of semen in cervicovaginal secretions. J AIDS Human Retrovirol 1995;8:236–238.

7. Belec L, Gherardi R, Payan C, Prazuck T, Malkin J-E, Benissan CT, Pillot J. Proinflammatory cytokine expression in cervicovaginal secretions of normal and HIV-infected women. Cytokine 1995;7 (6):568–574.

8. Belec L, Georges AJ, Hallouin M-C, Mohamed AS, Morand-Joubert L, Goerges-Coutbot M-C. Human T-lymphotropic virus type I excretion and specific antibody response in paired saliva and cervicovaginal secretions. AIDS Res Human Retrovir 1996;12:157–167.

9. Sha BE, D'Amico RD, Landay AL, Spear GT, Massad S, Rydman RJ, Warner NA, Padnick J, Ackatz L, Charles LA, Benson CA. Evaluation of immunologic markers in cervicovaginal fluid of HIV-infected and uninfected women: implications for the immunologic response to HIV in the female genital tract. JAIDS 16:161–168, 1997.

10. Ginsburg KA, Wolf NA, Fidel PL. Potential effects of midcycle cervical mucus on mediators of immune reactivity. Fertil Steril 1997;67:46–50.

11. Gargiulo AR, Fichorova RN, Hill JA, Anderson DJ. Cervicovaginal lavages of fertile women throughout ovulatory menstrual cycles contain detectable levels of cytokines im-

plicated in blastocyst implantation: a normative series of potential non-invasive implantation markers. Abstract presented at the 1997 meeting of the Society for Gynecologic investigations, San Diego, CA.

12. Gargiulo AR, Haimovici F, Fichorova R, Hill JA, Anderson DJ. Cytokines implicated in blastocyst implantation are detectable in cervicovaginal lavages. J Soc Gynecol Invest 1997, 4(1):240A.

13. Anderson DJ, Politch JA, Tucker LD, Fichorova R, Haimovici F, Tuomala RE, Mayer KH. Quantitation of mediators of inflammation and immunity in genital tract secretions and their relevance to HIV transmission. AIDS Res Human Retrovir, 1998;14: S-43–S-49.

14. Steinborn A, Kuhnert M, Halberstadt E. Immunmodulating cytokines induce term and preterm parturition. J Perinat Med 1996;24:381–390.

15. Lockwood CJ, Ghidini A, Wein R, Lapinski R, Casal D, Berkowitz RL. Increased interleukin-6 concentrations in cervical secretions are associated with preterm delivery. Am J Obstet Gynecol 1994, 171:1097–1102.

16. Inglis SR, Jeremieas J, Kuno K, Lescale K, Peeper Q, Chervenak FA, Witkin SS. Detection of tumor necrosis factor-α, interleukin-6, and fetal fibronectin in the lower genital tract during pregnancy: relation to outcome. Am J Obstet Gynecol 1994;171:5–10.

17. Platz-Christensen JJ, Mattsby-Baltzer I, Thomsen P, Wiqvist N. Endotoxin and interleukin 1-α in the cervical mucus and vaginal fluid of pregnant women with bacterial vaginosis. Am J Obstet Gynecol 1993;169:1161–1166.

18. Naz RK, Butler A, Witt BR, Barad D, Menge AC. Levels of interferon-γ and tumor necrosis factor-A in sera and cervical mucus of fertile and infertile women: implication in infertility. J Reprod Immunol 1995; 29:105–117.

19. Naz RK, Butler A. Interleukins-6 and -8 levels in sera and cervical mucus of fertile, idiopathic infertile and immunoinfertile women: implication in infertility. Am J Reprod Immunol 1996;35:534–540.

20. Belec L, Meillet D, Levy M, Georges A, Tevi-Benisan C, Pillot J. Dilution assessment of cervicovaginal secretions obtained by vaginal washing for immunological assays. Clin Diagn Lab Immunol 1995;2:57–61.

21. Cox SM, King MR, Linette Casey M, MacDonald PC. Interleukin-1ß, -1α, and -6 and prostaglandins in vaginal/cervical fluids of pregnant women before and during labor. J Clin Endocrinol Metabol 1993;77:805–815.

22. Rizzo G, Capponi A, Vlachopoulou A, Angelini E, Grassi C, Romanini C. Interleukine↑-6 concentrations in cervical secretions in the prediction of intrauterine infection in preterm premature rapture of the membranes. Gynecol Obstet Invest 1998;46:91–95.

23. Hill JA. Production and effect of cytokines on local immunoendocrine reproductive events in the female reproductive tract. In: Griffin PD, Johnson PM, eds. Local Immunity in Reproductive Tract Tissues. Oxford University Press, Oxford, 1993;245–254.

24. Anderson D, Fichorova R, Haimovici F, Gargiulo A, Hill J. Cytokine levels in cervicovaginal secretions of women throughout the menstrual cycle. J Reprod Immunol 1997;34 (1):41 (Abstract No. 24).

25. Srivastava MD, Lippes J, Srivastava BIS. Cytokines of the human reproductive tract. Am J Reprod Immunol 1996;36:157–166.

26. Depuydt CE, Bosmans E, Zalata A, Schoonjans F, Comhaire FH. The relation between reactive oxygen species and cytokines in andrological patients with or without male accessory gland infection. J Androl 1996;17:699–707.

27. Naz RK, Kaplan P. Increased levels of interleukin-6 in seminal plasma of infertile men. J Androl 1994;15:220–227.

28. Naz RK, Chaturvedi MM, Aggarwal BB. Role of cytokines and protooncogenes in sperm cell function: relevance to immunologic infertility. Am J Reprod Immunol 1994; 32:26–37.

29. Comhaire F. Bosmans E, Ombelet W, Pujabi U, Schoonjans F. Cytokines in semen of normal men and patients with andrological diseases. Am J Reprod Immunol 1994;31:99–103.

30. Shimoya K, Matsuzaki N, Ida N, Okada T, Taniguchi T, Sawai K, Itah S, Ohashi K, Saji F, Tanizawa O. Detection of monocyte chemotactic and activating factor (MCAF) and interleukin (IL)-6 in human seminal plasma and effect of leukospermia on these cytokine levels. Am J Reprod Immunol 1995;34:311–316.

31. Yasumoto R, Kawano M, Tsujino T, iwai Y, Hayashi S, Nishisaka N, Horii A, Kishimoto T. Seminal plasma cytokines in nonbacterial prostatitis: changes following sparfloxacin treatment. Hinuokika Kiyo 1995;41:771–774.

32. Zalata A, Hafez T, Van Hoecke MJ, Comhaire F. Evaluation of beta-endorphin and interleukin-6 in seminal plasma of patients with certain andrological diseases. Hum Reprod 1995;10:3161–3165.

33. Gruschwitz MS, Brezinschek R, Brezinschek H-P. Cytokine levels in the seminal plasma of infertile males. J Androl 1996;17:158–163.

34. Rajasekaran M, Hellstrom W, Sikka S. Quantitative assessment of cytokines (GRO alpha and IL-10) in human seminal plasma during genitourinary inflammation. Am J Reprod Immunol 1996;36:90–95.

35. Rajasekaran M, Hellstrom WJ, Naz RK, Sikka SC. Oxidative stress and interleukins in seminal plasma during leukocytospermia. Fertil Steril 1995;64:166–171.

36. Paradisi R, Capelli M, Mandini M, Bellavia E, Focacci M, Flamigni C. Interleukin-2 in seminal plasma of fertile and infertile men. Arch Androl 1995;35:35–41.

37. Hussenet F, Dousset B, Cordonnier JL, Foliguet B, Grignon G, Nabet P. Interleukin-2 and human seminal fluid. Contracept Fertil Sex 1993;21:376–377.

38. Hussenet F, Dousset B, Cordonnier JL, Jacob C, Foliguet B, Grignon G, Nabet P. Tumor necrosis factor alpha and interleukin 2 in normal and infected human seminal fluid. Human Reprod 1993;8:409–411.

39. Miska M, Mahmoud M. determination of soluble interleukin-2 receptor in human seminal plasma. Arch Androl 1993;30:23–28.

40. Shimonovitz S, Barak V, Zacut D, Ever-Hadani P, Ben Chetrit A, Ron M. High concentration of soluble interleukin-2 receptors in ejaculate with low sperm motility. Human Reprod 1994;9:653–655.

41. Huleiheil M, Lunenfeld E, Levy A, Potashnik G, Glezerman M. Distinct expression levels of cytokines and soluble cytokine receptors in seminal plasma of fertile and infertile men. Fertil Steril 1996;66:135–139.

42. Kelly RW, Carr GG, Critchley HO. A cytokine switch induced by human seminal plasma: an immune modulation with implications for sexually transmitted diseases. Human Reprod 12:1997:677–681.

43. Robertson SA, Mau VJ, Hudson SN, Tremellen KP. Cytokine-leukocyte networks and the establishment of pregnancy. Am J Immunol. 1997;37:438–442.

44. Eschenbach DA. Bacterial vaginosis: emphasis on upper genital tract complications. Obstet Gynecol Clin North Am 1997;16 (3):593–611.

45. Rizzo G, Capponi A, Rinaldo D, Tedeschi D, Arduini D, Romanini C. Interleukin-6 concentrations in cervical secretions identify microbial invasion of the amniotic cavity in patients with preterm labor and intact membranes. Am J Obstet Gynecol 1996;175:812–817.

46. Imseis HM, Greig PC, Livengood CH, Shunior E, Durda P, Erikson M. Characterization of the inflammatory cytokines in the vagina during pregnancy and labor and with bacterial vaginosis. J Soc Gynecol Invest 1997;4:90–94.

47. Mattsby-Baltzer I, Platz-Christensen JJ, Hosseini N, Rosen P. Il-1 beta, Il-6, TNF alpha, fetal fibronectin, and endotoxin in the lower genital tract of pregnant women with bacterial vaginosis. Acta Obstet Gynecol Scand 1998;77:701–706.

48. Svanborg C, Agace W, Hedges S, Linder H, Svensson M. Bacterial Adherence and epithelial cell cytokine production. Zbl. Bakt 1993;278:359–364.

49. Agace WW, Hedges SR, Ceska M, Svanborg C. Interleukin-8 and the neutrophil response to mucosal gram-negative infection. J Clin Invet 1993;92:780–785.

50. Jung HC, Eckmann L, Yang S-K, Panja A, Fierer J, Morzycka-Wroblewska E. A distinct array of proinflammatory cytokines is expressed in human colon epithelial cells in response to bacterial invasion. J Clin Invest 1995;95:55–65.

51. Eckman L, Kagnoff MF, Fierer J. Intestinal epithelial cells as watchdogs for the natural immune system. Trends Microbiol 1995;3:118–120.

52. Royce RA, Sena A, Cates W Jr., Cohen MS. Sexual transmission of HIV. New Engl J Med 1997;336:1072–1078.

53. Meyaard L, Schuitemaker H, Miedema F. Cytokines in HIV-1 Infection. In: Remick DG, Friedland JS, eds. Cytokines in Health and Disease. Marcel Dekker, 1997; 623–635.

54. Tan X, Pearce-Pratt R, Phillips DM. Productive infection of a cervical epithelial cell line with human immunodeficiency virus: implication for sexual transmission. J Virol 1993;67:6447–6452.

55. Furuta Y, Eriksson K, Svennerholm B, Fredman P, Horal P, Jeansson S, Vahlne A, Holmgren J, Czerkinski C. Infection of vaginal and colonic epithelial cells by the human immunodeficiency virus type 1 is neutralized by antibodies raised against conserved epitopes in the envelope glycoprotein gp 120. Proc Natl Acad Sci USA 1994;91:12559–12563.

56. Granelli-Piperno A, Moser B, Pope M et al. Efficient interaction of HIV-1 with purified dendritic cells via multiple chemokine receptors. J Exp Med 1996;184:2433–2438.

57. Iversen AK, Fugger L, Eugen-Olsen J, Balslev U, Jensen T, Wahl S, Gerstoft J, Mullins JI, Skinhoj P. Cervical human immunodefficiency virus type 1 is associated with genital beta-chemokine secretion. J Infect Dis 1998;178:1334–1342.

58. Spear GT, Sha BE, Saarloos MN, Benson CA, Rydman R, Massad LS, Gilmore R, Landay AL. Chemokines are present in the genital tract of HIV-seronegative women: correlation with other immune mediators. J AIDS Human Retrovirol 1998;18:454–459.

59. Cocchi F, DeVico AL, Garzino-Demo A, Arya SK, Gallo RC, Lusso P. Identification of RANTES, MIP-1α, and MIP-1ß as the major HIV-suppressive factors produced by CD8+ T cells. Science 1995;270:1811–1815.

60. Anderson DJ, Fichorova R, Wang YM, Pudney J. ß-chemokines and their receptors in human reproductive tract secretions and tissues. Abstract presented at the 1997 meeting of the Society for Gynecologic investigations, San Diego, CA.

61. Labeit D, Labeit S, Berger M, Gallati H, Rosenberg R, Friese K. Interferon-alpha controls HPV infection in cervix epithelium. Zentrabl Gynakol 1995;117 (11):566–577.

62. Clerici M, Merola M, Ferrario E, Trabattoni D, Villa MC, et al. Cytokine production patterns in cervical intraepithelial neoplasia: assiciation with human papillomavirus infection. J Natl Cancer Inst 1997;89:245–250.

63. Kyo S, Inoue M, Hayasaka N, Inoue T, Yutsudo M, Tanizawa O, Hakura A. Regulation of early gene expression of human papillomavirus type 16 by inflammatory cytokines. Virology 1994;200:130–139.

64. Pao Cc, Lin CY, Yao DS, Tseng CJ. Differential expression of cytokine genes in cervical cancer tissues. Biochem Biophys Res Commun 1995;214:1146–1151.

65. Bornemann MAC, Vernoff J, Peterson PK. Macrophages, cytokines and HIV. J Lab Clin Med 1997;129:10–16.

66. Dragic T, Litwin V, Allaway GP, Martin SR, Huang Y, Nagashima KA, Cayanan C, Maddon PJ, Koup RA, Moore JP, Paxton WA. HIV-1 entry into CD4[+] cells is mediated by the chemokine receptor CC-CKR-5. Nature 1996;381:667–673.

5

CYTOKINES AND GROWTH FACTOR NETWORKS IN HUMAN ENDOMETRIUM FROM MENSTRUATION TO EMBRYO IMPLANTATION

Nasser Chegini and R. Stan Williams

University of Florida, Gainesville, Florida

During the menstrual cycle, human endometrium undergoes extensive cyclic architectural modifications in preparation for embryo implantation. This process, which begins with degenerative signals resulting in menstrual bleeding and endometrial shedding, integrates many overlapping and dynamic events to regenerate and become receptive to such an event. The endometrial regenerative process is initiated by an inflammatory reaction and is followed by a rapid cell proliferation, angiogenesis, differentiation (tissue formation), and tissue remodeling. If conception is not established, the next cycle begins. The process of endometrial regeneration remarkably resembles that of wound healing in that the tissue repairs rather than regenerates. The importance of ovarian steroids in the regenerative and receptive processes and in embryo implantation and development is well established. However, emerging evidence

Cytokines in Human Reproduction, Edited by Joseph A. Hill
ISBN 0-471-35242-X   Copyright © 2000 Wiley-Liss, Inc.

suggests that local expression and synthesis of various autocrine/paracrine growth factors and cytokines in the endometrium (Table 5.1) also play a critical role in these events. The relative low rate of successful implantation in humans suggests that the expression of these molecules and their biologic signals must be optimal, precise, and synchronized. The correct and timely progression of expression and interactions of these signals provides a receptive endometrial environment for the embryo. Aberrations of some of these factors may be responsible for inappropriate preimplantation embryonic development (tubal factor), and failure in implantation (endometrial factor). Despite a lack of direct evidence to support cytokine involvement in normal physiological and pathophysiological processes affecting the endometrium, in this chapter we attempt to present the current understanding regarding their expression and potential involvement in events leading to menstruation, endometrial regeneration (proliferation, differentiation, angiogenesis, and remodeling), and embryo implantation.

Table 5.1. The Effect of Genetic Knockouts on Embryo Implantation and Development

Geno	Overall Phenotype	Effect	Reference
Estrogen R	Viable	Females infertile; males have reduced fertility	Lubahn DB et al. PNAS 1993;90:11162
Progesterone R	Viable	Defect in reproductive tissues, hyperplasia, inflammation	Lydon JP et al. Genes Dev 1995;9:2266
TGF-α	Viable	Hair follicle and eye defect	Mann GB et al. Cell 1993;73:249
EGF-R	Viable (lethal E7.5)	Implantation chamber is filled with maternal blood, no distinct endoderm	Threadgill DW et al. Science 1995;269:230
IGF-I	Viable	Perinatal lethality, infertile	Baker J et al. Cell 1993;75:73
IGF-II	Viable	Growth retardation at birth	DeChiara TM et al. Nature 1990;345:78
IGF-I + IGF-II	Viable	Growth retardation	Liu JP et al. Cell 1993;75:59
IGF-IR	Viable (die in utero)	Organ hypoplasia	Liu JP et al. Cell 1993;75:59
IGF-I + IGF-IR	Viable	Perinatal lethality, infertile	Liu JP et al. Cell 1993;75:59
IGF-II + IGF-IR	Viable (die in utero)	Perinatal lethality, infertile	Liu JP et al. Cell 1993;75:59
PDGF B	Viable (die prenatally)	Several anatomic and histological abnormalities	Levee P et al. Genes Dev 1994;8:1875

(continued)

Table 5.1. The Effect of Genetic Knockouts on Embryo Implantation and Development (*Continued*)

Gene	Overall Phenotype	Effect	Reference
PDGF ßR	Viable (die prenatally)	Kidney defect, hemorrhagic anemic thrombocytopenia	Soriano P et al. Genes Dev 1994;8:1888.
TGF-ß1	Viable (neonatally lethal)	Neonatal lethal multifocal inflammation	Christ M et al. J. Immunol 1994;153:1936
TGF-ß1	Viable	Humoral autoimmunity	Dang N et al. J Immunol 1995;155:3205
TGF-ß3	Viable (neonatally lethal)	Undeveloped lung	Kaartinen V et al. Nat Genet 1995;11:415
FGF-4	Viable	Embryo does not develop (lethal E4–6)	Feldman B et al. Science 1995;267:246
HGF	Viable E13–E16.5)	Impaired placental labyrinth	Schmidt C et al. Nature 1995;373:699
VEGF (het)	Viable (lethal E11–12)	Impaired angiogenesis	Ferrara N et al. Nature 1996;380:439
VEGF (hom)	Viable (lethal E10.5)	Impaired vascular development	Carmeliet P et al. Nature 1996;380:435
NGF	Viabale (perinatal death)	Impairment in sensory and sympathetic ganglia	Crowley C et al. Cell 1994;76:1001
NGFR	Viable	Decreased sensory innervation	Davies AM et al. Neuron 1993;11:565
Angiotensin 1	Viable	Lesions in the renal cortex	Niimura F et al. J Clin Invest 1995;96:2947
IL-1ß	Viable	Delay typed and contact hyper-sensitivity	Zheng H et al. Immunity 1995;3:9
IL-1ß convertase	Viable	Low IL-1 production resistance to endo-toxic shock	Li P et al. Cell 1995;80:401
IL-1 IR	Viable	Sensitization of cytokines	Leon LR et al. Am J Physiol. 1996;271:1668
IL-1Ra	Viable	Decreased body mass	Hirsch E et al. PNAS 1996;93:11008
IL-2	Viable	Reject islet allografts	Steiger J et al. J Immunol 1995;155:489
IL-2R γ chain	Viable	Lymphopenia	DiSanto JP et al. PNAS 1995;92:377

(*continued*)

Table 5.1. The Effect of Genetic Knockouts on Embryo Implantation and Development
(*Continued*)

Gene	Overall Phenotype	Effect	Reference
IL-2 + IL-4	Viable	Increased T cell proliferation	Sadlack B et al. Eur J Immunol 1994; 24:281
IL-3 R α chain	Viable	No response to IL-3	Ichihara M et al. EMBO J 1995;14:939
IL-3R ß chain	Viable	Lung pathology	Nishinakamura R et al. Immunity 1995;2:211
IL-4	Viable	CD4 -produced cytokines reduced	Kopf M et al. Nature 1993;362:245.
IL-6	Viable	Impaired immune response	Poli V et al. EMBO J 1994;13:1189
IL-7	Viable	Severe lymphoid abnormality	von Freeden-Jeffrys U et al. J Exp Med 1995;181:1519
IL-7 R	Viable	Impaired lymphocyte expansion	Peschon JJ et al. J Exp Med. 1994;180:1955
IL-8 R	Viable	Lymphoadenopathy	Cacalano G et al. Science 1995;270:794
IL-10	Viable	Reduced growth	Kuhn R et al. Cell 1993;75:263
IFN-γ	Viable	Fertile, with multiple immune disorders	Dalton DK et al. Science 1993;259:1739
IFN-γ R	Viable	Normal except with defective natural resistance	Eng VW et al. J Exp Med 1995;181:1893
Lymphotoxin A (TNF-β)	Viable	Defect in secondary lymphoid organs	Banks TA et al. J Immunol 1995;155:1685
TNF-ß	Viable	No lymph nodes, increased IgM + B cells	De Togni P et al. Science 1994;264:703
TNF-R1 (P55)	Viable	Resistance to endotoxic shock	Rothe J et al. Nature 1993;364:798
TNF-R2 (P75)	Viable	Resistance to TNF-induced necrosis and death	Erickson SL et al. Nature 1994;372:560
p55/p75	Viable	Combination of both	Erickson SL et al. Nature 1994;372:560
GM-CSF	Viable	Pulmonary pathology	Dranoff G. et al. Science 1994;264:713

(continued)

TTable 5.1. The Effect of Genetic Knockouts on Embryo Implantation and Development (*Continued*)

Gene	Overall Phenotype	Effect	Reference
M-CSF	Viable	Abnormal brain stem auditory	Michaelson MD et al. Development 1996;122:3661
G-CSF	Viable	Chronic neutropenia, defect granulopoiesis	Lieschke GJ et al. Blood 1994;84:1737
LIF	Viable (no implantation in homozygous mother)	Decreased hematopoietic stem cells	Stewart CL et al. Nature 1992;359:76
CNTF	Viable (die prenatally	Defect in peripheral nervous system	Sariola H et al. Ann Med 1994;26:355
NT (neurotrophin)	Viable	Defect in peripheral nervous system	Sariola H et al. Ann Med 1994;26:355
gp-130	Viable (die E12.5–term)	Myocardial and hematopoiesis defect	Yoshida K et al. PNAS 1996;93:407
Src/fyn/yes	Viable	No defect	Kiefer F et al. 1994; Curr Opin Biol 4:100
Egr-1	Viable	Female infertile, reduced uterine weight	Lee SL et al. Science 1996;273:1219
Retinoblastom	Viable (lethal E14)	Neural/hematopoietic defect	Wiman KG. FASEB J 1993;7:841
V-rel	Viable	Develop multicentric leukemia	Carrasco D et al EMBO J. 1996;15:3640
Fas	Viable	Accumulation of abnormal T cells	Adachi M et al. PNAS 1996;93:213
P53	Viable	Susceptible to tumor formation	Doenhower LA et al. Nature 1992:356:215
c-myc	Viable (lethal E9.5)	Growth retardation	Davis AC et al. Gen Dev 1993;7:671
Jak-3	Viable	Severe block in B cell development	Thomis DC et al. Science 1995;270:794
Stat4	Viable	Fail to respond to IL-12	Kaplan MH et al. Nature 1996;382:174
Stat6	Viable	IL-4-mediated function	Shimoda K et al. Nature 1996;380:630
p-Selectin	Viable	Leukocyte defects	Mayadas TN et al. Cell 1993;74:541
L-Selectin	Viable	Defective delayed-type hypersensitivity	Xu J. et al. J Exp Med. 1996;92:12426
Vitronectin	Viable	Normal (low PAI-1)	Zheng X et al. PNAS 1995;183:589

(*continued*)

Table 5.1. The Effect of Genetic Knockouts on Embryo Implantation and Development
(*Continued*)

Geno	Overall Phenotype	Effect	Reference
Fibronectin	Viable (lethal E 9–10)	Defects in mesoderm, neural tube, and blood vessel development	George EL et al. Development 1993;119:1079
Tenassin-C	Viable	Normal	Forsberg E et al. PNAS 1996;93:6594
E-Catherin	Viable (die around the time of implantation	Fail to form trophec-toderm	Larue L et al. PNAS 1994;91:8263
S-laminin	Viable (neonatally lethal)	Proteinuria, neuro-muscular junction defects	Noakes PG et al. Nature 1995;374:258
Desmin	Viable (fertile)	Defect in muscle tissue organization	Milner DJ et al. J Cell Biol; 1996:134:1255
ß catenin	Viable	Defect in ectodermal cell layer; lack of mesoderm	Haegel H et al. Development 1995;121:3529
Collagen α 1	Viable	Degenerative inflammatory joint disorder	Fassler R et al. PNAS 1994;91:5070
Collagen α2 (V)	Viable (neonatal death)	Abnormalities in spine, skin, and eyes	Andrikopoulous K et al. Nature Genet 1995;9:31
Procollagen type V	Viable (postnatal death)	Abnormalities in spine, skin, and eyes	Andrikopoulos K et al. Nature Genet 1995;9:31
Collagen 4A3	Viable	Normal	Cosgrove D et al. Genes Dev 1996;10:2981
Integrin α3	Viable		
Integrin α4	Viable (lethal E11)	Severe heart defect and facial abnormalities	Yang JT et al. Development 1995;121:549
Integrin α5	Viable (lethal E10–11)	Mesodermal defect	Yang JT et al. Development 1993;119:1093
Integrin α6	Viable (neonatally lethal)	Loose and easily detachable skin	Georges-Labouesse E et al. Nature Genet 1996;13:370
Integrin αv	Viable	Die after birth due to hemorrhage	
Integrin ß1	Viable (lethal E5.5)	No extensive invasion of decidua periimplantation lethality	Stephens LE et al. Genes Dev 1995;9:1883

(*continued*)

Table 5.1. The Effect of Genetic Knockouts on Embryo Implantation and Development
(*Continued*)

Geno	Overall Phenotype	Effect	Reference
Integrin ß2	Viable	Progressive dermatitis	Bullard DC et al PNAS 1996;93:2116
Integrin ß4	Viable (neonatally lethal)	Detachment of epidermis and other squamous epithelia	Van der Neut R et al. Nature Genet 1996;13:366
Integrin ß7	Viable	Hypoplasia of the gut associated with lymphoid tissue	Wagner N et al. Nature 1996;382:366
ICAM-1	Viable	Leukocytosis, impaired immune response	Xu H et al. J Exp Med 1994;180:95
VCAM-1	Viable (lethal E8–10)	Chorioallantoic fusion disrupted	Gurtner GC et al. Genes Dev 1995;9:1
CD43	Viable	Enhancement in homotypic adhesion	Manjunath N et al. Nature 1995;377:535
CD45	Viable	Increased B cell number	Byth KF et al. J Exp Med. 1996;183:1707
Sialomucin CD34	Viable	Normal	Cheng J et al. Blood 1996;87:479
CD28	Viable	Decreased T cell response to lectins	Green J et al. Immunity 1994;41:501
COX-2	Viable	Ovarian defect-infertile	Dinchuck JE et al. Nature 1995;378:406
AP-2	Viable (die at) birth	Cranial neural defect	Zhang J et al. Nature 1996;381:238
Plasminogen	Viable	Fertile, but pre-disposed to severe thrombosis	Bugge TH et al. Genes Dev 1995;9:794
uPA	Viable	Occasional fibrin deposition	Carmeliet P et al. Nature 1994;368:419
tPA	Viable	Impaired clot lysis	Carmeliet P et al. Nature 1994;368:419
tPA/uPA	Viable	Extensive fibrin deposition	Carmeliet P et al. Nature 1994;368:419
PAI-I	Viable	Mildly hyper-fibrinolytic	Carmeliet P et al. J Clin Invest. 1993;92:2746
TF	Viable (lethal E8.5)	Defect in blood vessel formation	Carmeliet P et al. Nature 1996;383:75
TIMP-1	Viable	Normal	Nothnick WB et al. Biol Reprod 1997;56:1181

CYTOKINES, GROWTH FACTORS, AND CYCLIC ENDOMETRIAL REGENERATION

From infancy to menarche, except for normal body growth, the endometrium undergoes little morphological change. However, with the onset of puberty, remarkable morphological and biochemical alterations begin that are unique to the endometrium and are unmatched by any other tissue in the body. These events, which begin with the proliferation of endometrial cells are governed by the action of estrogen which initiate the cyclic changes that ultimately lead to the establishment of the menstrual cycle. Upon the establishment of regular ovulatory cycles, the endometrium, under the influence of ovarian steroids, undergoes cyclic morphological and biochemical changes that are remarkably consistent during each cycle and throughout the reproductive years. Despite the ill defined boundaries between functionalis, and basalis regions, the most dramatic changes that occur in the endometrium take place in the functionalis, which sheds during menstruation. This is assumed to be due to differences in response to ovarian steroid action in that the basalis responds to the mitogenic actions of estrogen, whereas the functionalis responds to both estrogen and progesterone actions (1). During the preovulatory phase of the menstrual cycle, estrogen acts as a mitogen for various endometrial cells. As estrogen levels fall, progesterone acts on the estrogen primed endometrium, inducing differentiation and secretory changes in the glandular epithelial cells. Progesterone also causes stromal decidualization and acts to prepare the endometrium for embryo implantation during the postovulatory phase. In the event of pregnancy, progesterone is responsible for the implantation process; however, a sudden decline in progesterone production at the end of the luteal phase leads to constriction of the endometrial spiral or coiled arteries, which initiates menstrual bleeding and denudation of the functionalis region (1).

After the disruption and loss of normal tissue architecture in higher vertebrates, the tissue undergoes many overlapping and dynamic processes in order to repair or regenerate to return to its normal function. These processes include the inflammatory response, cell growth and differentiation, angiogenesis, extracellular matrix turnover, tissue remodeling, and apoptosis. Commonly these processes occur during endometrial regeneration and wound healing; however, there is a lack of perfect tissue regeneration in the adult wound. A comparison of adult and fetal wound healing reveals that in a site specific manner the fetal wound can heal with nearly perfect regeneration or scarless healing (2). In fetal wound healing, the extent of trauma, degree of inflammation, and level of inflammatory cytokines appear to be important determinants and are linked to fetal tissue regeneration (2). Thus, fetal wound healing may closely resemble the regeneration of endometrium following menstruation. The regulating mechanisms of endometrial tissue regeneration, a process that does not normally occur in other tissues, is unknown. A well orchestrated expression of cytokines, potentially regulated by ovarian steroids, may play an important role.

Inflammatory Cytokines and Menstruation

Menstruation begins with vasodilation and the disruption of blood vessels resulting in endometrial blood flow and shedding of the endometrial functionalis. This event lasts for a few days and creates trauma to the endometrial tissue, which must undergo a rapid regeneration, appropriate for embryo implantation. The identity of the factors that initiate normal menstrual bleeding and their molecular mechanisms is virtually unknown; however, it begins with a sharp decline in plasma progesterone levels (1). Immediately following menstrual bleeding, coagulation and platelet aggregation are initiated to prevent excess blood loss. These events are initiated by cell surface activation of Hageman factor, a tissue procoagulant factor released from damaged cells, surface membrane coagulation factors, and phospholipids that are expressed by activated platelets and vascular endothelial cells (3, 4). At the same time, clots must begin to lyse as a requirement to allow the initiation of endometrial regeneration. Both clot formation and degradation require the adsorption and the activation of coagulation proenzymes and the production of many intrinsic blood vessel substrates. These include production of eicosanoids such as prostacyclin (a major vasodilator and inhibitor of platelet aggregation), thromboxane (a vasoconstrictor), antithrombin III (inhibits thrombin activity), protein C (degrades coagulation factors V and VIII), plasminogen activators (convert plasminogen to plasmin and limits the extent of clotting by initiating clot to lysis), and plasminogen activator inhibitors (inhibit plasminogen activity) (3–13).

Many of these activities are regulated by the local release of various soluble factors produced by platelets and inflammatory cytokines, which in turn are synthesized and released by infiltrating and activated inflammatory cells. Platelet secretory products are stored in their α-granules and are the immediate network of highly active substances that are released in the endometrial environment during menstruation. They are also the source of many proteins with adhesive properties, including fibrinogen, fibronectin, thrombospondin, and von Willebrand factor VIII (14). These adhesion molecules act as ligands for platelet aggregation, whereas von Willebrand factor VIII also mediates platelet adhesion to fibrillar collagens through interaction with integrin and subsequent platelet activation (14–17). The activated platelets are known to release leukocyte chemotactic factors, platelet derived growth factor (PDGF), transforming growth factor alpha (TGF-α), heparin binding epidermal growth factor (HB-EGF), transforming growth factor beta (TGF-ß), and an interleukin (IL-7) (18–22). The fibrin clot, which provides an early form of extracellular matrix (ECM), contains many of the platelet-derived factors that potentiate the migration of inflammatory cells into the region (14–18).

The induction of a local inflammatory reaction is an important feature of soft tissue repair and is essential for continued endometrial regeneration. Animals depleted of macrophages have defective tissue debridement, fibroblast proliferation, and wound repair (23). Infiltration of peripheral blood neutrophils and monocytes initiates the inflammatory process. Their recruitment into the tissue is further sustained in part by the action of platelet-derived cytokines as well as other chemoattractant factors (18). These chemoattractant factors may include fibrinopeptides which are cleaved from fibrinogen by thrombin; degradation products of fibrin produced by plasmin; platelet factor 4 (PF4) released from platelets; eicosanoids (LTB$_4$, LTC$_4$, and PG$_2$E) and platelet-activating factor (PAF) released from endothelial cells or activated neutrophils (18). The recruitment of inflammatory cells is also facilitated by adhesive molecules such as fibrin, fibronectin, and vitronectin, which are present in the fibrin clot (provisional matrix), as well as the integrin receptors that recognize these molecules (16, 17, 25, 26). The infiltrating monocytes become activated and differentiate into macrophages, which have the capability of synthesizing well over 100 distinct biological regulators such as growth factors and cytokines, including those initially released by platelets (27–31). Macrophage-derived factors include interleukins (ILs), granulocyte macrophage colony stimulating factor (GM-CSF), granulocyte stimulating factor (G-CSF), colony stimulating factor 1 (CSF-1) or macrophage stimulating factor (M-CSF), tumor necrosis factors (TNFs), leukemia inhibitory factor (LIF), oncostatin M (OSM), ciliary neurotrophic factor (CNTF), and interferons (IFNs). In addition, macrophages express growth factors such as epidermal growth factor (EGF), TGF-α, HB-EGF, PDGFs, TGF-ßs, insulin-like growth factors (IGFs), fibroblast growth factors (FGFs), and vascular endothelial growth factor (VEGF) that are synthesized and released after their activation (19–22, 26–31).

Cytokines such as IL-1, CSF, TNF-α, IFNs, TGF-ß, and PDGF regulate eicosanoid (prostaglandins, thromboxane and leukotrienes) production, which is an essential part of the coagulation cascade and inflammatory response (19–22, 26–33). It appears that cytokine and growth factor induced eicosanoid production through the cyclooxygenase pathway antagonizes, whereas the products of the lipoxygenase pathway mediate or amplify the effect of cytokine activation. For example, PGE_2 inhibits CSF-1 production, and CSF-1 is induced by TNF-α (34), whereas LTB_4 can stimulate IL-1 and TNF-α release by macrophages (35). TGF-ß, EGF, and TNF-α stimulatory action on fibroblasts has also been shown to be augmented in the presence of cyclooxygenase inhibitors but reduced in the presence of PGE_2, PGE_1, and PGI_2 (36). In addition, eicosanoids, such as PGs, act as intracellular mediators of cytokine and growth factor actions in various cell types (34–36).

Collectively the platelet and macrophage derived cytokines and growth factors appear to be essential for degradative as well as reparative processes. These processes occur simultaneously in the endometrium following the initiation of menstruation. These cytokines and growth factors are involved in the transition of the endometrium from an inflammatory to a reparative environment similar to that which occurs during wound repair. The resolution of the inflammatory reaction is also essential for the repair process to proceed. This process begins with diminished neutrophil infiltration. Those neutrophils already present in the tissue are removed by their entrapment within the clot and desiccated tissue, which then becomes senescent and phagocytosed by macrophages (37–40). A number of cytokines including GM-CSF, IL-1ß, TNF-α, and IFN-γ have also been shown to promote the uptake of neutrophils by macrophages (37–40). The mechanism involved in the clearance of macrophages after the completion of their function in the inflammatory reaction has not been defined, although macrophages can undergo apoptosis under in vitro conditions (37–40).

It has become clear in recent years that many cytokine receptors are detectable in naturally occurring soluble forms, often representing the ligand binding domain of the receptor complex. These soluble receptors are detected in serum, plasma, urine, and in various cell culture conditioned media and include IL-1, IL-2, IL-4, IL-5, IL-6, IL-7, IL-9, LIF, G-CSF, M-CSF, GM-CSF, and TNF-α as well as EGF and PDGF

(41–47). The alternative mRNA splicing of these receptors with a truncated region encoding the transmembrane domain, or proteolytic cleavage of the extracellular domain of the receptor, has been proposed as a mechanism for production of these soluble receptor molecules (41, 45, 46, 48). The in vivo functions of these soluble receptors are not known; however, they may have the potential property of restricting the biologic activities of their receptive ligand by acting as antagonists, or scavengers, thereby controlling the availability of these cytokines to their cell surface receptors. Although evidence is lacking, such a scenario may also take place in the endometrium at various stages of the menstrual cycle including menstruation.

Much information is available regarding the expression and influence of cytokines in human endometrium during the postmenstrual period; however, our current understanding of their expression and involvement in normal menstruation, as well as pathological conditions associated with dysfunctional uterine bleeding, spotting, and breakthrough bleeding, is lacking. It would not be surprising to find that many of these cytokines are expressed in the endometrium during menstruation. Nonetheless, it is essential to establish the relationship, if any, between the cytokines and normal menstrual bleeding by implementing some of the recent advances in the nature and function of cytokines and growth factors. This may in turn help us understand the nature of pathologic menstrual-like bleeding that 30% of women encounter sometime during their lives (11–13, 49, 50). These include anovulatory bleeding in adolescents, dysfunctional uterine bleeding during reproductive years, and bleeding in postmenopausal women taking hormone replacement therapy (49, 50).

Cytokines, Growth Factors, and Angiogenesis

In the healthy adult, angiogenesis occurs only in the corpus luteum, the placenta during development, the endometrium during the menstrual cycle, and during wound healing (51–53). Angiogenesis is a self-limiting and strictly regulated event. It occurs in a sequential manner involving degradation of the vascular basement membrane and interstitial matrix by endothelial cells, migration and proliferation of endothelial cells, and finally tubulogenesis and formation of capillary loops (51–53). Production of proteolytic enzymes in response to angiogenic factors is fundamental to angiogenesis, not only for the degradation of perivascular ECM and tissue stroma, but for the migration and proliferation of the endothelial cells. During angiogenesis in wound healing, the initial migration and proliferation of endothelial cells occurs in a fibronectin rich ECM, whereas vascular maturation, which takes place at the later stages, is laminin rich (54, 55). These processes also involve the integrin molecules, which are essential for cell migration and other cellular interactions (56, 57). At the initial stage of angiogenesis, induction of type I collagenase, plasminogen activators (tPA and uPA), stromalysin, and other matrix metalloproteinases (MMPs) in endothelial cells is necessary to degrade ECM including fibronectin and laminin (4– 6, 10, 51, 52). These proteases are produced in inactive forms and can become locally activated by plasmin, which is coordinately expressed with uPA (4–6, 10, 51, 58, 59). The proteolytic activity of these enzymes is regulated by several protease inhibitors that include plasminogen activator inhibitor (PAI-I) and tissue inhibitor of MMPs

(TIMPs) (4-6, 10, 58, 59). These proteolytic enzymes and their inhibitors are expressed in human endometrium and, as in other systems, their expression is reported to be regulated by various cytokines and growth factors, as well as ovarian steroids (4, 11–13, 60–63). Cytokines and growth factors such as IL-1, IL-8, TNF-α, GM-CSF, VEGF, FGFs, EGF, TGF-α, TGF-ß, PDGF, and IGF-I are considered angiogenic enhancing factors owing to their ability to regulate the expression of proteolytic enzymes and their inhibitors, and at the same time modulate the endothelial cell proliferation and migration (51–53, 64–67). Human endometrial capillaries and arteriole endothelial cells express mRNA and protein for these growth factors with specific receptors that respond to their mitogenic actions.

In situ hybridization of mRNA encoding VEGF has been reported not to be restricted to vascular smooth muscle, but to be present in endometrial epithelial and stromal cells, and its distribution changes during the course of the menstrual cycle (68–70). However, in a recent study VEGF mRNA and protein are reported to be focally expressed in glandular epithelial cells, with their highest expression occurring in the secretory endometrium (69). Vascular endothelial cells express VEGF and VEGF receptors, which are abundant during their proliferation (64, 68). Lack of VEGF expression in endometrial vascular endothelial cells suggests that VEGF expressed by other endometrial cell types and inflammatory cells (macrophages) may affect endothelial cell proliferation in a paracrine manner. In fact four species of mRNA encoding VEGFs have been identified in the human endometrium throughout the menstrual cycle (VEGF 189, 165, 145, and 121), arising by alternative splicing of the exons encoding the C-terminal of the VEGF (64). Two species, VEGF165 and VEGF121, are expressed by peripheral leukocytes, indicating tissue-specific splicing of the VEGF189 and 145 transcripts in the human endometrium (68). Neither of these studies examined the discrimination between the splice variants of VEGF expression and cellular distributions in human endometrium. Furthermore, the endometrium also expresses VEGF receptors and the fms-like tyrosine kinase (flt), which is in the family of type III receptor kinases that include *c-kit* and the PDGF α and ß receptors (64, 68). Another receptor that is similar to *flt* is the KRD receptor. Although the biologic action of VEGF in human endometrium has not been investigated, VEGF expression during menstruation reflects its potential role in coagulation, fibrinolytic, and angiogenic activities.

Additional growth factors with multiple biological activities including angiogenesis are the FGF family, composed of at least nine structurally related polypeptides (65, 66). The FGF family includes acidic and basic FGF, int-2 protein, HST/K-FGF, FGF-4, FGF-6, keratinocyte growth factor (KGF), androgen-induced growth factor (AIGF), and glia-activating factor, which are numbered FGF-1 through FGF-9, with a 35–55% structural homology (65, 66). The FGFs are expressed by a wide variety of cells and tissues. Their expression and biologic activities in the human endometrium are limited to only aFGF (FGF-1) and bFGF (FGF-2), demonstrated at the level of mRNA and immunoreactive protein localization (70–73). Both FGF-1 and FGF-2 are in fact synthesized by various cell types that are involved in wound repair including monocytes/macrophages, T lymphocytes (both CD-4 and CD-8), vascular endothelial cells, and fibroblasts (65, 66). Although FGF-1 and FGF-2 lack the classical secretory signal peptides implicating cell association, they are detected in the extracellular matrix with an unknown cellular origin (65, 66). However, FGFs can be released as a result of cellular injury as shown by mechanically induced injury of the endothelial cells in culture (74). If the FGFs are not secreted by either endometrial or infiltrating inflammatory cells during menstruation, they may be released after cellular damage during the menses. KGF (FGF-7) has been shown to be expressed in primate endometrium (75). It is a highly active mitogen for epithelial cells and has been shown to stimulate keratinocyte uPA expression (65, 66).

The angiogenic property of these growth factors such as VEGF is also reflected in their ability to induce the expression of both uPA and tPA and their inhibitors PAI-1 in microvascular endothelial cells, in addition to stimulating their invasion into collagen gel (4, 5, 51, 52, 64). Furthermore, VEGF can stimulate von Willebrand and tissue factors in endothelial cells. FGF, VEGF, EGF, and TGF-α, by stimulating PA expression, provide an activation factor for the conversion of TGF-ß from its latent to active form (51, 52, 76, 77). The active TGF-ß inhibits PA expression, thus interacting through a feedback loop through FGF, VEGF, TGF-α, and PA. In fact, FGF-2 and TGF-ß appear to have an opposing effect on PA activity of endothelial cells, with FGF acting as a potent inducer of uPA expression with a relatively modest effect on PAI-I synthesis, whereas TGF-ß downregulates uPA and upregulates PAI-I synthesis. bFGF and VEGF can synergistically enhance endothelial cell PA expression, and M-CSF and GM-CSF can upregulate the expression of PAI-I, whereas IL-4 is ineffective (64, 65, 78, 79). In addition to VEGF and FGF, EGF/TGF-α has also been shown to be angiogenic in human omental microvascular endothelial cells. TNF-α can stimulate angiogenesis by a receptor mediated mechanism (51, 52).

Angiogenesis depends on a balance between the angiogenic factors and their inhibitors. Among the angiogenic suppressors reported are cytokines such as TGF-ß, TNF-α, IFNs, and several other agents (51, 52, 80–82). These include collagen synthesis modifiers, protamine, which is an arginine rich protein and inhibits the mitogenic action of FGF, cyclosporin, PF-4, placental RNase inhibitors, hyaluronic acid, although its degradative products may be angiogenic, and thrombospondin, which is released by platelets and is present around mature quiescent vessels but absent from actively growing sprouts (51, 52, 80–82). Recently isolation of a tumor suppressor led to identification of an angiogenic inhibiting factor referred to as angiostatin (80). Angiostatin has considerable homology with plasminogen and hepatocyte growth factor (HGF), which is also an angiogenic factor (51). The action mechanism of angiostatin is not known; however, it has been proposed that it competes with HGF for its receptor c-met (51). In addition, an endogenous estrogen metabolite, 2-methoxyestradiol, has been shown to inhibit angiogenesis in vivo and prevents endothelial cell proliferation and migration in vitro (81, 82). Although 2-methoxyestradiol interacts minimally with estrogen receptors, it induces uPA in endothelial cells, suggesting that modulation of the fibrinolytic system is in part responsible for its inhibitory action (51, 81, 82). The vascular endothelial cells, including those in the endometrium, contain receptors for ovarian steroids, suggesting their potential regulatory action of vascular activities. Although their potential role in neovascularization in the early stage of endometrial regeneration may be limited, owing to low levels of plasma estrogen during menstruation, they may become active participants when the plasma estrogen level rises. Such complex interactions among these factors imply that angiogenesis is regulated both directly and indirectly by various factors. Many aspects of neovascularization in endometrium await investigation, in particular the role of cytokines. This is particularly important in the area of dysfunctional uterine bleeding in which the endometrium undergoes repetitive breakdown and repair.

POSTMENSTRUAL CYTOKINE EXPRESSION AND POTENTIAL FUNCTION

The regeneration of denuded endometrium begins well before the cessation of overt menstrual bleeding. Interestingly, the plasma level of estrogen is low during menstruation, implying that factors other than estrogen initiate the endometrial repair process. Cytokines and growth factors, along with their specific receptors or binding proteins, appear to have the potential property of orchestrating such rapid and dramatic tissue reorganization which results in endometrium regeneration. Remarkably few inflammatory cells, such as macrophages, are seen in the endometrium immediately after menstruation (83). The mechanism that regulates the clearance of the inflammatory cells in the endometrium following menses remains totally unclear. However, before their clearance, inflammatory cells provide the continued production of essential cytokines and many other biologically active substances after the initial levels of platelet derived cytokines subside. These cytokines are the initial mitogenic factors that begin the proliferation of various endometrial cell types, ultimately leading to tissue regeneration. At the same time, the rising plasma level of estrogen, corresponding to ovarian follicular development and maturation (follicular phase of the menstrual cycle), results in increased mitotic activity in both endometrial glandular and stromal cell compartments, with maximal activity occurring during the preovulatory peak in plasma estrogen. These mitotic activities continue for about 3 days postovulation. With the rise in the level of plasma progesterone, these cells undergo differentiation with an increase in secretory activities. The plasma estrogen levels, which had declined, now begin to rise to reach a new peak at about the seventh to eighth day postovulation.

Using three different methods of detection, northern blot analysis, RNAse protection assay, and standard or quantitative RT-PCR, mRNAs for many cytokines and growth factors and their receptors have been detected in endometrial cells and tissue. Northern blot analysis is often used when the mRNA under study is moderately abundant and the quantity of the specimen is not limited. However, owing to its sensitivity RNAse protection assay allows the sub-picogram levels of mRNA/µg of total RNA to be assayed in a fairly quantitative manner. Competitive quantitative RT-PCR, which utilizes tandemly linked primer sets constructed in a single multicompetitor plasmid, provides a far more sensitive (estimated to be 1000-fold over northern blot analysis) and quantitative detection of various RNA from minute samples of cells or tissues (84–88). This is particularly important in regard to the use of small tissue biopsies obtained from women to determine uterine receptivity. Using these biopsies allows the detection of as many as 20 messages in such a small amount of tissue. Utilizing tandemly linked primer sets for cytokines, growth factors, fibrinolytic enzymes, integrins, and ovarian steroid receptors constructed in several single multicompetitor plasmids in our laboratory, we have just begun analyzing not only their levels, but also the pattern of their expression in the endometrium throughout the menstrual cycle.

Through these approaches, the expression of most cytokines and growth factors such as ILs, LIF, GM-CSF, CSF-1, G-CSF, TNF-α, EGF, TGF-α, TGF-ßs, PDGFs, VEGF, and IGFs, and to a limited extent, the expression of their receptors, has been documented in human endometrium during the postmenstrual period (68–73, 85–102). However, efforts to date have resulted in only limited information regarding the proliferation, differentiation, angiogenesis, and other cellular activities of cytokines in various human endometrial cell types. To overcome this limitation, efforts have been made to correlate various aspects underlying the mechanism of steroid hormone action in endometrium to the steroid mediated expression of these cytokines and their receptors. The assumption is that the level of expression of these cytokines may in turn reflect their distinct biologic activities in various endometrial cell types at various stages of the menstrual cycle. Despite the inconsistency of the evidence supporting their menstrual cycle dependency, the pattern of mRNA and protein expression for some cytokines appears to correspond to the plasma levels of estrogen and progesterone, implying their regulation by these hormones (68–72, 85–105). However, in addition to ovarian steroid regulatory actions, many of these cytokines are capable of regulating their own expression or that of other cytokines, independent of ovarian steroids. Collectively, the local expression of these cytokines and their specific receptors acting in an autocrine/paracrine or juxtacrine manner, along with the ovarian steroids, coordinates various endometrial biologic activities. The signaling pathways by which the cytokine receptors mediate their biologic activities in the endometrium remain largely unknown; however, the activation of several phosphorylated proteins have been implicated in mediating the signaling processes for these cytokines in other cell systems, which may imply a similar mechanism in endometrial cells (106, 107).

In addition to their role as inflammatory and immune regulating cytokines, ILs are presumed to play a role in a number of other cellular activities in various tissues. It appears that postmenstrual human endometrium expresses mRNA for all ILs from IL-1 to IL-17 (Chegini N, Expression of interleukines mRNA in human endometrium throughout the menstrual cycle; unpublished data). Although menstrual cycle dependency and specific cellular distribution of mRNA and protein, as well as their respective receptors, await analysis, this observation suggests the potential role of ILs in various endometrial biologic activities. IL-1, which consists of IL-1α and IL-1ß, is encoded by two different genes and is expressed by a variety of cell types including monocytes, macrophages, mast cells, fibroblasts, and T and B lymphocytes (108). IL-1α and IL-1ß utilize the IL-1 receptors types I and II to mediate biologic activities (type I transduces signals in immune cells) and are expressed in the human endometrium with levels increasing during the late secretory phase (93, 108–112). Despite IL-1 expression by both endometrial epithelial and stromal cells, it does not appear to be a mitogen for these cells in vitro (110). However, IL-1 maximal expression during the late luteal phase may correspond with endometrial preparation for menses or it may cause an incomplete decidualization of stromal cells by inhibiting the expression and release of prolactin and IGFBP-1, which are regarded as markers of stromal decidualization (93, 110, 111). IL-1 also stimulates prostaglandin (PG) production, FGF-2 expression, and production of TNF-α, similar to that caused by IL-6 (110, 111).

IL-2, originally referred to as T cell growth factor, is synthesized by activated T helper cells and is a mitogen for T, NK, and B cells (113, 114). IL-2, through its receptor, which appears to share a common chain with IL-4, IL-7, IL-9, and IL-15, stimulates the release of IFN-γ, IL-3, IL-4, IL-5, and GM-CSF, and it also enhances the expression of class II MHG molecules by the T cells (113, 114). IL-3, which is referred to as multi-CSF, is another product of activated T cells and mast cells and stimulates eosinophils and B cell differentiation, whereas it inhibits lymphokine-activated killer (LAK) cell activity. IL-3 shares several biologic activities including its ß receptor with GM-CSF. IL-4 is produced by and stimulates CD4+ (TH) cells, mast cells, and basophils and regulates the CD4+ T cell differentiation into TH2 cells, while suppressing the development of TH1 cells (115). IL-4 enhances class II MHC expression of B cells and immunoglobulin class switching to IgG1 and IgE, an effect that is downregulated by IFN-γ. Because of IL-4 stimulatory action on collagen and IL-6 production by human dermal fibroblasts, and inhibition of IL-1, IL-6, IL-8, and TNF-α, IL-4 may play a role in the pathogenesis of fibrotic disorders and anti-inflammatory agents, respectively (116–118). IL-5, also known as B cell growth factor II (BCGFII) and T cell replacing factor (TRF), is produced by CD4+ T helper and NK cells and regulates eosinophil differentiation, increases B cell proliferation, enhances T cell cytotoxicity, and stimulates immunoglobulin class switching to IgA. The combined production of IL-4 and IL-5 by CD4+ TH2 cells results in IgE and IgA production and mast cell and eosinophil stimulation (114, 118).

IL-6 is produced by a variety of cells including mononuclear phagocytes, T cells, and fibroblasts and is a mitogen for mature B cells and their maturation into antibody producing plasma cells (119). It is involved in T cell activation and differentiation and can induce IL-2 and IL-2 receptor expression, but inhibits TNF production, providing negative feedback for limiting the acute inflammatory response. Upregulation of IL-6 production has been observed in a variety of chronic inflammatory and autoimmune disorders (114, 119, 120). The expression of IL-6 mRNA and the presence of immunoreactive IL-6, the IL-6 receptor, and gp130, the associated signal transducing component for IL-6, IL-11, LIF, OM, and CNTF receptors, implicates another member of the IL family in human endometrial activities (98, 99, 111, 119). IL-6 has been reported in the endometrium during the entire menstrual cycle, with IL-6 receptor and gp130 present primarily in the endometrial glands, and to a lesser extent in the stromal cells. The immunoreactivity of these proteins has been reported not to change in the endometrial cells during the entire menstrual cycle with the exception of gp130, which is reduced in the glands in the menstrual phase, and IL-6, which is increased in stromal cells in the upper functionalis during the late secretory/menstrual phases (98). Interestingly, IL-6 expression at both mRNA and protein levels is positively regulated by IL-1, TNF-α, OSM, and PDGF (120–122), whereas it is inhibited by IL-4 and IL-10 through a mechanism involving activator protein 1

(AP-1), c-fos, and c-jun (123). IL-6 may also be involved in angiogenesis owing to its stimulatory action of endothelial cell proliferation (124) and VEGF expression in various cell lines (125). IL-6 expression is reported to be inhibited by IL-5 in human lymphocytes (126). IL-7 is synthesized by bone marrow and thymic stromal cells. It stimulates the development of pre-B and pre-T cells and acts as a growth factor for B cells, T cells, and early thymocytes. It has been recently reported that IL-7 was detected in the blood derived from activated platelets (R & D publication # 1996) (128). We have also shown that IL-7 mRNA is expressed in human endometrium (Chegini N, unpublished observations).

IL-8, which belongs to the chemotactic cytokine family, is the main chemotactic factor for neutrophils and stimulates granulocyte activity (129). IL-8, by upregulating cell-surface adhesion molecule expression (such as endothelial leukocyte adhesion molecule, ELAM-1, and intracellular adhesion molecule, ICAM-1), enhances neutrophil adherence to endothelial cells and facilitates their diapedesis through vessel walls. IL-8 is also expressed in human endometrium (100, 104). However, information regarding its cellular distribution in this tissue is lacking. The expression of IL-8 in endometrial stromal cells is upregulated by IL-1 and TNF-α. Progesterone and a synthetic progestin, medroxyprogesterone acetate (MPA), enhance the action of IL-1 principally through mRNA stabilization (104). The receptor for IL-8, which is in a family of cytokine receptors that includes the receptors for IFNs, IL-1, and TNF-α, has not yet been identified in human endometrium. These receptors are distinct and differ from the receptors for IL-2, IL-3, IL-4, IL-5, IL-6, IL-7, IL-9, G-CSF, GM-CSF, LIF, and CNTF, which belong to a superfamily of hematopoietic cytokine receptors, including growth hormone and prolactin receptors (41–48). High-affinity binding is required for these cytokines to mediate their biologic activities. This is achieved in some cases through the formation of heterodimeric association of the α and ß subunits seen with IL-3, IL-5, and GM-CSF receptors associated with common ß and unrelated α subunits (41–48).

IL-9, previously known as mast cell growth enhancing activity (MEA) and T cell growth factor (P40), is another secretory product of TH2 and B lymphoma cells. IL-9 inhibits lymphokine production by IFN-γ-producing CD4+ T cells, enhances the growth of CD8+ T and mast cells, and promotes the production of immunoglobulins by B cells. IL-9 expression is enhanced by IL-2, IL-4, and IL-10 (130). IL-10, or as previously referred to as B cell derived T cell growth factor and cytokine synthesis inhibitory factor (CSIF) owing to its inhibitory action on IFN-γ production by activated T cells, is expressed by a variety of cell types, including CD4+, CD8+ T cells, and activated B cells. IL-10 reduces antigen-specific T cell proliferation, inhibits IL-2 induced IFN-γ production by NK cells, and IL-4 and IFN-γ induced MHC class II expression on monocytes (131). Because IL-10 is produced by TH2 cells and inhibits TH1 function by preventing TH1 cytokine production (such as IFN-γ), it is considered a T cell cross-regulatory factor, or "anticytokine." IL-11 is produced by bone marrow stromal cells and by some fibroblasts, and includes stimulation of T cell-dependent B cell immunoglobulin secretion, increased platelet production, and induction of IL-6 expression by CD4+ T cells. IL-11 is a functional homologue of IL-6 and can replace IL-6 in the proliferation of certain plasmacytoma cell lines and in the induction of acute phase protein secretion in the liver (132). IL-12, previously known as natural killer cell stimulatory factor (NKSF) and cytotoxic lymphocyte maturation factor (CLMF), is produced by activated B cells, macrophages, and other antigen presenting cells (133). Its biologic activities include enhancement of cytotoxic T cells and lymphokine activated killer cell generation and activation, increased NK cell cytotoxicity, induction of activated T cell and NK cell proliferation, induction of IFN-γ production by NK cells and T cells, and inhibition of IgE synthesis by IL-4 stimulated lymphocytes via IFN-γ dependent and independent mechanisms. IL-4 and IL-10 can inhibit IL-12 production by these cells, whereas the stimulatory effect of IL-12 on TH1 development is antagonized by IL-4 promoting TH2 cell development. Thus IL-12 is an important cell mediated inflammatory agent and may contribute to the regulation of immunoglobulin production.

IL-13 was originally identified as a protein produced by activated murine TH2 lymphocytes and referred to as P600. IL-13 acts as an anti-inflammatory agent by inhibiting the production of inflammatory cytokines, such as IL-1ß, TNF-α, IL-8, and IL-6 by human peripheral blood monocytes induced with LPS (134). IL-14, similar to IL-4, has been referred to as B cell growth factor (BCGF) owing to its ability to induce B cell proliferation while inhibiting immunoglobulin secretion (135). IL-15, one of the recently discovered interleukins, is structurally related to IL-2 and appears to bind to the same receptor as IL-2 (136). It is a mitogen for T cells and is expressed in skeletal muscle, placenta, and various other cell types. IL-16, which was originally identified as a chemotactic factor also referred to as lymphocyte chemoattractant factor or lymphotactin and T cell produced protein, is a mitogen for these cells; however, it can act on a variety of other cell types owing to its widespread receptor expression (137). IL-17 has been shown to induce the expression of IL-6 and IL-8 by fibroblasts (138, 139). Another recently identified IL termed IFN-γ inducing factor (IGIF) is related to IL-1 and has been termed IL-1γ or potentially IL-18 (140). We have shown that human endometrium expresses IL-15, IL-16, and IL-17; however, like other ILs, their cellular distribution, menstrual cycle dependency, and biologic activity remain to be investigated.

In the case of LIF, it is expressed in the endometrium most abundantly during the mid and late luteal phases, and is associated primarily with endometrial epithelial cells (96, 105). The endometrial expression of LIF, OM, and CNTF, which are a family of related cytokines, as well as LIF receptor ß and glycoprotein gp130, has been examined and reported to be detectable only in the endometrium of women of proven fertility, with expression restricted to the glands during the secretory phase, but absent during the proliferative phase (141). LIF receptor ß, however, appears to be expressed during the proliferative and secretory phases and is restricted to the luminal epithelium, whereas gp130 is expressed in both the luminal and glandular epithelium throughout the cycle (141). Interestingly, LIF is the only cytokine whose expression is required for embryo implantation as shown in LIF knockout mice. Unlike IL-8, LIF expression by endometrial stromal cells appears not to be affected by estradiol and progestins; however, IL-1, TNF-α, PDGF, EGF, and TGF-ß are potent inducers, whereas IFN-γ inhibits LIF expression induced by these cytokines (105). In contrast, the glandular epithelial cells have a high constitutive level of LIF mRNA which is relatively less regulated (105). Such constitutive expression of LIF in endometrial epithelial cells argue against LIF involvement in women with infertility as suggested by Arici et al. (105). In addition, evidence suggests that the LIF expression in the rhesus monkey is detectable in endometrium from progesterone but not estrogen dominated stages (142). In breast, kidney, and prostate tumors, LIF regulates their proliferation in the presence of estrogen (143). However, LIF suppresses trophoblast production of hCG and ß hCG mRNA, and increases oncofetal fibronectin mRNA and protein expression, but not progesterone production by these cells (144). Human trophoplasts' oncofetal fibronectin expression has also been shown to be highly regulated by TGF-ß (145). Furthermore, IL-1ß and TNF-α were reported to induce LIF expression in human lung fibroblasts and umbilical vein endothelial cells (146).

In regard to TNF-α, which is a potent proinflammatory cytokine with similar functions as IL-1 and IL-6, is expressed in human endometrium with cellular distribution reported to be within both stromal/epithelial cells (32, 90, 91, 147–149). Endometrial epithelial cells from the late proliferative phase (day 12) appear to express higher levels of TNF-α (111) similar to that observed in endometrial tissue by Hunt et al. (147), which is in contrast to that reported by Philippeaux and Piguet (148) and Tabizzadeh et al. (149). TNF-α immunoreactive protein has been detected only in epithelial rather than stromal cells in culture and is induced by IL-1 and placental protein 14 (109). At pharmacological levels, progestins either alone or in the presence of estradiol stimulate TNF-α production in endometrial epithelial cells prepared from proliferative phase tissue, but decrease TNF-α production in cells prepared from secretory tissue (109). Using quantitative RT-PCR, we have demonstrated that TNF-α mRNA appears to be expressed more than 100-fold higher in endometrium during the proliferative than secretory phase (149a). Interestingly, the expression of TNF-α receptor mRNA was inversely related to its ligand. Although the biologic significance of such inverse expression of TNF-α and its receptor in endometrium is not known, it is possible that TNF-α expression may be regulated differently from that of its receptor. In fact, the most intriguing action of TNF-α is its ability to induce apoptosis in a variety of cell types, which is related to its toxic effect (32). TNF-α binds to TNF-α receptors of 55kDa and 75 kDa with similar affinity, with 55 kDa required for transduction of a signal induced by TNF-α (32). Mice lacking the 55 kDa are moderately resistant to the lethal effect LPS; however, mice lacking the 75 kDa receptor are moderately resistant to the lethal effect of TNF-α itself. Mice lacking both receptors have the sum of both effects without any gross developmental abnormality, suggesting that the two receptors function differently in vivo (32). Although TNF-α appears not to have any effect on endometrial epithelial and stromal cell growth, low expression of TNF-α receptor during the proliferative phase of the menstrual cycle may potentially serve to reduce or prevent the action of TNF-α at the time extensive regeneration is underway. However, at the later stage of the menstrual cycle, in which endometrium is prepared for menstruation, higher TNF-α receptor content may facilitate TNF-α apoptotic action. Other cytokines such as IL-10 and IFN-γ may facilitate upregulation of TNF-α expression (150).

CSF-I (also known as M-CSF), G-CSF, and GM-CSF are other members of the hematopoietic cytokine family that are synthesized by activated monocytes and macrophages with mitogenic activities for multipotential progenitor cells and activation of granulocytes and macrophages (151–156). The primary transcript for CSF-I encodes a precursor peptide in which the mature secreted form is generated by proteolytic cleavage of a transmembrane domain as a disulfide-bonded homodimeric proteoglycan. At least five forms of CSF-1 are generated by alternative splicing in which four are within a single exon. CSF-I mediates its action through CSF-1 receptors which are encoded by the c-fms proto-oncogene, considered a member of the PDGF family of growth factors. Human endometrium expresses CSF-1 and receptor throughout the menstrual cycle with maximal levels occurring during proliferative and early to mid luteal phase (94). Although the potential biologic activity of CSF-1 has not been investigated in human endometrium, it stimulates placental cells and their differentiation into syncytiotrophoblasts and hCG production (154). The expression of M-CSF in human endometrium and its regulation in stromal cells by progesterone has been demonstrated whereas estradiol treatment has no effect (155). In the case of GM-CSF, using quantitative RT-PCR, immunohistochemistry, and ELISA, we have demonstrated that GM-CSF, as well as GM-CSF α and ß receptor mRNA and protein, are expressed in human endometrial tissue throughout the menstrual cycle, and isolated endometrial epithelial and stromal cells in cultures (86, 87, 97). GM-CSF mRNA and protein are predominantly expressed by epithelial cells, whereas GM-CSF α receptor was restricted to the stromal and vascular endothelial cells, but was either absent or expressed at low levels in the glandular epithelium. GM-CSF receptors belong to the cytokine receptor superfamily with α receptors appearing to be ligand specific, whereas the ß receptor is commonly shared with IL-3 and IL-5 (157, 158). GM-CSF receptor ß is expressed without any restriction with a pattern similar to that seen with its ligand GM-CSF.

GM-CSF also appears not to be a mitogen for either stromal or glandular epithelial cells in vitro, but in an interactive manner, it induces the expression of TGF-ß1 (86, 87). However, GM-CSF expression in both endometrial epithelial and stromal cells is downregulated by TGF-ß1. Both GM-CSF and TGF-ß are able to induce their own expression by these cells. Interestingly, TGF-ß is a potent chemoattractant factor for macrophages and fibroblasts, whereas GM-CSF promotes the macrophages' uptake of apoptotic neutrophils, but the rate in which neutrophils undergo apoptosis is inhibited by GM-CSF (37). If such an interaction occurs between TGF-ß and GM-CSF in the endometrium, GM-CSF may function as an important regulator of inflamation reaction and TGF-ß immunosuppressive activity similar to that which occurs at the time of implantation. IL-5, which is also expressed by human endometrium (unpublished data), has also been shown to have a similar activity without affecting neutrophil longevity (37). Furthermore, the expression of TGF-α by macrophages is markedly stimulated after exposure to GM-CSF (159).

POSTMENSTRUAL GROWTH FACTOR EXPRESSION AND POTENTIAL FUNCTION

Many platelet and macrophage derived growth factors including EGF, TGF-α, HB-EGF, TGF-ßs, IGFs, FGFs, VEGF, and PDGFs along with their receptors or respective binding proteins are expressed by human endometrium. EGF was among the first growth factors to be identified in human endometrium, with later characterization of other members of the EGF family, TGF-α, and HB-EGF along with their common receptor, the EGF receptor (68–72, 160). The expression and cellular distribution of EGF, TGF-α, and HB-EGF as well as their receptors in the endometrium revealed a widespread association, lacking a clear menstrual cycle dependency. This suggests that the EGF family of growth factors along with their receptors can potentially affect a wide range of endometrial activities throughout the menstrual cycle. Consistent with these data, EGF was found to act as a mitogenic factor for endometrial epithelial cells, but weakly influence stromal cell proliferation, which is synergistically enhanced by IGF and PDGF (68, 92, 161). IGFs with insulin-like growth promoting activities and their unique class of binding proteins (IGFBPs), which regulate IGF-I availability, are present in circulation as well as in tissue fluids in association with IGFBPs through high affinity binding (162). The IGFs, IGF receptors, and the six distinct forms of IGFBPs have been identified at mRNA and protein levels in human endometrium throughout the cycle, with the highest level of expression occurring during the proliferative phase for IGF-I and IGF-II (92, 161). IGF-I acts as a mitogen for many cell types but, similar to EGF, is not a particularly strong mitogen for endometrial cells and requires interaction with other growth factors such as EGF and PDGF (68, 92, 161). The requirement for synergistic interaction between various growth factors has been demonstrated under culture conditions in which stromal cells were exposed to serum before their exposure to EGF, IGF, or PDGF. The mitogenic action of EGF, IGF, or PDGF may have been due to their interactions with other factors that are present in the serum.

The requirement for growth factor interactions is demonstrated in a variety of cell types in culture and is related to the ability of individual growth factors to act as a competence (PDGF) or progression (EGF and IGF) factor. This interaction allows the cells to become competent to enter the cell cycle and subsequently progress through the cell cycle. In fact, PDGF, TGF-α, HB-EGF, and IGF-1, which are expressed and released by platelets and macrophages, can potentially act in this manner influencing endometrial cell proliferation at the earliest stages of menstruation. Human platelets release PDGF-AB, but PDGF-AA and PDGF-BB are produced by other cell types (20, 21). Interestingly, PDGFs differ in their secretory behavior, for PDGF-AA and PDGF-AB are rapidly secreted after synthesis, whereas PDGF-BB remains to a large extent associated with the producer cells (20, 21). Whether a similar phenomenon exists in human endometrium is not known, although it expresses PDGF-A and PDGF-B mRNA and protein. PDGFs bind to PDGF receptors consisting of α α, ß ß, and α ß. PDGFs have a tendency to bind the α α and ß ß receptors, with PDGF-BB binding to ß ß with high affinity and PDGF-AB binding to ß ß with a lower affinity, whereas PDGF-AA does not bind to ß ß or α ß receptors (20, 21). PDGF-B mRNA and PDGF-AB protein appear to be expressed with similar relative abundance in both phases of the menstrual cycle; however, PDGF ß receptor was higher in the proliferative than the secretory phase (102, 163). Only recently have we begun reexamining the expression of PDGFs and PDGF receptors using quantitative RT-PCR. Using such a technique, we have demonstrated that endometrial tissues as well as isolated glandular epithelial and stromal cells in primary culture express PDGF-AA, PDGF-BB, and

PDGF α and ß receptors (102: Chegini N, unpublished data). Additionally, radio-receptor assay (RRA) and cross-linking revealed the presence of specific binding sites for[125] I-PDGF-AA,[125] I-PDGF-AB, and[125] I-PDGF-BB in endometrial stromal cells, with highest levels (binding sits/cell) for PDGF-AB, which were 2.2- and 7-fold higher than PDGF-BB and AA, respectively (Chegini N, unpublished data).

Both PDGF-AB and PDGF-BB are mitogens for endometrial stromal cells, with maximum activity occurring in synergistic interaction with EGF and IGF-1 (102). Although PDGF is a potent monocyte chemotactic factor, PDGF receptor expression is not detected in macrophages (164), and thus macrophages are essentially refractory to stimulation by this growth factor. This suggests that macrophage-derived PDGFs are capable of binding to endometrial cells that contain PDGF α and ß receptors. The stimuli for PDGF expression by macrophages have not been systematically investigated, but other cytokines, including IL-1ß (165) and IFN-γ (166), have been shown to induce PDGF expression. Data generated from in vitro experiments also indicate that TNF-α, which has some growth promoting activity, induces the expression of PDGF by fibroblasts, IGF-I by macrophages, and IL-6, which also induces PDGF expression (167). As indicated above, four species of mRNA encoding VEGFs (VEGF189, 165, 145, and 121) as well as FGF-1 and FGF-2 expression are reported in human endometrium. In situ hybridization and immunohistochemical data indicate VEGF mRNA expression in endometrial epithelial and stromal cells throughout the cycle, and the distribution changed during the course of the cycle (68–70). Immunoreactive FGF-1 and FGF-2 are localized in human endometrial luminal and glandular epithelial cells throughout the menstrual cycle without any changes in their expression (68, 71–73). Endometrium also expresses the VEGF receptor, a fms-like tyrosine kinase (flt).

Unlike other growth factors whose activities are generally stimulatory, TGF-ßs are bifunctional in respect to cell growth and differentiation. TGF-ßs are part of a family of structurally related polypeptides that include activin, inhibin, and mullerian inhibitory substance (19, 77). Among the five TGF-ß isoforms (TGF-ßs 1–5), only TGF-ß1–3 are prevalent in mammals and are found in a variety of normal and transformed cells and tissues. TGF-ß is secreted as a high molecular weight latent dimer complex consisting of the mature TGF-ß subunits noncovalently associated with the precursor segment, referred to as latency associated protein (LPA) (77). In vivo, TGF-ß released by cells is stored at the cell surface and in association with extracellular matrix proteins, which further regulate TGF-ßs activity. However, TGF-ß must be activated before binding to TGF-ß receptor. The mechanisms that accomplish this conversion in vivo remain unknown, but transient acidification, heating, or exposure to plasmin results in activation of latent TGF-ß in vitro (77). Platelets are the richest source of TGF-ßs, but they are synthesized in large quantity by activated macrophages (77). Human endometrium expresses TGF-ß1-3 mRNA and protein and their cellular distribution reveals that the epithelial cells are their major site of expression, although other cell types including stromal and arteriole compartments express TGF-ßs (101). Indeed, the level of TGF-ß1 produced by the epithelial cells is approximately threefold higher than that produced by stromal cells, with a significant portion released as an inactive form (168). TGF-ß1 and TGF-ß2 production by human endometrial stromal cells are regulated differently by ovarian steroids, for TGF-ß2 secretion is inhibited by progesterone and estradiol, whereas TGF-ß1 production is slightly enhanced by E2 (155).

The nearly identical biologic activities of the TGF-ßs are mediated through at least three specific cell surface receptors, types I, II, and III (77, 169, 170). Unlike EGF, PDGF, and IGF receptors with tyrosine kinase activities, TGF-ß type I and II receptors contain the cytoplasmic protein serine/threonine kinase domain and interact to form a signaling complex that is necessary for TGF-ß activity (77, 169, 170). TGF-ß type III receptor, betaglycan, may not be directly involved in signal transduction, but rather present TGF-ßs to the signaling receptors. TGF-ß receptors (type I, II, and III) are expressed in the endometrium throughout the menstrual cycle with maximal expression occurring during the luteal phase (101). TGF-ßs have been found to have multiple effects depending on cell type and the environment. In regard to their actions in endometrium, we have found that TGF-ß1, TGF-ß2, and TGF-ß3 in a biphasic manner stimulate the rate of thymidine incorporation at low concentrations (>1 ng/mL) and retain the cells in a half-stimulated stage at higher concentrations, without affecting their proliferation (168). This is in contrast to other reports implicating TGF-ß1 as a mitogen to these cells; this effect may be due to differences in culture conditions, including preexposure to serum (171). In fact the mitogenic action of TGF-ß has been reported to be indirect and due to PDGF and PDGF-α receptor expression, which mediates the mitogenic effect of TGF-ß on different cell types (20, 21, 172–175). TGF-ß has also been reported to enhance the synthesis and expression of the EGF receptor and synergize the stimulation of EGF in c-fos and actin genes expression and DNA synthesis in several cell types (19, 77, 176, 177). EGF has been shown to induce synthesis of TGF-ß1 but not TGF-ß2 in NRK-49F and A549 cells (177). TGF-ß1 in turn decreases the number of high-affinity EGF receptors such as that shown in a variety of endothelial cell types (77, 177, 178). This interaction may serve as a mechanism for EGF inhibition of stromal cells at high concentration (102) as well as prevention of the EGF mediated induction of several growth regulatory genes. Moreover, TGF-ß can be upregulated by its own expression, as shown in a variety of cell types (77) including endometrial cells (178) and by the ovarian steroids (179). TGF-ß is also a potent stimulant for ECM expression and an inhibitor of their degradation (77).

Therefore, upon tissue trauma such as menstrual bleeding, platelet derived TGF-ß becomes immediately available and by the time it is lost from the site, TGF-ß derived from macrophages replaces it. We have demonstrated that the inflammatory cells in postmenstrual human endometrium express IGF-I, IGFBPs, TGF-ßs, and TGF-ß receptors as well as GM-CSF and GM-CSF receptors (101, 161). These inflammatory cells express a higher estrogen receptor mRNA than other cell types in the rhesus monkey uterine tissue (180). A human monocytic leukemia cell line J111 and rat peritoneal macrophages have been shown to contain specific estrogen receptors (181). However, U937 cells, another human monocytic cell line that expresses a wide variety of cytokines and growth factors and is used as a model for investigating the role of macrophages in uterine and intraperitoneal environments (182, 183), appear not to contain progesterone receptors (184). Unlike the situation with TGF-ß where macrophages both express and respond to TGF-ß, macrophages can only be considered a source of PDGF.

In addition to modulation of their own and other cytokine expression, the ECM components are important in regulating the expression of cytokines in an interactive manner (185–188). This is evident from in vitro experiments indicating that the expression of TNF-α, which is a potent pro-inflammatory cytokine, PDGF, which is a potent chemoattractant and mitogen for fibroblasts such as endometrial stromal cells, CSF-1, which is necessary for monocyte-macrophage survival, and c-fos and c-jun, transactivating factors necessary for many activation signals, depend on the existence of ECM (54, 166, 185–188). However, the expression of TGF-ß, which is constitutive, IL-1, which is stimulated by bacterial endotoxin, and leukocyte antigen-D-related (HLA-DR), which is stimulated by IFN-γ, are independent of the presence of ECM (166, 187). The importance of ECM becomes further apparent when we consider the association of many cytokines and growth factors with soluble receptors with this compartment (41–46). Various biologic activities induced by cytokines and growth factors are initiated by binding to their specific cell surface receptors. Such specific ligand–receptor interactions in some cases involve either a single or a complex of two or more subunits commonly shared among some cytokines to initiate a cascade of intracellular signal transduction (107, 108). However, it has become clear that many of these receptor molecules, often representing the ligand binding domain of the receptor complex, are detectable in naturally occurring soluble forms in serum, plasma, urine, and in various cell culture conditioned media (41–46, 77). These include soluble receptors for ILs, LIF, G-CSF, M-CSF, GM-CSF, and TNF-α, as well as EGF, TGF-α, TGF-ß, PDGF, and IGFBPs. Although all TGF-ß isoforms bind to the same set of receptors, the soluble type II receptor associates only with TGF-ß1 and TGF-ß3, whereas the LAP associates with all TGF-ßs (77). In vitro association of TGF-ß with decorin, as well as other ECM components such as biglycan and fibromodulin, results in inactivation of TGF-ß (77). Also, in most cases TGF-ß can downregulate the expression of decorin while upregulating biglycan. Although the in vivo functions of these soluble receptors are unknown, they have the potential to restrict the biologic activities of their receptive ligand (antagonists), act as scavengers, and control the physiological levels of these cytokines, or function as transport proteins to be presented to the cell surface receptors.

ENDOMETRIUM DERIVED CYTOKINES AND IMPLANTATION

The attachment of the blastocyst to the endometrial surface epithelium, or embryo implantation, occurs during a limited time period referred to as the receptive phase or window of implantation, corresponding to postovulatary day 5–7, after which the endometrium becomes refractory (189, 190). Experience gained from assisted reproductive technology indicates that the optimal time frame for a 4–16 cell stage embryo transfer in women undergoing in vitro fertilization is between days 17 and 19 of the artificial cycle, but not on days 20–24 (190). In fertile women, the well orchestrated regenerative events prior to the receptive phase have optimally prepared the endometrium with respect to the expression of biologically active substances to receive the blastocyst for implantation (90–92, 189–191). Little is known about the molecular markers that distinguish the stages immediately prior, during, or after the receptive phase. However, the event begins with the physical engagement between the blastocyst and the receptive endometrial epithelial cells and appears to involve specific adhesion molecules and their receptors (integrins and ECM) (190, 191). Such interaction establishes a direct biochemical dialogue between the embryo and endometrium that later results in a gradual invasion of the trophoplasts into the underlaying stromal cells.

In recent years, accumulating evidence has emerged that implicates many factors including cytokines, growth factors, and their receptors as communicating signals critical for embryo implantation (89–92, 189–195). These assumptions are based on the experimental data showing the occurrence of maximal expression of these factors in human endometrium during the receptive phase, as well as those generated from animal models most noticeably in rodents with normal and delayed implantation (89–92, 189–195). However, the endometrial expression of such a large number of factors, including cytokines and growth factors prior to and during the receptive phase, makes one wonder if the event has specificity in respect to an individual factor. Despite the persuasive assumption generated from studies performed in rodents regarding the impact of cytokines/growth factors in implantation, lessons learned from knockout mice with specific gene deletion failing to affect implantation consistently suggest otherwise. This failure has been suggested to be due to the redundancy among many cytokines and growth factors with overlapping biologic activities. As far as other factors such as integrins ($\alpha v \beta 3$), ECM (fibronectin, vitronectin) and proteoglycan (Muc-1) are concerned, the failure of specific gene deletions affecting implantation also implies a similar redundancy in their involvements in this process. However, deletion of E-Cadherin gene causes failure of terophoectoderm formation in homozygous animals and vesatage around the time of implantation.

Considering the low rate of successful implantation in humans, this event most likely is an interactive process involving many of these factors. However, it is reasonable to assume that among these cytokines and growth factors exist a selective few with putative properties to act as master regulators. An analogy to such a selectivity is with that of a member of an orchestra who is directed by the conductor, the one interpreting the musical notes. The conductor has the ability of orchestrating different instruments, as well as using selective members to act as soloists. With this analogy, cytokines and growth factors with a wide range of interactive functions could act as the potential members of such a biologic orchestra, with some having the ability to act as soloist. This notion is supported by data indicating that in female mice with disrupted cytokines or growth factors, only a selective few show inhibition or interruption in embryo implantation. However, mice with disrupted estrogen receptor genes are infertile, implicating ovarian steroids as the conductor of this event (196). In addition to its requirement in fertility, estrogen receptors appear to be essential for female sexual receptivity (197), whereas mating stimuli may activate progestin receptor in a progesterone-independent manner in the absence of progesterone (198). Interestingly, in the absence of the conductor (ovarian steroids), the endometrium of postmenopausal women and ovariectomized cycling animals (possibly mice lacking estrogen receptors) still express many of the other gene products (cytokines), but at substantially lower levels than during the normal cycle.

Among the cytokines so far examined only the interruption of the LIF gene results in the failure of blastocyst implantation (199), making it an attractive molecule to be considered as a soloist of this event. In humans, data suggest that LIF is expressed only in the endometrial tissue during the receptive phase in fertile, but not infertile women (141), although LIF mRNA expression has been reported during proliferative as well as secretory phase endometrium (96, 105). These results tend to suggest that as in mice, uterine expression of LIF in humans may have a role in regulating embryo implantation. However, mice lacking type I IL-1 receptor do not exhibit any profound alteration in their reproduction, similar to that shown for IL-6, IL-12, IFN-γ, GM-CSF, TNF-α, TNF-α receptors, EGF, and TGF-α (200). In contrast, repeated administration of IL-1 receptor antagonist (IL-1Ra), which interferes with IL-1 binding to IL-1 type I receptor, blocks implantation in superovulated mice (201). GM-CSF is also reported to have a potentially important function in early embryonic development and throughout the pregnancy (89, 192). Furthermore, administration of GM-CSF to a mouse model of pregnancy failure during pre- and postimplantation periods restores normal embryo development in vivo (89, 192) Morula or blastocyst stage embryos collected from GM-CSF treated animals were able to develop further in vitro and implant, and the action of GM-CSF was reversed by using anti GM-CSF neutralizing antibody. The absence of other factors such as CSF-1 results in a reduction of fertility. Furthermore, immunoreactive IL-6 was weakly expressed during the proliferative phase, increased during the putative "implantation window," was most pronounced by far in both the glandular and surface epithelial cells, and was present in stromal cells only in the upper functionalis during the late secretory/menstrual phases. The menstrual cycle-dependent expression of IL-6 suggests that this cytokine may play a role in changes in the endometrium that prepare this tissue for implantation (190).

In regard to growth factors, in vitro studies have demonstrated that EGF, TGF-α, PDGF, TGF-ß, and IGF play an important role in embryogenesis and early embryo development (92, 191–194). However, normal embryo development and implantation is not affected in mice lacking a functional TGF-α gene, or mutation in EGF receptor, but the embryos are lost soon after implantation in mice having mutated EGF receptor genes (191). Mouse embryos with a null mutation in functional TGF-ß1 genes are able to develop normally, and in the homozygous mouse, 30% to 50% of the embryos reach parturition, though they die at 2–3 weeks of age with an inflammatory disorder (195, 202). The fact that 50% to 70% of the TGFβ1 *null* mice die in utero would suggest that there might be developmental abnormalities in the majority of these mice. Preimplantation mouse embryos at all stages express IGFBPs, and blastocysts also express IGFBP6, but IGFBP5 is not detected in any preimplantation stage embryo (92). Despite their potential involvement, mice with either single IGF-I, IGF-II, IGF-I receptor and IGF-II receptor gene deletion or double deletions of either IGFs or their receptors had normal embryonic growth and implantation (162). However, these mice all had a very low postnatal growth rate and in the case of IGF-I and II receptors, the animals died either postnatally or in utero, respectively. Possible explanations that may account for the occurrence of normal development in mice lacking genes for cytokines and growth factors such as IL-1, IL-6, IFN-γ, TNF-α, EGF, TGF-α, and FGF, and other factors such as integrins, TIMP-1, Muc-1, tenascin, fibronectin, and vitronectin are as follows: (1) the maternal (oviductal, uterine, and placental) transfer of the factors is not being expressed by the embryo; (2) there is functional redundancy between these factors, such as TGF-ß1-3, EGF, TGF-α, and HB-EGF, and various ILs; (3) if factors such as TGF-ß2 or TGF-ß3 as well as EGF or HB-EGF do not compensate for lack of TGF-ß1 or TGF-α, respectively, there is functional redundancy at a point distal to receptor signaling and perhaps less likely; (4) these cytokines and growth factors have no function in early embryonic development and implantation.

It is not known whether the presence of the preimplantation embryo is required for priming the maternal environment. However, no matter how receptive the endometrium is, the establishment and maintenance of a viable embryo prior to reaching the endometrium is essential for successful implantation, in part because more than 65% of the embryos that reach the endometrium do not implant. Although controversial, data from Assisted Reproductive Technology Programs suggest that the highest rate of pregnancy is achieved by tubal procedures such as gamete intrafallopian transfer (GIFT) followed by zygote intrafallopian transfer (ZIFT) and tubal embryo transfer (TET), whereas lower success rates are achieved following transcervical transfer during a stimulated cycle with exogenous hormonal preparations. This is particularly important because more than 28% of female infertility cases are of tubal origin. This may also be due to the fact that embryo growth media is not yet maximum. During the journey, which takes more than 4–5 days, the sperm, egg, fertilized egg, and embryo, until they reach the morula stage, are in direct contact with the tubal epithelial lining and their secretory products. Tubal secretory products, which include endometrium derived cytokines and growth factors may provide the milieu that influences final oocyte maturation, sperm capacitation, fertilization, and early embryo development (203).

The preimplantation embryo itself also expresses specific growth factors and their receptors, which may receive the tubal derived growth factors. Direct co-culturing of early stage embryos with isolated oviductal epithelial cells or, for that matter, other cell types as a feeder layer, or direct exposure to these factors enhances embryo development possibly through exchange of growth factors and cytokines derived from the feeder cells. CSF-1 and Steel factor (SF) transcripts that are not detected in early preimplantation embryos are expressed in cumulus cells, oviduct, and uterus. Therefore interactive networks of cytokines with many diverse but overlapping biologic activities may regulate the necessary events, which include proliferation, angiogenesis, and differentiation, that transform the proliferative endometrium into a receptive condition for embryo implantation. Moreover, the influence of cytokines and growth factors on embryonic development may begin with their preexposure to these factors in the fallopian tubes, and may serve as inducers of memory and later survival in the uterine environment. If a successful pregnancy is not established, the endometrial environment is prepared for another cycle of destructive, regenerative, and receptive phases utilizing these same molecules.

PROSPECTIVE

Classical endocrinology, assisted reproductive technology, cloning of estrogen and progesterone receptors, as well as the recent advancement in the use of knockout mice lacking estrogen and progesterone receptors document the vitality of ovarian steroids in various aspects of endometrial biologic and physiological functions. Moreover, the unprecedented advancement in molecular biologic approaches during the past decade has led to the identification and action of many biologically active substances in the endometrium, including cytokines, which were initially discovered and identified as the products of inflammatory and immune cells. The central role of ovarian steroids in endometrial integrity was further established by their ability to regulate the expression of these growth factors and cytokines, which is now accepted as a characteristic of ovarian steroid action in their target tissues. In turn, these growth factors and cytokines, working in concert and in an interactive manner, regulate various aspects of endometrial biological activity in preparation for its vital role, embryo implantation, during the reproductive years.

Despite all this information, the gene knockout experiments in mice indicate that the majority of generated phenotypes with disrupted cytokine genes do not have a profound effect on embryo implantation. However, many were found to be neonatally or postnatally lethal. Although these cytokines appear to be developmentally important, these findings suggest the possibility of their involvement during embryo implantation. The common and overlapping biologic functions among many cytokines, which are evolved from the recruitment of multiple signaling molecules with similar downstream pathways and their ability to use alternative pathways to trigger the full-scale activation of cellular responses, may compensate for the function of deleted gene product. Such functional pleiotropy and redundancy, a characteristic feature of cytokines, have been attributed to the molecular structure of their receptor system. For example, disruption of the LIF gene results in impairment of embryo implantation, whereas the gp-130, shared by LIF, IL-6, IL-11, OM, and CNTF receptors as a common signal transducer, was found not to be essential for implantation, but was for early embryo development.

Despite the growing list of cytokines expressed in human endometrium, and increasing insight into their importance in human reproductive tract tissues, their major roles in endometrial biological function are speculative and come from data generated in rodents. With regard to the involvement of cytokines, in particular those associated with acute and chronic inflammation, we do not know, even at the basic level, their role during menses. This information is essential and may lead to a better understanding and potential therapy of abnormal uterine bleeding, which is unique and affects every woman sometime during her lifetime. In addition, there are virtually no data currently available regarding the cytokine receptor system and signal pathways in human endometrium throughout the menstrual cycle. It is particularly important to elucidate data on how the signaling pathways cooperate and interact with each other and to identify the molecules that are involved in the downstream signaling cascades. This may allow us to distinguish the potentially vital cytokines in the endometrial environment during regeneration and receptive phases, as well as during the period in which endometrium is preparing for the new menstrual cycle.

The recent discovery of the new estrogen receptor, type ß, has opened another direction for the role of estrogen action in target tissue including the uterus. Until this discovery, it was generally accepted that the biologic action of estrogen was mediated through the existence of one form of estrogen receptor, type α. Although both estrogen α and ß receptors have virtually identical DNA binding domains, suggesting similar interaction with estrogen response elements, their A/B domains and activation function-1 are different. The question then arises whether the pattern of endometrial and blastocyst cytokine expression differs in estrogen receptor α knockout mice that are infertile, compared to the estrogen receptor ß. Identifying the pattern of estrogen α and ß receptors expression and its correlation with endometrial and oviductal cytokines and growth factor expression in fertile and infertile women may lead to a better understanding of the regulation and importance of these receptors, not only in postmenstrual uterine preparation for embryo implantation, but also in oocyte maturation, fertilization, and early embryonic development.

ACKNOWLEDGMENTS

We would like to acknowledge the research contributions of Drs. Rossi, Tang, Dou, Zhao, and Pfiefer performed in our laboratory.

REFERENCES

1. Strauss JF, Gurpide E. The endometrium: regulation and dysfunction. In: Yen SSC, Jaffe RB, eds. Reproductive Endocrinolgy. 3rd ed. Philadelphia: WB Saunders, 1991;309–356.
2. McCallion RL, Ferguson MWJ. Fetal wound healing and the development of antiscarring therapies for adult wound healing. In: Clark RAF, ed. The Molecular and Cellular Biology of Wound Repair. 2nd ed. New York: Plenum Press, 1996:561–600.
3. Furie B, Furie BC. The molecular basis of blood coagulation. Cell 1988;53:505–518.
4. Collen D, Lijnen HR. Basic and clinical aspects of fibrinolysis and thrombolysis. Blood 1991;78: 3114– 3124.
5. Carmeliet P, Collen D. Targeted gene manipulation and transfer of the plasminogen and coagulation systems in mice. Fibrinolysis 1996;10:195–213.
6. Kane KK. Fibrinolysis: a review. Ann Clin Lab Sci 1984;14:443–449.
7. Van der Walt JG. Eicosanoids: a short review. J S Afr Vet Assoc 1989;60:65–68.
8. Stern DM, Nawroth PP, Marcum J, et al. Interaction of antithrombin III with bovine aortic segments. J Clin Invest 1985;75:272–279.
9. Loedam JA, Meijers JCM, Sixma JJ, et al. Inactivation of human factor VIII by activated protein C: Cofactor activity of protein S and protective effect of von Willebrand factor. J Clin Invest 1988; 82:1236–1243.

10. Dear AE, Medcalf RL. The cellular and molecular biology of plasminogen activator inhibitor type-2. Fibrinolysis 1995;9:321–330.

11. Lockwood CJ, Schatz F. A biological model for the regulation of peri-implantational hemostasis and menstruation. J Soc Gynecol Invest 1996;3:159–165.

12. Lockwood CJ, Krikun G, Aigner S, et al. Effects of thrombin on steroid-modulated cultured endometrial stromal cell fibrinolytic potential. J Clin Endocrinol Metab 1996; 81:107–112.

13. Lockwood CJ, Krikun G, Papp C, et al. The role of progestationally regulated stromal cell tissue factor and type-1 plasminogen activator inhibitor (PAI-1) in endometrial hemostasis and menstruation. Ann NY Acad Sci 1994;734:57–79.

14. Ruggeri ZM. von Willebrand factor and fibrinogen. Curr Opin Cell Biol 1993;5:898–906.

15. Ginsberg MH, Loftus JC, Plow EF. Cytoadhesins, integrins, and platelets. Thromb Haemost 1988;59:1–6.

16. Ruosiahti E. Integrins. J Clin Invest 1991;87:1–5.

17. Hynes RO. Integrins: Versatility, modulation, and signaling in cell adhesion. Cell 1992;69:11–25.

18. Weksler BB. Platelets in Inflammation: In: Gallin JI, Goldstein IM, Snyderman R, eds. Basic Principle and Clinical Correlates. New York: Raven Press, 1992:727–746.

19. Sporn MB, Roberts AM. Transforming growth factors: recent progress and new challenges, J Cell Biol 1992;119:1017–1021.

20. Ross RR, Raines EW. Platelet-derived growth factor and cell proliferation. In: V. R. Sara et al., eds. Growth Factors: From Genes to Clinical Application. New York: Raven Press, 1990;193–199.

21. Westermark B. The molecular and cellular biology of platelet-derived growth factor. Acta Endocrinologica (Copenh) 1990;123:131–142.

22. Iida N, Haisa M, Igarashi A, et al. Leukocyte-derived growth factor links the PDGF and CXC chemokine families of peptides. FASEB J 1996;10:1336–1345.

23. Leibovich SJ, Ross R. The role of the macrophage in wound repair: a study with hydrocortisone and antimacrophage serum. Am J Pathol 1975;78:71–100.

24. Lanir N, Ciano PS, Van de Water L, et al. Macrophage migration in fibrin gel matrices 11. Effects of clotting factor XIII, fibronectin, and glycosaminoglycan content on cell migration, J Immunol 1988;140:2340–2349.

25. Ciano PS, Colvin RB, Dvorak AM, et al. Macrophage migration in fibrin gel matrices. Lab Invest 1986;54:62–70.

26. Cavaillon JM, Haeffner-Cavaillon N. Cytokines and inflammation. Rev Prat 1993; 43:547–552.

27. Lowry SF. Cytokine mediators of immunity and inflammation. Arch Surg 1993;128: 1235–1241.

28. Wahl SM, Wong H, McCartney-Francis N. Role of growth factors in inflammation and repair. J Cell Biochem 1989;40:193–199.

29. Higashiyama S, Abraham JA, Miller J, et al. A heparin-binding growth factor secreted by macrophage-like cells that is related to EGF. Science 1991;251:936–939.

30. Nathan C, Sporn M. Cytokines in context. J Cell Biol 1991;113:981–986.

31. Rappolee DA, Werb Z. Macrophage-derived growth factor. Curr Top Microbiol Immunol 1992;181:87–140.

32. Bazzoni F, Beutler B. The tumor necrosis factor ligand and receptor families. Semin Med Beth Israel Hos Boston 1996;334:1717–1725.

33. Peplow PV. Actions of cytokines in relation to arachidonic acid metabolism and eicosanoid production. Prostaglandins Leukot Essent Fatty Acids. 1996;54:303–317.

34. Sherman M, Weber B, Datta R, et al. Transcriptional and posttranscriptional regulation of macrophage-specific colony stimulating factor gene expression by tumor necrosis factor. Involvement of arachidonic acid metabolites. J Clin Invest 1990;85:442–447.

35. Gagnon L, Filion L, Dubois et al. Leukotrienes and macrophage activation: augmented cytotoxic activity and enhanced interleukin 1, tumor necrosis factor, and hydrogen peroxide production. Agent Action 1989;26:142–147.

36. Hori T, Yamanaka Y, Hayakawa M, et al. Prostaglandin antagonize fibroblast proliferation stimulated by tumor necrosis factor. Biochem Biophys Res Commun 1991;174:758–766.

37. Lee A, Whyte MBK, Haslett C, et al. In hibition of opoptosis and prolongation of neutrophil functional longevity by inflammatory mediators. J Leuk Biol 1993;54:283–288.

38. Savill JS, Fadok V, Hersar PM, et al. Phagocyte recognition of cell undergoing apoptosis. Immunol Today 1993;14:131–136.

39. Savill JS, Dransfield I, Hogg N, et al. Macrophage recognition of "senescent self." The vitronectin receptor mediates phagocytosis of cells undergoing apoptosis. Nature 1990;342:170–173.

40. Collins MKL, Perkins GR, Rodriguez-Tarduchy G, et al. Growth factors as survival factors: Regulation of apoptosis. Bioassays 1994;16:133–138.

41. Ramanathan M. A pharmacokinetic approach for evaluating cytokine binding macromolecules as antagonists. Pharm Res 1996;13:84–90.

42. Arend WP. Inhibiting the effects of cytokines in human diseases. Adv Intern Med 1995;40:365–394.

43. McCarthy PL. Down-regulation of cytokine action. Baillieres Clin Haematol 1994;7:153–177.

44. Layton MJ, Owczarek CM, Metcalf D, et al. Complex binding of leukemia inhibitory factor to its membrane-expressed and soluble receptors. Proc Soc Exp Biol Med 1994;206:295–298.

45. Jacobs CA, Beckmann MP, Mohler K, et al. Pharmacokinetic parameters and biodistribution of soluble cytokine receptors. Int Rev Exp Pathol 1993;34:123–135.

46. Gehr G, Braun T, Lesslauer W. Cytokines, receptors, and inhibitors. Clin Invest 1992;70:64–69.

47. Austgulen R, Arntzen KJ, Vatten LJ, et al. Detection of cytokines (interleukin-1, interleukin-6, transforming growth factor-ß) and soluble tumor necrosis factor receptors in embryo culture fluids during in vitro fertilization. Human Reprod 1995;10:171–176.

48. Fernandez-Botran R. Soluble cytokine receptors: their role in immunoregulation. FASEB J 1991;5:2567–2574.

49. Bayer SR, DeCherney AH. Clinical manifestations and treatment of dysfunctional uterine bleeding. JAMA 1993;269:1823–1828.

50. Wathen PI, Henderson MC, Witz CA. Abnormal uterine bleeding. Med Clin North Am 1995;79:329–344.

51. Cockerill GW, Gamble JR, Vadas MA. Angiogenesis: models and modulators. Int Rev Cytol 1995:159:113–160.

52. Folkman J, Shing T. Angiogenesis. J Biol Chem 1992;267:10931–10934.

53. Kuwano M, Ushiro S, Ryuto M, et al. Regulation of angiogenesis by growth factors. Gann Monogr Cancer Res 1994;42:113–125.

54. Knox P, Crooks S, Rimmer CS. Role of fibronectin in the migration of fibroblasts into plasma clots. J Cell Biol 1986;102:2318–2323.

55. Kubota Y, Kleinman, HK, Martin J. Role of laminin and basement membrane in the morphological differentiation of human endothelial cells into capillary-like structures. J Cell Biol 1988;107:1589–1598.

56. Brooks PC, Clark RAF, Cheresh DA. Requirement of vascular integrin αvβ3 for angiogenesis. Science 1994;264:569–571.

57. Brooks PC, Montgomery AMP, Rosenfeld M, et al. Integrin (αvβ3 antagonists promote tumor regression by inducing apoptosis of angiogenic blood vessels. Cell 1994;79:1157–1164.

58. Matrisian LM. Matrix metalloproteinases gene expression. In: Greenwald RA, Goublm LM, eds. Inhibition of matrix metalloproteinases: therapeutic potential. Ann New York Acad Sci, 1994;732:42–50.

59. Overall CM. Regulation of tissue inhibitor of matrix metalloproteins expression. In: Greenwald RA, Goublm LM, eds. Inhibition of matrix metalloproteinases: therapeutic potential. Ann NY Acad Sci 1994;732:51–64.

60. Hulboy DL, Rudolph LA, Matrisian LM. Matrix metalloproteinases as mediators of reproductive function. Mol Human Reprod 1997;3:27–45.

61. Rodgers WH, Matrisian L, Guidice LC, et al. Pattern of matrix metalloproteinase expression in cycling endometrium imply differential functions and regulation by steroid hormones. J Clin Invest 1994;94:946–953.

62. Osteen KG, Rodgers WH, Gaire M, et al. Stromal-epithelial interaction mediated steroidal regulation of matrix metalloproteinase expression in the human endometrium. Proc Natl Acad Sci USA 1991;91:10129–10133.

63. Bruner K, Rodgers WH, Gold LI, et al. Transforming growth factor ß mediates the progesterone suppression of an epithelial metalloproteinase by adjacent stroma in the human endometrium. Proc Natl Acad Sci USA 1995;95:7362–7366.

64. Ferrara N, Houck K, Jakeman L. Molecular and biological properties of the vascular endothelial growth factor family of proteins. Endocrin Rev 1992:13;18–32.

65. Klagsbrun M. The fibroblast growth factor family: structural and biological properties. Prog Growth Factor Res 1990;1:207–235.

66. Abraham JA, Klagsbrun M. Modulation of wound repair by membranes of the fibroblast growth factor family. In: Clark RAF, ed. The Molecular and Cellular Biology of Wound Repair. New York: Plenum Press, 1996;195–248.

67. Koch AE, Polverini PJ, Kunkel S, et al. Interleukin-8 as a macrophage-derived mediator of angiogenesis. Science 1982;258:1798–1801.

68. Smith SK. Growth factors in the human endometrium. Human Reprod 1994;9:936–946.

69. Shifren JL, Tseng JF, Zaloudek IP, et al. Ovarian steroid regulation of vascular endothelial growth factor in human endometrium: Implication for angiogenesis during menstrual cycle and in the pathogenesis of endometriosis. J Clin Endocrinol Metabol 1996;81:3112–3118.

70. Charnock-Jones DS, Sharkey AM, Rajput-Williams, J et al. Identification and localization of alternately spliced mRNAs for vascular endothelial growth factor in human uterus and estrogen regulation in endometrial carcinoma cell lines. Biol Reprod 1993;48:1120–1128.

71. Rusnati M, Casarotti G, Pecorelle E, et al. Basic fibroblast growth factor in ovulatory cycle and postmenopausal human endometrium. Growth Factors 1990;3:299–307.

72. Ferriani R, Charnock-Jones D, Prentice A, et al. Immunohistochemical localization of acidic and basic fibroblast growth factors in normal human endometrium and endometriosis and the detection of their mRNA by polymerase chain reaction. Human Reprod 1993;8:11–16.

73. DiBlasio AM, Centinaio G, Carniti C, et al. Basic fibroblast growth factor messenger ribonucleic acid levels in eutopic and ectopic human endometrial stromal cells as assessed by competitive polymerase chain reaction amplification. Mol Cell Endo 1995;115:169–175.

74. McNeil PL. Cellular and molecular adaptation to injurious mechanical stress. Trend Cell Biol 1993;3:302–307.

75. Koji T, Chedid M, Rubin JS, et al. Progesterone-dependent expression of keratinocyte growth factor mRNA in stromal cells of the primate endometrium: keratinocyte growth factor as a progestromedin. J Cell Biol 1994;125:393–401.

76. Sato Y, Tsuboi R, Luons R, et al. Characterization of the activation of latent TGF-ß by co-culture of endothelial cells and pericytes or smooth muscle cells: A self-regulating system. J Cell Biol 1990;111:757–763.

77. Roberts AR. Transforming growth factor ß: activity and efficacy in animal models of wound healing. Wound Rep Reg 1995;3:408–418.

78. Hamilton JA, Whitty GA, Wojta J, et al. Regulation of plasminogen-activator inhibitor-1 levels in human monocyte. Cell Immunol 1993;152:7–17.

79. Hamilton JA, Whitty GA, Atanton H, et al. Macrophage colony stimulating factor and granulocyte colony stimulating factor stimulate the synthesis of plasminogen-activator inhibitor-1 by human monocyte. Blood 1993;82;3616–3621.

80. O'Reilly MS, Holmgren L, Shing Y, et al. Angiostatin: A novel angiogenesis inhibitor that modulates the suppression of metastases by a Lewis Carcinoma. Cell 1994;79:315–328.

81. Fotsis T, Pepper MS, Aldercrutz H, et al. Genistein, a deitry-derived inhibitor of in vivo angiogenesis. Proc Natl Acad Sci USA 1993;90:2690–2694.

82. Fotsis T, Zhang Y, Pepper MS, et al. The endogenous oestrogen metabolite 2-methoxy-oestradiol inhibits angiogenesis and suppress tumor growth. Nature 1994:368:237–239.

83. Robertson W. The Endometrium. London: Butterworths. 1981.

84. Souaze F, Ntodou-Thome A, Tran CY, et al. Quantitative RT-PCR: Limits and accuracy. Biotechnique 1996;21:280–285.

85. Dou Q, Zhao Y, Tarnuzzer RW, et al. Suppression of TGF-ßs and TGF-ß receptors mRNA and protein expression in leiomyomata in women receiving gonadotropin releasing hormone agonist therapy. J Clin Endocrinol Metab 1996;81:3222–3230.

86. Tang X-M, Zhao Y, Dou Q, et al. Regulation of TGF-ß1 mRNA and protein expression by granulocyte- macrophage colony stimulating factor (GM-CSF) in human endometrium. J Soc Gynecol Invest 1995;2:Abst#P399.

87. Dou Q, Tang X-M, Kipersztock S, et al. The interactive relationship between transforming growth factor ß and granulocyte-macrophage stimulating factor in human uterus. J Soc Gynecol Invest 1996;3:Abstract NoP261.

88. Dou Q, Williams RS, Chegini N. The expression of integrin messenger RNA in human endometrium. A quantitative RT-PCR study. Fertil Steril 1999;71:347–353.

89. Hill JA. Cytokines considered critical in pregnancy. Am J Reprod Immunol 1992: 28:123–126.

90. Tabibzadeh S, Sun XZ. Cytokine expression in human endometrium throughout the menstrual cycle. Human Reprod 1992;7:1214–1221.

91. Chard T: Cytokines in implantation. Human Reprod (Update) 1995;1:385–396.

92. Tazuke SI, Gudice LC. Growth factors and cytokines in endometrium, embryonic development, and maternal embryonic interactions. Semin Reprod Endocrinol 1996;14:231–245.

93. Kauma S, Matt D, Strom S, et al. Interleukin 1ß, human leukocyte antigen HLA-DR and transforming growth factorß expression in endometrium, placental membranes. Am J Obstet Gynecol 1990;163:1430–1437.

94. Pamper S, Arceci RJ, Pollard JW. Role of colony stimulating factor-1 and other lymphohematopoietic growth factors in mouse pre-implantation development. BioEssays 1991;10:535–540.

95. Kojima K, Kanzaki H, Iwai M, et al. Expression of leukemia inhibitory factor in human endometrium and placenta. Biol Reprod 1994;50:882–887.

96. Charnock-Jones DS, Sharkey AM, Fenwick P, et al. Leukaemia inhibitory factor mRNA concentration peaks in human endometrium at the time of implantation and the blastocyst contains mRNA for the receptor at this time. J Reprod Fertil 1994;101:421–426.

97. Zhao Y, Tang XM, Chegini N. The expression of granulocyte-macrophage colony stimulating factor (GM-CSF), GM-CSF α and ß receptors mRNA and immunoreactive gene product for GM-CSF in human uterine tissue. Society for Gynecologic Investigation 41st Annual Meeting, 1994; Abstract No. O117.

98. Tabibzadeh S, Kong QF, Babaknia A, et al. Progressive rise in the expression of interleukin-6 in human endometrium during menstrual cycle is initiated during the implantation window. Human Reprod 1995;10:2793–2799.

99. Vandermolen DT, Gu Y. Human endometrial interleukin-6 (IL-6): in vivo messenger ribonucleic acid expression, in vitro protein production, and stimulation thereof by IL-1ß. Fertil Steril 1996;66:741–747.

100. Arici A, Head J, MacDonald P, et al. Regulation of interleukin-8 gene expression in human endometrial cells in culture. Mol Cell Endocrinol 1993;94:195–204.

101. Chegini N, Zhao Y, Williams RS, et al. Human uterine tissue throughout the menstrual cycle expresses TGF-ß1, TGF-ß2, TGF-ß3 and TGF-type II receptor mRNA and proteins and contain ^{125}I-TGF-ß1 binding sites. Endocrinology 1995;135:439–449.

102. Chegini N, Rossi MJ, Masterson BJ. Platelet-derived growth factor, epidermal growth factor and EGF and PDGF ß receptors in human endometrial tissue: Localization and in vitro action. Endocrinology 1992;130:2763–2775.

103. Kanzaki H, Hatayama H, Narukawa S, et al. Hormonal regulation in the production of macrophage colony-stimulating factor and transforming growth factor-beta by human endometrial stromal cells in culture. Horm Res 1995;44:30–35.

104. Arici A, MacDonald PC, Casey ML. Progestin regulation of interleukin-8 mRNA levels and protein synthesis in human endometrial stromal cells. J Steroid Biochem Mol Biol 1996;58:71–76.

105. Arici A, Engin O, Attar E, et al. Modulation of leukemia inhibitory factor gene expression and protein biosynthesis in human endometrium. J Clin Endocrinol Metab 1995;80:1908–1915.

106. Dinarello CA. Interleukin-1. In: Thomson A, ed. The Cytokine Handbook. San Diego: Academic Press, 1994:434–443.

107. Tronick SR, Aaronson SA. Growth factors and signal transduction. In: Ruddon RW, ed. Cancer Biology. 3rd ed. New York:Oxford University Press, 1995:117–140.

108. Chao MV. Growth factor signaling: where is the specificity? Cell 1992;68:995–997.

109. Laird SM, Tuckerman EM, Saravelos H, et al. The production of tumor necrosis factor α (TNF-α) by human endometrial cells in culture. Human Reprod 1996;11:1318–1323.

110. Frank GR, Brar AK, Jikihara H, et al. Interleukin-1 beta and the endometrium: an inhibitor of stromal cell differentiation and possible autoregulator of decidualization in humans. Biol Reprod 1995;52:184–191.

111. Laird SM, Tuckerman EM, Li TC, et al. Stimulation of human endometrial epithelial cells interleukin-6 production by interleukin-1 and placental protein 14. Human Reprod 1994;9:1339–1343.

112. Simon C, Frances A, Piquette GN, et al. Interleukin-1 system in the materno-trophoblast unit in human implantation: immunohistochemical evidence for autocrine/paracrine function. J Clin Endocrinol Metabol 1994;78:847–858.

113. Arai KI, Lee F, Miyajima A, et al. Cytokines: coordinators of immune and inflammatory responses. Ann Rev Biochem 1991;59:783–836.

114. Cohen MC, Cohen S. Cytokine function. a study in biologic diversity. Am J Clin Pathol 1996;105:589–598.

115. Schrader JW. Interleukin-3 In: Thomson A, ed. The Cytokine Handbook. San Diego: Academic Press, 1994:81–98.

116. Miossec P. Interleukin 4. A potential anti-inflammatory agent. Rev Rheum 1993;60:119–124.

117. Beckmann MP, Cosman D, Fanslow W, et al. The interleukin-4 receptor: structure, function, and signal transduction. Chem Immunol 1992;51:107–134.

118. Yokota T, Arai N, De Vries J, et al. Molecular biology of interleukin 4 and interleukin 5 genes and biology of their products that stimulate B cells, T cells, and hemopoietic cells. Immunol Rev 1988;102:137–187.

119. Hirano T. The biology of interleukin-6. Chem Immunol 1992;51:153–180.

120. Brown TJ, Rowe JM, Liu JW, et al. Regulation of IL-6 expression by oncostatin. M J Immunol 1991;147:2175–2180.

121. Rifas L, Kenney JS, Marcelli M, et al. Production of interleukin-6 in human osteoblasts and human bone marrow stromal cells: evidence that induction by interleukin-1 and tumor necrosis factor-α is not regulated by ovarian steroids. Endocrinology. 1995;136:4056–4067.

122. Donnelly RP, Crofford LJ, Freeman SL, et al. Tissue-specific regulation of IL-6 production by IL-4. Differential effects of IL-4 on nuclear factor-kappa B activity in monocytes and fibroblasts. J Immunol 1993;151:5603–5612.

123. Dokter WHA, Koopmans SB, Vellenga E. Effects of IL-10 and IL-4 on LPS-induced transcription factors (AP-1, NF-IL6 and NF-kappa B) which are involved in IL-6 regulation. Leukemia 1996;10:1308–1316.

124. Motro B, Itin A, Sachs L, et al. Pattern of interleukin 6 gene expression in vivo suggests a role for this cytokine in angiogenesis. Proc Natl Acad Sci USA 1990;87:3092–3096.

125. Cohen T, Nahari D, Cerem LW, et al. Interleukin 6 induces the expression of vascular endothelial growth factor. J Biol Chem 1996;271:736–741.

126. Enokihara H, Nakamura Y, Nagashima S, et al. Regulation of interleukin-5 production by interleukin-4, interferon-alpha, transforming growth factor-ß and interleukin-6. Int Arch Allergy Immunol 1994;104:44–45.

127. Fenton MJ, Buras JA, Donnelly RP. IL-4 reciprocally regulates IL-1 and IL-1 receptor antagonist expression in human monocytes. J Immunol 1992;149:1283–1288.

128. Namen AE, Williams DE, Goodwin RG. Interleukin-7: a new hematopoietic growth factor. Prog Clin Biol Res 1990;338:65–73.

129. J Van Damme. Interleukin-8 and related chemotactic cytokines. In: Thomson A, ed. The Cytokine Handbook. San Diego: Academic Press, 1994:186–208.

130. Kelleher K, Bean K, Clark SC, et al. Human interleukin-9: genomic sequence, chromosomal location, and sequences essential for its expression in human T-cell leukemia virus (HTLV)-I-transformed human T cells. Blood 1991;77:1436–1441.

131. de Waal Malefyt RH, Yssel MG, Roncarolo H, et al. Interleukin-10. Curr Opin Immunol 1992;4:314–320.

132. Paul SR, Schendel P. The cloning and biological characterization of recombinant human interleukin 11. Int J Cell Cloning 1992;10:135–143.

133. Scott P. IL-12: initiation cytokine for cell-mediated immunity. Science 1993;260:496–507.

134. Minty A, Chalon P, Derocq JM, et al. Interleukin-13 is a new human lymphokine regulating inflammatory and immune responses. Nature 1993;362:248–250.

135. Ford R, Tamayo A, Martin B, et al. Identification of B-cell growth factors (interleukin-14; high molecular weight-B-cell growth factors) in effusion fluids from patients with aggressive B-cell lymphomas. Blood 1995;86:283–293.

136. Giri JG, Anderson DM, Kumaki S, et al. IL-15, a novel T cell growth factor that shares activities and receptor components with IL-2. J Leukoc Biol 1995;57:763–766.

137. Laberge S, Cruikshank WW, Beer DJ, et al. Secretion of IL-16 (Lymphocyte chemoattractant factor) from serotonin-stimulated CD8+ T cells in vitro. J Immunol 1996;156:310–315.

138. Yao Z, Painter SL, Fanslow WC, et al. Human IL-17: a novel cytokine derived from T cells. J Immunol 1995;155:5483–5486.

139. Yao Z, Fanslow WC, Seldin MF, et al. Herpesvirus Saimiri encodes a new cytokine, IL-17, which binds to a novel cytokine receptor. Immunity 1995;3:811–821.

140. Shimpei U, Motoshi N, Takanri O, et al. Cloning of the cDNA for human IFN-γ inducing factor, expression in Escherichia coli, and studies on the biologic activities of the protein. J Immunol 1996;156:4274–4279.

141. Cullinan EB, Abbondanzo SJ, Anderson PS, et al. Leukemia inhibitory factor (LIF) and LIF receptor expression in human endometrium suggests a potential autocrine/paracrine function in regulating embryo implantation. Proc Natl Acad Sci USA 1996;93:3115–3120.

142. Ace CI, Okulicz WC. Differential gene regulation by estrogen and progesterone in the primate endometrium. Mol Cell Endocrinol 1995;115:95–103.

143. Kellokumpu-Lehtinen P, Talpaz M, Harris D, et al. Leukemia-inhibitory factor stimulates breast, kidney and prostate cancer cell proliferation by paracrine and autocrine pathways. Int J Cancer 1996;66:515–519.

144. Nachtigall MJ, Kliman HJ, Feinberg RF, et al. The effect of leukemia inhibitory factor (LIF) on trophoblast differentiation: a potential role in human implantation. J Clin Endocrinol Metab 1996;81:801–806.

145. Fienberg RF, Kilman HJ, Wang CL. Transforming growth factor ß stimulates trophoblast oncofetal fibronectin synthesis in vitro: implications for trophoblast implantation in vivo. J Clin Endocrinol Metabol 1994;78:1241–1248.

146. Lubbert M, Mantovani L, Lindemann A, et al. Expression of leukemia inhibitory factor is regulated in human mesenchymal cells. Leukemia 1991;5:361–365.

147. Hunt JS, Chen HL, Hu XL, et al. Tumor necrosis factor α mRNA and protein in human endometrium. Biol Reprod 1992;47:141–147.

148. Philippeaux MM, Piguet PF. Expression of tumor necrosis factor-α and its mRNA in the endometrial mucosa during the menstrual cycle. Am J Pathol 1993;143:480–486.

149. Tabibzadeh S, Babaknia A, Liu R, et al. Site and menstrual cycle-dependent expression of proteins for the TNF receptor family, and BCL-2 oncoprotein and phase specific production of TNF-α in human endometrium. Hum Reprod 1995:10:277–286.

149a. Chegini N, Dou Q, Williams RS. An inverse relation between the expression of tumor necrosis factor alpha (TNF-α) and TNF-α receptor in human endometrium. Am J Reprod Immol 1999; In press.

150. Donnelly RP, Freeman SL, Hayes MP. Inhibition of IL-10 expression by IFN-γ up-regulates transcription of TNF-α in human monocytes. J Immunol 1995;155:1420–1427.

151. Metcalf D. The colony stimulating factors. Discovery, development, and clinical applications. Cancer 1990;65:2185–2195.

152. Nagata S. Granulocyte colony stimulating factor and its receptor. In: Thomson A, ed. The Cytokine Handbook. San Diego: Academic Press, 1994:

153. Nicola NA. Hemopoietic cell growth factors and their receptors. Ann Rev Biochem 1989;58:45–77.

154. Garcia-Lloret MI, Morrish DW, Wegmann TG, et al. Demonstration of functional cytokine-placental interactions: CSF-1 and GM-CSF stimulate human cytotrophoblast differentiation and peptide hormone secretion. Exp Cells Res 1994;214:46–54.

155. Kanzaki H, Hatayama H, Narukawa S, et al. Hormonal regulation in the production of macrophage colony-stimulating factor and transforming growth factor-beta by human endometrial stromal cells in culture. Horm Res 1995;44 (Suppl 2): 30–35.

156. Kanzaki H, Crainie M, Lin H, et al. The in situ expression of granulocyte macrophage colony stimulating factor (GM-CSF) mRNA at the maternal-fetal interface. Growth Factors 1991;5:69–74.

157. Brown MA, Gough NM, Willson TA, et al. Structure and expression of the GM-CSF receptor α and ß chain genes in human leukemia. Leukemia 1993;7:63–74.

158. Kastelein RA, Shanafelt AB. GM-CSF receptor: Interaction and activation. Oncogene 1993;8:231–236.

159. Zhu JQ, Wu J, Zhu DX, et al. Recombinant human granulocyte macrophage colony stimulating factor (rhGM-CSF) induces human macrophage production of transforming growth factor-alpha. Cell Mol Biol 1991:37;413–419.

160. Ishikawa M, Takashima S, Stewart EA, et al. Heparin-binding epidermal growth factor and its receptor are differentially expressed in human endometrium. myometrium and leiomyomas. J Soc Gynecol Invest 1995; 2: Abstract No. 402.

161. Tang XM, Rossi MJ, Masterson BJ, et al. Insulin-like growth factor I (IGF-I), IGF-I receptors and IGF binding proteins 1-4 in human uterine tissue: tissue localization and IGF-I action in endometrial stromal and myometrial smooth muscle cells *in vitro*. Biol Reprod 1994;50:

162. Jones J, Clemmons D. Insulin-like growth factors and their binding proteins, biological actions. Endocrine Rev 1994;16:3–34.

163. Boehm KD, Daimon M, Gorodeski IG, et al. Expression of the IGF and PDGF genes in human uterine tissues. Mol Reprod Dev 1990;27:93–101.

164. Reuterdahl C, Sundberg C, Rubin K, et al. Tissue localization of ß receptors for platelet-derived growth factor and platelet-derived growth factor B chain during wound repair in humans. J Clin Invest 1993;91:2065–2075.

165. Raines EW, Dower SK, Ross R. Interleukin-1 mitogenic activity for fibroblasts and smooth muscle cells is due to PDGF-AA. Science 1989;243:393–396.

166. Shaw RJ, Benedict SH, Clark RAF, et al. Pathogenesis of pulmonary fibrosis in interstitial lung disease: Alveolar macrophage PDGF (B) gene activation an up-regulation by interferon gamma. Am Rev Respir Dis 1991;143:167–173.

167. Riches DWH. Macrophages involvement in wound repair, remodeling and fibrosis. In: Clark RAF, ed. The Molecular and Cellular Biology of Wound Repair. 2nd ed. New York: Plenum Press, 1996:95–141.

168. Tang XM, Zhao Y, Rossi MJ, et al. Expression of TGF-ß isoforms and TGF-ß type II receptor mRNA and protein, and the effect of TGF-ßs on endometrial stromal cells growth and protein degradation *in vitro*. Endocrinology 1994;135:450–459.

169. ten Dijke P, Yamashita H, Ichijo H, et al. Characterization of type I receptors for transforming growth factor-ß and activin. Science 1994;264:101–104.

170. Wrana JL, Attisano L, Wieser R, et al. Mechanism of activation of the TGF-ß receptor. Nature 1994;370:341–347.

171. Hammond MG, Oh ST, Anners J, et al. The effect of growth factors on the proliferation of human endometrial stromal cells in culture. Am J Obstet Gynecol 1993;168:1131–1138.

172. Leof EB, Proper JA, Goustin AS, et al. Induction of *c-sis* mRNA and activity similar to PDGF by TGF-ß: A proposed model for indirect mitogenesis involving autocrine activity. Proc Natl Acad Sci USA 1986;83:2453–2457.

173. Janat MF, Liau G. TGF-β1 is a powerful modulator of PDGF action in vascular smooth muscle cells. J Cell Physiol 1992;150:232–242.

174. Ishikawa O, LeRoy EC, Trojanowska M. Mitogenic effect of TGF-ß1 on human fibroblasts involves the induction of PDGF α receptors. J Cell Physiol 1990;145:181–186.

175. Gronwald RGK, Seifert RA, Bowen-Pope DF. Differential regulation of expression of two PDGF receptor subunits by TGF-ß. J Biol Chem 1989;264:8120–8125.

176. Ranganathan G, Getz MJ. Cooperative stimulation of specific gene transcription by EGF and TGF-ß1. J Biol Chem 1990;265:3001–3004.

177. Danielpour D, Kim KY, Winokur TS, et al. Differential regulation of the expression of TGF-ß1 and ß2 by retinoic acid, EGF and dexamethasone in NRK-49F and A549 cells. J Cell Physiol 1991;148:235–244.

178. Tang X-M, Ghahary A, Chegini N. The interaction between transforming growth factor ß and relaxin leads to modulation of matrix and matrix metalloproteinases expression in human uterus. J Soc Gynecol Invest 1996; 3:Abstract No. 205.

179. Arici A, MacDonald PC, Casey ML. Modulation of the levels of transforming growth factor beta messenger ribonucleic acids in human endometrial stromal cells. Biol Reprod 1996;54: 463–469.

180. Koji T, Brenner RM. Localization of estrogen receptor messenger ribonucleic acid in rhesus monkey uterus by nonradioactive in situ hybridization with digoxigenin-labeled oligodeoxynucleotides. Endocrinology 1993;132:382–392.

181. Gulshan S, McCruden AB, Stimson WH. Oestrogen receptors in macrophages. Scand J Immunol 1990;31:691–697.

182. Juneja SC, Pfeifer TL, Tang XM, et al. Modulation of mouse sperm-egg interaction, early embryonic development and trophoblastic outgrowth by activated and unactivated macrophages. Endocrine 1995;3:69–79.

183. Dou Q, Williams RS, Chegini N. Inhibition of promonocytic TGF-ß1 expression by antisense oligonucleotides alters their growth, anchor-dependent colonogenity and integrins mRNA expression: implication to endometriosis and peritoneal adhesion formation. Mol Human Reprod 1997;3:383–391.

184. Schust DJ, Anderson DJ, Hill JA. Progesterone-induced immunosuppression is not mediated through the progesterone receptor. Human Reprod 1996;11:980–985.

185. Iozzo RV, Murdoch AD. Proteoglycans of the extracellular environment: clues from the gene and protein side offer novel perspectives in molecular diversity and function. FASEB 1996;10:598–614.

186. Raghow R. The role of extracellular matrix in postinflammatory wound healing and fibrosis. FASEB 1994;8:823–831.

187. Shaw RJ, Doherty DE, Ritter AG, et al. Adherance-dependent increase in human monocyte PDGF (B) mRNA is associated with increases in c-fos, c-jun and EGR-2 mRNA. J Cell Biol 1990;111:2139–2148.

188. Juliano RI, Haskill S. Signal transduction from the extracellular matrix. J Cell Biol 1992;120:577–589.

189. Enders AC. Implantation (embryology). Encyc Human Biol 1991;4:423–430.

190. Cross JC, Werb Z, Fisher SJ: Implantation and placenta: key pieces of the development puzzle. Science 1994;266:1508–1518.

191. Tabibzadeh S, Babaknia A. The signals and molecular pathways involved in implantation, a symbiotic interaction between blastocyst and endometrium involving adhesion and tissue invasion. Human Reprod 1995;10:1579–1602.

192. Robertson SA, Seamark RF, Guilbert L, et al. The role of cytokines in gestation. Crit Rev Immunol 1994;14:239–292.

193. Adamson ED: Activities of growth factors in preimplantation embryo. J Cell Biochem 1993;52:280–287.

194. Schultz GA, Heyner S. Growth factors in preimplantation mammalian embryos. Oxf Rev Reprod Biol 1993;15:43–81.

195. Akhurst RJ. The transforming growth factor ß family in vertebrate embryogenesis. In: Growth Factors and Signal Transduction in Development. New York: Wiley-Liss, 1994:97–122.

196. Korach KS. Insights from the study of animals lacking functional estrogen receptor. Science 1994;266:1524–1527.

197. Rissman EF, Early AH, Taylor JA, et al. Estrogen receptors are essential for female sexual receptivity. Endocrinology 1997;138:507–510.

198. Auger AP, Moffatt CA, Blaustein JD. Progesterone-independent activation of rat brain progestin receptors by reproductive stimuli. Endocrinology 1997;138:511–514.

199. Stewart CL, Kasper P, Brunel LJ, et al. Blastocyst implantation depends on maternal expression of leukaemia inhibitory factor. Nature 1992;359:76–79.

200. Abbondanzo SJ, Cullinan EB, McIntyre K, et al. Reproduction in mice lacking a functional type 1 IL-1 receptor. Endocrinology 1996;137:3598–3601.

201. Simon C, Frances A, Piquette GN, et al. The immune mediator interleukin-1 receptor antagonist (IL-1ra) prevents embryonic implantation. Endocrinology 1994;134;521–528.

202. Shull MM, Ormsby I, Kier AB, et al. Targeted disruption of the mouse transforming growth factors ß-1 gene results in multifocal inflammatory disease. Nature 1992;359:693–699.

203. Chegini N. Oviductal-derived growth factors and cytokines: Implication in preimplantation. Semin Reprod 1996;14:219–229.

6

IMPLICATION OF GROWTH FACTOR AND CYTOKINE NETWORKS IN LEIOMYOMAS

Nasser Chegini

University of Florida, Gainesville, Florida

Leiomyomas are benign uterine tumors that occur in 20% to 25% of women during the reproductive years. The majority of leiomyomas are asymptomatic, requiring no intervention; however, they are the leading indication and account for more than 30% of all hysterectomies (160–180 thousand) performed in the United States annually (1–5). Symptoms caused by the presence of tumors include abnormal vaginal bleeding, pelvic pain, pelvic mass, and infertility in 20% to 50% of these woman (2–5).

Histologically leiomyomas are well encapsulated tumors primarily consisting of smooth muscle cells, considered to arise from a single normal myometrial smooth muscle cell. Leiomyomas have limited vascularization and malignant transformation potential (<1%), and despite the presence of multiple tumors seen in the same uterus, they occur independently of metastasis (6–9). Cytogenetic analysis has revealed the occurrence of several nonrandom chromosomal alterations such as duplications, deletions, and translocations in leiomyoma smooth muscle cells. These chromosomal ab-

Cytokines in Human Reproduction, Edited by Joseph A. Hill
ISBN 0-471-35242-X Copyright © 2000 Wiley-Liss, Inc.

normalities have been suggested to account for leiomyoma tumorigenesis and growth; however, owing to inconsistency of their occurrence and lack of identity of their gene products it is most unlikely that they are directly responsible for these tumors (6, 10–12). Nonetheless, factors that initiate the conversion of normal myometrial smooth muscle cells into leiomyoma and orchestrate their subsequent growth and regression are unknown. However, considerable data exist that implicate ovarian steroids and various growth regulatory factors whose expression are in part regulated by ovarian steroids in leiomyoma growth.

THE ROLE OF OVARIAN STEROIDS

Overexpression of estrogen and progesterone receptors, leiomyomas' rapid growth and increase in mitotic activity during hyperestrogenic states such as pregnancy and luteal phase of the menstrual cycle, and their regression with menopause implicate ovarian steroids as a key regulator of leiomyoma growth (12–17). In the myometrium estrogen receptor levels are low throughout the menstrual cycle although they increase, reaching a maximum at midluteal phase. However, leiomyomas appear to have elevated levels of estrogen receptors throughout the menstrual cycle compared to unaffected myometrium (12–17). In leiomyomas the estrogen receptor mRNA and protein levels are reported to be 1.4–12.6- and threefold higher, respectively, compared to unaffected myometrial tissue (17). Scatchard analysis of 17ß-estradiol binding to cell-free extracts also indicates a higher binding capacity in leiomyomas than myometrium without any differences in their binding affinity (17).

Induction of a hyperestrogenic state in a rodent model that forms leiomyoma-like tumors in myometrium further implicates estrogen in the growth of these tumors (18–21). Furthermore, it has been shown that estrogen stimulates, whereas antiestrogen, tamoxifen, inhibits the proliferation of Eker rat leiomyoma-derived cell line in vitro and in vivo (19). However, unlike in humans, these tumors have a significantly higher mitotic activity, which also occurs in the adjacent myometrial tissue (18). It has recently been reported that transgenic mice expressing the simian virus 40 T antigen driven by the promoter of the Calbindin-D9K (CaBP9K) gene develop uterine smooth muscle tumors (22). These tumors are reported to occur in different parts of the reproductive tract, usually in the corpus, as well as in the horn of the uterus, and in the vagina. Because the CaBP9K regulatory sequences directing the expression of the Tag gene contains an estradiol responsive element, the development of these tumors has been considered to be estrogen dependent (22). In addition, the data suggest that expression of Tag gene is necessary for the initiation as well as development and maintenance of these tumors. Compared with the other animal models these transgenic mice could potentially serve as a useful model for studying the pathobiology of uterine leiomyomas and to help design new therapeutic approaches to this disease (22).

Local estrogen biosynthesis has also been suggested to play a role in promoting leiomyoma growth (23). Leiomyomas have been shown to express cytochrome p19 and its product aromatase p450 mRNA at levels similar to those detected in adipose tissues.

However, P450arom transcripts were not detectable in myometrium of women without leiomyomas, whereas myometrium adjacent to leiomyomas expressed these transcripts with levels 1.5- to 25-fold lower than the tumors. Furthermore, the aromatase activity of leiomyoma smooth muscle cells and explant cultures was stimulated by cAMP, whereas dexamethasone or platelet derived growth factor (PDGF) did not have any effect. It has been shown that leiomyomas convert androstenedione to estrone (23).

Progesterone receptor overexpression, increase in mitotic activity, and tumor enlargement during the progesterone dominated luteal phase implicates progesterone as an important factor in leiomyoma growth (13, 24). Progesterone exists in A and B forms, which are both expressed in leiomyomas and myometrium, with A form expression predominant (25–27). The level of progesterone receptor mRNA and protein has been reported to be significantly higher in leiomyomas compared to myometrium obtained from the same patient (13, 24). Progesterone A form is reported to repress the progesterone induced gene expression (26) and its absence has been associated with various gynecologic malignancies (25). Clinical studies have produced conflicting results regarding the effect of progesterone or synthetic progestins on leiomyoma growth (13, 28, 29). Under in vitro conditions progestin did not appear to influence the expression of connexin 43 gene expression in leiomyoma and myometrial primary cell cultures (30), suggesting that progesterone action in both tissues is mediated through a similar pathway. Data also exist in regard to estrogen receptor mediated transcriptional response in primary cultures of leiomyoma and myometrial smooth muscle cells in particular cells derived from estrogen dominated period (31). The identification of a new estrogen receptor, the type ß, as well as the differences in the expression and function of progesterone receptors A and B, raises new questions yet to be elucidated in regard to the role of ovarian steroids and steroid mediated regulatory factors in leiomyoma growth.

Creating a hypoestrogenic state by gonadotropin releasing hormone (GnRH) agonists (GnRHa) therapy often results in tumor regression, similar to that observed following menopause (32, 33). GnRHa therapy causes a reduction in uterine/leiomyomas steroid receptors content, volume, arteriole size and blood flow (32–36). However, because of adverse cardiovascular and skeletal side effects of GnRHa-induced hypoestrogenism prolonged therapy cannot be continued indefinitely, and discontinued therapy also results in tumors returning to their original size over a matter of months (33). This limitation has led to an approach called "add back therapy, " in which GnRHa is administered along with low doses of cyclic or continuous estrogen and progesterone, allowing the therapy to continue for a longer period (37). It has been demonstrated that the predominant change in uterine volume due to GnRHa therapy is on nonmyoma uterine tissue, and co-administration of medroxyprogesterone acetate (MPA) with GnRHa reverses the beneficial effect of GnRHa-induced hypoestrogenism and uterine/leiomyomas regression (28).

It has also been reported that daily administration of antiprogesterone (mifepristone:RU486) induced a significant decrease in leiomyomas/uterine volume, which was 20% greater than that induced by GnRHa therapy (38, 39). Although the number of subjects who have undergone mifepristone therapy is low and the work must be confirmed by others, its effect on leiomyomas appears to be clinically significant.

Because the hormonal milieu to which leiomyomas/uterus is exposed under RU-486 therapy is that of unopposed estrogen, the reduction in uterine blood flow has been suggested not to be mediated by a hypoestrogenic condition (38, 39). Similar arguments have been raised by others with regard to the effect of RU-486 on the endometrium (38, 39). RU-486 causes a significant reduction in leiomyoma progesterone receptor content, without affecting the estrogen receptor levels (38). The mechanism of RU-486 induced leiomyoma regression is unclear and requires detailed investigation. Antiprogestins are effective antagonists of progesterone that by either binding to progesterone–DNA complex such as RU-486 (type II antiprogestin) or blocking the progesterone receptor binding to progesterone receptor element such as ZK98299 (type I antiprogestin), interfere with progesterone actions (40). In addition, RU-486 can act as a weak agonist in the absence of progesterone. It has been shown that unlike progesterone B receptors, the A receptors are not transcriptionally activated by progesterone antagonists, suggesting that when both receptors are present the A receptor can annul the inappropriate transcription by B receptors (40). Immunoreactive progesterone A and B forms are present in leiomyomas and myometrium, with the A form being predominant (25). Interestingly, it has been shown that the level of progesterone A and B receptor expression can differ with respect to each other in certain target tissues, and the ratio of B to A receptors influences the direction of a tissue's response to progesterone antagonists (40). RU-486 has been shown to suppress prolactin production in both leiomyomas and myometrium in vitro (25), and various other progestin-induced biologic functions in other systems (27, 40). Preliminary data from our laboratory suggest that RU-486 and ZK98299 alter the rate of DNA synthesis and growth factor expression in primary cultures of myometrial and leiomyomas smooth muscle cells and leiomyosarcoma cell lines (Chegini N, unpublished data).

Although the predominant site of GnRHa action is central, extrapituitary GnRH receptors have been found in several tissues including human uterus and leiomyomas, implicating GnRHa direct action in these tissues (41–52). GnRH receptors detected in these tissues, as well as endometrial carcinoma and several cancer cell lines such as breast, ovarian, endometrial, and hepatoma, are of low affinity/high capacity; however, GnRH analogues have been shown to modulate the growth, as well as the expression, of EGF, IGF, TGF-ß, and receptors in these cells in (42, 44–49). It has also been reported that GnRH has a direct effect on enzymatic activities in the ovary, uterus, and placenta, and GnRHa has a stimulatory effect on spontaneous contraction of human myometrium and fallopian tubes in vitro (51, 52). Data obtained in our laboratory indicate that leiomyomas, myometrium, and myometrial smooth muscle cells in culture express GnRH and GnRH receptor mRNA, supporting the concept of GnRHa action in the uterus (53). We have further demonstrated that GnRHa inhibits myometrial smooth muscle cells rate of DNA synthesis, as well as TGF-ß1 mRNA and protein expression (53). Our in vitro data have also provided support for the concept of "add back therapy," demonstrating that 17ß-estradiol (E_2) and in particular MPA, and E_2 + MPA can partially override the GnRHa action (28, 37, 53). A comparable result has also been obtained using antiprogestins ZK98299 and RU 486 (Chegini N, unpublished data).

CELL PROLIFERATION, HYPERTROPHY, EXTRACELLULAR MATRIX ACCUMULATION, AND LEIOMYOMA GROWTH

A combination of mitotic activities, alterations in cellular hypertrophy, and extracellular matrix (ECM) accumulation has been speculated to play a major role in leiomyoma growth (6, 13). The rate of mitotic index, which reflects cellular proliferation, increases and remains high in leiomyomas throughout the luteal phase of the menstrual cycle and decreases during menses (6, 13, 54–59). The rate of mitotic activity is estimated to be as high as 40 mitotic figures/100 high-power fields in leiomyomas during the luteal phase, and significantly higher in tumors from younger (ages 30–34) than older (ages 45–49 or 50–54) women (6). During the proliferative phase leiomyomas appear to be quiescent, showing a mitotic index similar to that seen in the myometrium; however, in women who have received progestin therapy there is an increase in the rate of mitotic activity compared to untreated or estrogen/progestin treated groups (6, 55–59). Despite the inconsistency in the in vitro action of progesterone, isolated leiomyoma and myometrial smooth muscle cells are reported to have a higher rate of DNA synthesis and proliferation in response to progestin treatment (57, 60–62).

GnRHa induced leiomyoma regression is considered to be due to reduced tumor cellularity (10, 13, 63), although the mitotic index in these tumors is relatively too low to account for a rapid growth and conversely a rapid decrease in their size with GnRHa and RU-486 therapies (37, 38). Leiomyomas can undergo extensive growth with less than 10 mitotic index (6), implying the potential involvement of activities other than cell division to be responsible for leiomyomas growth in size. Thus alterations in cellular hypertrophy and extracellular matrix (ECM) accumulation have been speculated to play a major role in these processes (13, 64–66).

Leiomyomas are fibrotic tumors and accumulation of various ECM components must play a key role in their growth in size. The ECM is organized in a highly complex structure each consisting of different components including various collagens, fibronectin, vitronectin, laminin, elastin, and proteoglycans (67–69). Collagens are homo- or heterodimeric glycoproteins involving several α chains that are distinct gene products. All together 32 different α chains have been identified with common α repetitive motif Gly-X-Y that allows folding into a triple helix, and 19 different collagen types designated type I–XVIII have been identified and characterized in vertebrates so far (67, 68). Interstitial collagens I, II, III, V, and IX, which are synthesized in precursor form, are secreted after cleavage modification to form the collagen fibrils, with collagens V and XI representing the central core and collagens I, II, and III making most of the fibril mass. Only limited data are currently available regarding collagen expression and content in leiomyomas. The collagen content of leiomyomas is relatively high, with one report estimating the content to be as high as 50% more than unaffected myometrium, with an increase in the ratio of collagen I/III (65, 66). In addition, the relative level of collagens I and III mRNA expression, but not of fibronectin, has been reported to be higher in leiomyomas than normal myometrium, and in tissues from the proliferative phase of the menstrual cycle, suggesting their regulation by estrogen (66).

Besides providing the structural support for new tissue formation, collagens can have a profound effect on leiomyoma cell–cell and cell–matrix interactions. Collagens are chemoattractant factors for various cell types including the smooth muscle cells and fibroblasts, and they also alter the phenotypic nature and functions of these cells (69–71). These effects may be mediated in part through activation of integrin–collagen receptors such as α1ß1 and α2ß1, which are expressed by leiomyomas (72). Collagen matrix has been shown to reduce fibroblast proliferation and collagen expression while inducing procollagenase and integrin expression (68–71). The collagen rich environment of leiomyomas may contribute to maintenance of the smooth muscle cells' differentiated state and their phenotypic alterations. Under such conditions smooth muscle cells may assume a myofibroblast characteristic and fibroblasts switch from a migratory to a profibrotic phenotype. It has been shown that during granulation tissue formation these newly formed phenotypes produce abundant type I and type III collagens (69–71).

ECMs are also critical for tumor growth and tissue fibrosis. Among them is fibronectin, which is encoded by a single gene but exists in a number of variant forms generated from alternative splicing and is composed of two nearly identical chains that are linked by a single disulfhydryl bond (73, 74). Fibronectins are multifunctional cell adhesion proteins found in blood at 0.3 mg/mL concentration and expressed by a variety of cell types. They provide a provisional substratum for smooth muscle, fibroblast, and endothelial cell adhesion, migration, and ingrowth (73, 74). Fibronectin also provides a linkage for myofibroblasts and collagen fibrillogenesis and, owing to specific functional domains and cell binding sites it is capable of interacting with a wide variety of cell types, ECM, and cytokines, and may serve as a template for collagen deposition and modulate gene expression through integrin receptors activation (75–80). Fibroblasts cultured on the 120 kDa fibronectin fragment containing the RGD cell binding domain, but not other integrin recognition sites, or cultured on intact fibronectin containing the α4ß1 integrin recognition site, CS-1, enhances matrix metalloproteinase 1 (MMP-1) expression (81, 82). Such specificity in fibronectin and fibronectin fragment-induced signals may initiate feedback loop eliciting different proteolytic enzyme secretion that causes more fibronectin digestion or collagen deposition that are essential for cellular invasion, granulation tissue formation, and fibrosis (77–80).

Proteoglycans are diverse and heterogeneous molecules, found intracellularly in secretary granules, at the cell surface as intrinsic or extrinsic membrane proteins, and in the ECM (83). Proteoglycans have multiple tissue organizational functions that include extracellular organization, ECM growth factor storage, and promotion of growth factor receptor binding (83–85). Among proteoglycans are decorin, biglycan, and versican (83–85). Preliminary data obtained in our laboratory suggest that leiomyomas express mRNA and protein for decorin, biglycan, and versican (Chegini, unpublished data). Versican is a major contributor of tissue resilience (83) that by decreasing cell adhesion promotes cell migration (84); hyaluronan also modulates cell adhesion (85), whereas cell growth, that is, of smooth muscle cells, is inhibited by decorin, heparin, and heparan sulfate (86, 87). The ECM can also act as a reservoir for growth factors and cytokines such as FGF-I, FGF-4, FGF-7, PDGF, GM-CSF, IL-3,

TGF-ß1, and VEGF, as well as their soluble receptors, and leads to their cell surface receptor activations (86–95). ECM-bound growth factors and cytokines can be then released in an active form after degradation of ECM allowing the ligand to bind to their respective specific receptors. Furthermore, in some cases such as that with FGF, binding of FGF-2 to its receptor requires prior binding to a membrane-bound heparan sulfate (89), and matrix-associated TGF-ß that is inactive also becomes activated upon disassociation from ECM (93). Therefore leiomyoma's ECM may have a critical role in proper cell migration, proliferation, and gene expression, and act as a repository for growth factors and cytokines.

Owing to a lack of substantial cell division during leiomyoma growth and regrowth after GnRHa withdrawal, cellular enlargement (hypertrophy) is suggested as another possible mechanism in leiomyoma growth (13, 64). Cellular hypertrophy appears to result from incomplete growth stimulation by enlargement of existing cells with little or no change in cell number and occurs in a variety of cell types including terminally differentiated cells such as cardiac myocytes and smooth muscle cells (96–99). There are virtually no data available pertaining to this parameter and its stimuli in leiomyoma smooth muscle cells.

THE ROLE OF GROWTH FACTORS AND CYTOKINES IN LEIOMYOMA GROWTH

As discussed above, leiomyomas are hypersensitive to the action of ovarian steroids. However, it is generally accepted that the mitogenic actions of ovarian steroids in steroid-sensitive tissues such as uterus are mediated in part through the expression of autocrine/paracrine growth factors and cytokines. In regard to cytokine expression and actions there are no data currently available concerning leiomyomas. The growth factors IGF-I, IGF-II, EGF, heparin binding EGF, PDGFs, FGFs, and TGF-ßs are reported to be expressed in leiomyomas and myometrium as well as their isolated smooth muscle cells in primary cultures (6, 13, 60, 61, 100–120). These growth factors are pleiotropic and influence cell proliferation, angiogenesis, cellular hypertrophy, and ECM synthesis (93–95, 121–125), events that are important in leiomyoma growth and regression. These growth factors have multiple and individual activities with respect to tumor growth and tissue fibrosis. In addition, through their synergetic interactions these growth factors have been shown to modulate the growth of myometrial and leiomyoma smooth muscle cells in vitro (60, 61, 115, 116, 120).

The Implication of TGF-βs

Based on biochemical characterization and sequence analysis of cDNA clones, TGF-ß proteins consist of TGF-ß1–5 with considerable homology (from 82% between TGF-ß1 and TGF-ß4 to 64% between TGF-ß2 and TGF-ß4) in their sequences (93). TGF-ßs are synthesized as precursor proteins that, following homodimerization and proteolytic cleavage, form the mature TGF-ßs. It also appears that TGF-ß1 and TGF-ß2 may form a heterodimer of TGF-ß1.2 (93). TGF-ßs are synthesized and released as the latent or biologically inactive form, and must become activated before they can bind to TGF-ß receptors (93, 124). The processes that activate TGF-ßs in vivo are not known; however, various treatments including proteolytic processing, lysosomal cathepsin D, and plasmin result in their release from the latent protein complex (93). Hydrolysis with sialidase or interruption of carbohydrate interactions with mannose-6-phosphate or sialic acid have also been shown to activate TGF-ß (93).

TGF-ßs are bifunctional growth factors and can inhibit and stimulate cell growth depending on the cell types. Other biologic effects attributed to TGF-ßs include angiogenesis, cellular hypertrophy, and ECM turnover (93, 124, 125). TGF-ßs mediate their biologic activities by binding to three sets of receptors termed TGF-ß receptor (TGF-R) types I–III, of which type I and II are transmembrane proteins with a cytoplasmic serine/threonine kinase domain (126–131). TGF-ß type IR is also suggested to be the functional receptor, and its presence and interaction with type IIR is required for binding and receptor-mediated signaling (131). Types I and IIR bind with higher affinity to TGF-ß1 and TGF-ß3 than TGF-ß2 (93, 124). The type IIIR exists in both soluble and cell surface-associated forms and binds TGF-ßs with similar affinity, with the cell-associated form considered to be involved in presenting TGF-ßs to the signaling receptors, without influencing the signal transduction mechanism (124, 131).

Leiomyomas, unaffected myometrium, and their isolated smooth muscle cells express TGF-ßs and TGF-ß receptors mRNA and protein, with the highest relative level of expression occurring during the luteal phase (117–120). Using quantitative RT-PCR, in situ hybridization, and immunohistochemistry, we have demonstrated that leiomyomas express a significantly higher level of TGF-ß1 than TGF-ß2, with TGF-ß3 being least expressed, but they express a significantly higher level of TGF-ß type II than type I receptors (119). We have further demonstrated a significant reduction in the level of TGF-ß1, TGF-ß3, and TGF-ßR types I and II, but not TGF-ß2 mRNA and protein expression in leiomyomas from women receiving GnRHa therapy compared to untreated groups (119). TGF-ß1 and TGF-ß3 significantly stimulate the rate of DNA synthesis, but not proliferation of myometrial smooth muscle cells in vitro, with TGF-ß2 being least effective (120), suggesting their effect on cellular hypertrophy. Others have reported that leiomyomas and myometrium express similar levels of TGF-ß1 mRNA, and GnRHa therapy equally affected its expression in these tissues (118). A possible explanation for the difference between this study and ours is the sensitivity of quantitative RT-PCR used in our study, which has been estimated to be 1000 fold greater than northern blot analysis.

The effects of TGF-ß on ECM turnover are more complex and profound than that of any other growth factor, and are central to its effect on pathological matrix accumulation characteristic of fibrotic disease such as leiomyoma (93, 125, 132). The mechanisms leading to an increase in matrix abundance are many and varied, but include the following: (1) increased synthesis of a wide spectrum of matrix proteins including collagens, glycosaminoglycans, and fibronectin; (2) decreased synthesis of proteases that degrade ECM components such as matrix metalloproteinases (MMPs); and (3) increased synthesis of tissue inhibitor of MMPs (TIMPs) (93, 133–135). We have shown that TGF-ß1 upregulates the expression of α1 pro-collagen, fibronectin, and TIMP-1, whereas it reduces collagenase mRNA expression in these cells (136).

ECM turnover of the connective tissue matrix is important in tissue remodeling and is mediated by the action of MMPs that mediate collagen breakdown during collagen synthesis in a controlled fashion (78, 81, 82, 93, 133–135). The MMPs are classified according to their substrate specificity. MMP-1 (interstitial collagenase) degrades collagens I–III; MMP-2 (gelatinase A, or type IV collagenase) degrades collagens IV and V and fibronectin; MMP-3 (stromelysin) degrades collagens III and IV, fibronectin and laminin, and proteoglycans, and MMP-9 (gelatinase B or type V collagenase) degrades collagens IV and V and elastin (133, 135). MMP activities are kept in check by a number of inhibitors, including the TIMPs. TIMP-1 specifically inactivates MMP-1, MMP-2, MMP-3, and MMP-9, and TIMP-2, which binds the active form of these enzymes, also binds the latent form of MMP-2 (133–135). We have demonstrated that leiomyomas and unaffected myometrium express MMP-1, MMP-2, MMP-3, MMP-9, TIMP-1, and TIMP-2 mRNA and protein, with a very low number of copies of MMP-1, MMP-3, and MMP-9 mRNA expression in leiomyoma (137). A lower level of MMPs, but higher TIMP expression in leiomyoma, suggests the existence of a favorable condition that accommodates ECM accumulation compared to unaffected myometrium. Indeed, leiomyomas have been reported to contain a substantially higher amount of collagens with a greater ratio of collagens type I and III than myometrium (65, 66). Furthermore, we have shown that GnRHa therapy resulted in a significant increase in MMPs but a decrease in TIMP-1 mRNA and protein expression in leiomyomas and myometrium from GnRHa-treated subjects. This suggests that a wide spectrum of ECM is susceptible to proteolytic degradation by MMPs resulting in tumor regression (reduction in size).

Although a significant information is available with regard to the expression and regulation of MMPs and TIMPs in various other tissues and cells and to a limited extent in other reproductive tissues, factors that regulate their expression in leiomyoma during growth and GnRHa or antiprogestin-induced regression are presently unknown. A higher level of MMPs and TIMPs mRNA in leiomyomas and myometrium during the secretory phase and low expression of MMP-3 and MMP-9 during all phases of the menstrual cycle suggest a possible involvement of ovarian steroids, particularly progesterone, in their regulation. A significant change in TIMP-1 but not TIMP-2 mRNA expression in leiomyomas further suggests a distinct regulation between their expression in these tissues. Because of hypoestrogenism induced by GnRHa therapy we can conclude that ovarian steroids may stimulate TIMP-1, whereas they inhibit MMP expression in leiomyomas. In human endometrium the MMP mRNA expression throughout the menstrual cycle displays a highly specific pattern of cellular distribution (135, 138). Progesterone has been shown to inhibit the expression of collagenase and stromelysin in human endometrial stromal (139). In contrast, regulation of TIMPs by the ovarian steroid are contradictory as progesterone and 17ß-estradiol have been shown to affect TIMP-1 expression differently (139).

There are numerous examples of TGF-ß influence on expression and secretion of a variety of collagen genes, including collagen types I and III under in vitro conditions (93, 125, 140–145). Upregulation of collagen gene expression appears to be mediated in part by increased transcription of collagen mRNAs through effects of TGF-ß on nuclear factor I (NFI) and Spl binding sites in the collagen promoter and on stability of the procollagen mRNA (143–145). In addition, TGF-ß stimulates the synthesis and secretion of TIMP by IL-1ß stimulated human synovial fibroblasts (83), whereas it inhibits the expression of MMP-1 and MMP-2 and those induced by other factors including PDGF, IL-1ß, and TNF-α (134, 146–151). Thus TGF-ß increases ECM biosynthesis, by preventing their degradation by blocking the synthesis of ECM degrading enzymes and by increasing the synthesis of TIMPs. This condition creates an imbalance between collagen synthesis and collagen degradation resulting in tissue fibrosis. Besides the autocrine action of cellular TGF-ß, because the ECM serves as storage for the secreted TGF-ß, excess active TGF-ß can become available upon cleavage from the matrix and released for immediate action (93, 149, 150). Thus in response to a variety of stimuli and conditions, both the cellular expression of TGF-ßs and/or ECM-released TGF-ß can influence various leiomyoma cellular activities. Therefore, lowering of TGF-ßs/receptor expression in leiomyomas due to GnRHa or RU-486 therapy may in turn reduce the rate of ECM expression and deposition, and through differential regulation of MMPs and TIMPs accelerate the rate of ECM degradation leading to leiomyoma reduction in size (53, 136, 137). Because of these specific activities, TGF-ßs appear to have the essential property of acting as a major regulator of leiomyoma growth. Understanding the regulation of latent TGF-ß activation is likely to be key in providing insight into their role in fibrotic disease such as leiomyoma, since disregulation of the balance between active and latent TGF-ßs could result in excessive activity.

The Role of Platelet Derived Growth Factors

Platelet derived growth factor (PDGF) is a polypeptide of 30 kDa that consists of the A and B subunits, with approximately 60% homology (94). The PDGF A and B subunits through disulfide bonds form a homo- or heterodimer complex giving rise to three dimeric forms: PDGF-AA, PDGF-BB, or PDGF-AB, with different functional activities (94). Although platelets are the major source of PDGF, they are synthesized and released by a variety of other cell types. The PDGF isoforms bind to two distinct but closely related receptor molecules, the α and the ß subunits (94). Cross-competition binding studies with ^{125}I-PDGF isoforms and comparison of their binding properties has revealed the existence of two classes of PDGF receptors, the $\alpha\alpha$ and ßß forms, from dimerization of PDGF-R subunits (94). The PDGF $\alpha\alpha$ receptor binds all three PDGF isoforms, whereas the ßß receptor binds PDGF-BB with high affinity and PDGF-AB with a lower affinity, but does not bind PDGF-AA (94). The two receptors are expressed in varying numbers and proportions on different cell types and are differentially regulated (94). Therefore the capacity of PDGFs (AA, BB, and AB) to induce a biologic response depends on the expression of PDGF α or ß receptors in their target cells.

Only limited data are available regarding the expression of PDGFs and their receptors in uterine tissue of human and other species as well as leiomyomas (60, 101, 107). Human uterine tissue has been shown to express mRNA for the PDGF-B chain with similar relative abundance throughout the menstrual cycle (107). Human myometrium and primary cultures of myometrial smooth muscle cells also continue

PDGF-AB protein as well as PDGF ß receptor, but a low level of PDGF α receptors and their immunostaining intensity did not change throughout the menstrual cycle (60). In contrast, human gestational myometrium has been shown only to express the PDGF-AA, and the level of its transcript increased during the gestation and diminished during the puerperium (152). Northern blot analysis of leiomyoma and myometrial tissue revealed three RNA transcripts (2.8, 2.3, and 1.9 kb) for PDGF-A chain and one RNA transcript (4.0 kb) for PDGF-B chain (101). Western blot analysis and immunohistochemical analysis also revealed that PDGF proteins are present in these tissues and predominantly localized intracellularly in both vascular and myometrial smooth muscle cells (60, 101). Porcine myometrial smooth muscle cells appear to contain a low level of PDGF ß receptors, but following 24–48 h in culture a majority of the cells, and after 1 week all the cells, express the PDGF ß receptor mRNA and contain PDGF ß receptors (108). Using RT-PCR we have demonstrated that leiomyomas and unaffected myometrium from the same patients as well as isolated myometrial smooth muscle cells in primary culture express PDGF-AA, PDGF-BB, and PDGF α and ß receptors mRNA. The myometrial smooth muscle cells also express PDGF-AB, and PDGF ß, but not α, receptors, whereas leiomyomas were reported to contain more PDGF receptor sites than myometrial, but with lower affinity (115). Furthermore, using radioreceptor assay (RRA) and cross-linking experiments we have also demonstrated that myometrial smooth muscle cells contain specific binding sites for [125] I-PDGF-AA, [125] I-PDGF-AB, and [125] I-PDGF-BB with the level of binding sites/cell being highest for PDGF-AB, followed by BB and AA, respectively (Tang XM and Chegini N, unpublished data).

PDGFs have long been recognized to be potent stimuli of connective tissue cell proliferation and migration, such as fibroblasts and smooth muscle cells. PDGF-AB and PDGF-BB are mitogenic for myometrial smooth muscle cells obtained from both phases of the menstrual cycle, and their actions were synergistically enhanced by EGF and IGF-I (60, 61). PDGF either alone or in the presence of EGF and insulin also stimulates the rate of DNA synthesis by myometrial and leiomyomas cells (60, 61, 115). E_2 or P_4 (1 μM) or their combination did not have a significant effect on ^{3}H-thymidine incorporation either alone, or that induced by PDGFs, EGF, or IGF-I (60, 61). Myometrial smooth muscle cell proliferation was significantly stimulated by PDGF-BB in combination with IGF-I, EGF, or IGF + EGF in a time dependent manner (61). A requirement for growth factor interactions to stimulate cell cycle progression is that PDGF act as a competence factor to stimulate quiescent fibroblasts, whereas IGF-I and EGF act as a progression factor in stimulating these cells to progress through the cycle (94, 95). In tissue such as myometrium, which under normal conditions is quiescent, these growth factors may act as differentiation factors; however, in leiomyomas, overexpression and interactions of these growth factors may represent a condition that is ideal for tumor growth. Owing to upregulation of PDGF in myometrium during pregnancy and PDGF stimulation of DNA synthesis by myometrial smooth muscle cells PDGFs may regulate myometrial/leiomyoma cellular hypertrophy that occurs during pregnancy and leiomyomas growth, respectively.

As do TGF-ß, PDGFs regulate their own expression, and through the interactions with other growth factors and cytokines induce cellular proliferation and differentiation and other cellular activities (94). PDGF also stimulates the expression of TGF-ß1 and the mitogenic action of TGF-ß has been suggested to be mediated through the induction of PDGF receptors (65). The mitogenic actions of IL-1ß and IFN-γ have also been shown to be due to the induction of PDGF expression (153, 154). Although regulation of PDGF and PDGF receptors in leiomyomas and myometrium has not been investigated, data generated from other systems suggest that leiomyoma growth is modulated by a delicate balance and interaction of autocrine/paracrine mechanisms involving both positive (PDGFs, EGF/TGF-α, and IGFs) and negative (TGF-ßs) growth regulators.

The Implication of Insulin and Insulin-like Growth Factors

Insulin-like growth factors (IGFs) are polypeptides with insulin-like growth promoting activities that are expressed in a variety of tissues and promote a variety of biologic activities in a number of cell types (95). The biologic actions of IGFs are modulated through the specific and high-affinity cell surface IGF-I and IGF-II receptors and a unique class of proteins that regulate IGF-I availability, the IGF binding proteins (IGFBPs) (95). IGFs are present in circulatory as well as in tissue fluids in association with IGFBPs, which bind IGFs with high affinity (95). Six distinct forms of IGFBPs have been identified and are synthesized and secreted by a variety of cell types (95). In reproductive tract tissues the expression of IGFs, IGF receptors, and IGFBPs mRNA and proteins are well characterized in the ovary and uterus throughout the cycle and pregnancy with substantial data implicating the involvement of ovarian steroids in their regulation (95).

Myometrium and leiomyomas express various components of IGFs and IGFBPs (61, 109–115, 155). In leiomyomas the IGF-I mRNA expression is reported to be most abundant during the late proliferative phase of the menstrual cycle and undetectable during other stages of menstrual cycle. In contrast, the IGF-II expression was not cycle dependent and detectable throughout the menstrual cycle in leiomyomas and myometrium (109). However, IGF-II mRNA expression is reported to be higher in leiomyomas than in myometrium throughout the menstrual cycle (155). Leiomyomas also express IGFBPs mRNA with relative abundance, IGFBP-4 > IGFBP-3 > IGFBP-5 > IGFBP-2, without any menstrual cycle dependency (109). In another study it has been shown that leiomyomas compared to myometrium have a similar relative abundance of IGFBP-2, but IGFBP-1 mRNA was undetectable; however, there was an increase in the relative abundance of IGFBP-3 mRNA in myometrium (110). In addition, the relative abundance of IGBPs mRNA was reported to be similar in leiomyomas and myometrium in GnRHa-treated and untreated groups (155). However, leiomyoma explant cultures secrete more IGF-II than myometrium, without any differences detected between tissues obtained from women who received or did not receive GnRHa therapy (113). IGFBP synthesis has also been studied in explant cultures of leiomyomas and myometrium, with IGFBP-2 reported as being inconclusive and IGFBP-1 not being detectable (109). Despite these inconsistencies studies to date indicate that mRNAs encoding IGF-I, IGF-II, IGFBP-2, and IGFBP-3, as well as their proteins are expressed in both leiomyomas and myometrium (109, 110, 155).

IGF receptor type I and II are also expressed by leiomyomas in a manner independent of the menstrual cycle. The level of IGF-I binding sites in leiomyoma membrane preparations is reported to be higher than in unaffected myometrium (114). IGF-I like EGF is a progression factor for fibroblast proliferation allowing these and other cell types to progress through the G phase of the cell cycle and to synthesize DNA. Although IGF-I has been shown to be mitogenic for leiomyoma smooth muscle cells in primary cell cultures (116), insulin and IGF-I stimulate the rate of DNA synthesis in human myometrial and leiomyoma cells without altering their proliferation (60, 61, 115). The effect of IGF-I is synergistically enhanced through interaction with EGF and PDGFs (60, 61, 115). In addition, components of the ECM may also stimulate the expression of IGF-I (95).

The Role of Epidermal Growth Factor

Epidermal growth factor (EGF) is a member of a family of growth factors that include TGF-α, HB-EGF, ampheregulin, and poxyvirus growth factor (121). They are encoded by separate genes, but the mature forms of their proteins have a substantial sequence homology and are expressed by a variety of tissues and cells, and mediate their biologic activities by binding to a common receptor, the EGF receptor (121). EGF and TGF-α are potent mitogens for a number of cell types of ectodermal, mesodermal, and endodermal origin in vivo and in vitro (121). Other studies have also demonstrated that EGF has an inhibitory effect on cell growth, including human epidermoid carcinoma cells (A 431), which express an unusually high number of EGF receptors (156–160). Although promoting proliferation, EGF inhibits the terminal differentiation of human keratinocytes (121). EGF, in addition to the above properties, stimulates hormone synthesis and secretion, phosphorylation of cellular proteins, changes in cellular morphology, pinocytotic activities, and a variety of other events (161–163).

EGF, TGF-α, and HB-EGF are also expressed in several reproductive tissues including uterus (60, 100–102). Using quantitative RT-PCR with a synthetic internal standard, EGF mRNA was reported to be expressed equally in human myometrium throughout the menstrual cycle (100). Northern blot analysis also revealed a 2.5 kb RNA transcript for HB-EGF in normal myometrium but little or no expression in the corresponding leiomyoma tissue (101). Immunoperoxidase staining showed that HB-EGF was a cell-membrane-associated protein in both normal myometrial and leiomyoma smooth muscle cells with more intense staining in normal myometrium. Furthermore, it has been shown that leiomyomas express a significantly higher level of EGF mRNA than myometrium only in tissues obtained during the luteal phase and its level of expression is significantly reduced in both leiomyomas and unaffected myometrium from women treated with GnRHa (100). Data obtained in our laboratory using a similar approach have confirmed these findings and have further shown a similar reduction in TGF-α and EGF receptor mRNA expression in leiomyomas and myometrium from women who have received GnRHa therapy (164) (Chegini, unpublished data). From these observations it was suggested that progesterone may be a more important hormone in fibroid growth, possibly through the induction of growth factors such as EGF (100). However, EGF has been shown to induce an estrogenic effect in ovariectomized rodent genital tract growth and differentiation, which further indicates that the mitogenic action of steroids in uterine tissue is most likely mediated through the induction of growth factors such as EGF. Furthermore, a number of studies have shown that ovarian steroids regulate the expression of EGF/TGF-α/HB-EGF and EGF receptor in uterine tissue (100). However, the level of EGF binding sites in leiomyoma and myometrial membrane preparation was reported to be similar with respect to the stage of the menstrual cycle and in women treated with GnRHa (104, 105).

The local production of EGF, TGF-α, and HB-EGF, as well as the presence of their receptors in these tissues, implies an autocrine/paracrine role for these peptides in leiomyomas and myometrial biologic processes. Myometrial and leiomyoma smooth muscle cells in culture also express EGF, TGF-α, and EGF receptor (60, 100–102). The primary action of EGF and TGF-α is identified by their ability to induce both DNA synthesis and the proliferation of specific target cells. However, EGF appears to act as a weak mitogen for leiomyomas and myometrium by increasing the rate of DNA synthesis in these cells (60, 115). Myometrial and leiomyoma smooth muscle cells respond similarly to mitogenic action of EGF, and as seen with PDGFs and IGFs require synergistic interaction for maximal activity (60, 115). Because of the importance of the EGF family of growth factors in various cellular activities, detailed investigation is essential to further our understanding of their role in leiomyoma growth.

The Role of Fibroblast Growth Factor

Fibroblast growth factors (FGF) are a family of growth factors comprising at least nine structurally related polypeptides (122). The FGF family includes acidic FGF (aFGF or FGF-1), basic FGF (bFGF or FGF-2), FGF-4, FGF-6, and keratinocyte growth factor (KGF or FGF-7) with a 35% to 55% structural homology (122). The FGFs are expressed by a wide variety of cells and tissues with multiple biologic activities including angiogenesis, through their mitogenic activities for vascular endothelial cells, fibroblasts, and smooth muscle cells. FGF-1 and FGF-2 lack the classic secretory signal peptides implicating cell association; however, they are detected in the ECM with an unknown cellular origin, where they interact with heparan sulfate (122). However, it is not yet clear how FGFs gain access to the ECM compartment in the absence of a classic signal peptide. Although in association with ECM, FGF appears to be incapable of stimulating cell proliferation. FGF-1 was initially found in the extract of brain and pituitary and its expression appears to be restricted to limited tissues, however, FGF-2 has been detected in many cells and tissues including uterus. Northern blot analysis of leiomyoma and myometrial tissue revealed two RNA transcripts (3.7 and 3.5 kb) for bFGF (101). RNase protection assay has shown elevated expression of the bFGF mRNA transcript in leiomyomas. Western blot analysis and immunohistochemistry further revealed that FGF-2 is primarily bound to the ECM of myometrium and fibroids, with leiomyomas showing much stronger staining for FGF-2, possibly due to the large areas of ECM in these tumors (101). It has been suggested that membrane associated urokinase-like plasminogen activator (uPA) plays an important role in releasing bFGF from ECM similar to that shown for TGF-ß (149, 150). Because TGF-ß, but not bFGF, TNF-α, or IL-1ß, stimulates the activity of the uPA, TGF-ß may further amplify the release of growth factors and/or cytokines from the ECM (149).

In addition, the expression of mRNAs for KGF (FGF-7) and its receptor has been evaluated in primate uterine tissues (165), and normal human myometrium and leiomyomas (166). The KGF mRNA expression was detected in the mRNA of myometrial smooth muscle cells and the walls of the spiral arteries, but the degree of expression did not differ with hormonal milieu as demonstrated with the endometrium (165). Although KGF, KGF receptor, and FGF receptor 2 mRNAs were detectable in endometrium, myometrium and leiomyomas express mRNA for KGF and FGF receptor 2, but not for KGF receptor (166). Selective expression of KGF receptor and closely related FGF receptor-2 occurs in the human uterus, with the latter being expressed predominantly in myometrium. FGF-2 has been shown to stimulate the rate of DNA synthesis in both myometrial and leiomyoma smooth muscle cells, with leiomyoma cells showing less responsiveness to FGF than matched myometrial cells (167). In addition, estradiol is reported not to interact synergistically with FGF in these cells. In addition to FGFs, four species of mRNA encoding vascular endothelial growth factor (VEGF) have also been identified in human endometrium and myometrium (168). In situ hybridization of mRNA encoding VEGF was not restricted to uterine vascular smooth muscle but was present in other cell types, however, expression in leiomyomas awaits investigation (168). Because of the importance of FGFs and VEGF as potent angiogenic factors, these growth factors may influence the initial vascularization of leiomyomas. Despite the inconsistency in the level of their expression and content of their receptors, the growing list of growth factors and cytokines in leiomyoma suggests that through an autocrine or paracrine mechanism, they regulate various aspects of leiomyoma biologic activity.

Other Polypeptide Factors

Recently a major mitogen for smooth muscle cell and fibroblast cell lines was isolated from leiomyoma extracts. Partial amino acid sequencing of these 18 kDa leiomyoma derived mitogen protein led to its identification as human cysteine-rich protein. The levels of expression of this protein were reported to be three to six times higher in leiomyomas than in myometrium; however, the protein is not mitogenic for leiomyoma smooth muscle cells despite its mitogenic activity on KW human uterine smooth muscle-like cells and NIH/3T3 fibroblast cells (169).

Several other polypeptide hormones including prolactin, growth hormone, relaxin, and parathyroid hormone-like peptide have been shown to be produced by leiomyomas and myometrial tissues (6, 170–175). It has been shown that leiomyomas and myometrium express prolactin with levels reported to be in excess of serum concentrations (170). However, unlike human endometrial and decidual tissues in which progesterone stimulates prolactin expression, leiomyoma and myometrial explant culture prolactin production is inhibited by progesterone (6, 170). In addition the explant cultures of leiomyomas and myometrium from women who have received GnRH-a therapy release significantly lower levels of prolactin compared to untreated controls (172). These data implicate ovarian steroids in regulating prolactin production by leiomyomas and myometrium. Furthermore, human chorionic gonadotropin (hCG) or the α subunit of hCG significantly stimulates prolactin production by these explant cultures compared to untreated and hCG-treated myometrium (172). The action of hCG in leiomyomas and myometrium is mediated through the presence of specific hCG receptors that are present in both leiomyomas and myometrium (176). Leiomyomas and myometrium have been reported to produce growth hormone and contain growth hormone receptors (6, 173). The significance of these findings are unknown; however, they are considered to influence uterine weight either alone or in synergistic interaction with estrogen (6).

Relaxin is a peptide hormone of about 6 kDa with similar structure to insulin (174). Although corpus luteum is the major site of relaxin production, relaxin has been shown to be expressed in several other reproductive tissues including uterus, which is known to be the primary target tissue for its action (174). Both myometrial and leiomyomas have been shown to contain relaxin binding sites; however, leiomyomas appear to have a higher capacity to bind relaxin than myometrium (6, 174). Previous studies have shown that relaxin binds to myometrial smooth muscle cells, with the assumption that the physiological response is to inhibit uterine muscle contraction. In addition, relaxin has been shown to inhibit proliferation, but not differentiation, of 3T3-L1 cells in culture (174). We have previously demonstrated that ^{125}I-human relaxin with two classes of specific binding sites binds with human myometrial smooth muscle cells that were undetectable in endometrial stromal cells (177). Insulin, IGF-I, and EGF did not compete with relaxin binding sites. The addition of either porcine or synthetic human relaxin to quiescent endometrial stromal and myometrial smooth muscle cells had no significant effect on the rate of ^{3}H-thymidine incorporation into these cells (177). However, in a dose-dependent manner relaxin inhibited the stimulatory action of EGF on DNA synthesis by the smooth muscle cells, but not stromal cells. Regardless of treatment, the cells did not initiate mitosis (177).

We have demonstrated that relaxin either alone or through interaction with TGF-ß1 modulates the expression of various extracellular matrix components in human myometrial smooth muscle cells as well as endometrial glandular and stromal cells in vitro (136). Northern blot analysis indicates that these cells express pro α1 collagen, collagenase, TIMP-1, fibronectin, and TGF-ß1 mRNA. Treatment with TGF-ß1, human recombinant relaxin, or TGF-ß1 + relaxin increased the level of pro α1 collagen transcripts compared to the control (136). However, the expression of collagenase in myometrial smooth muscle cells was downregulated by both relaxin and TGF-ß1, but not TGF-ß1 + relaxin as compared to the control. In addition, TIMP-1 and fibronectin expression was upregulated by TGF-ß1, relaxin, and their combination, whereas TGF-β1 upregulated its own expression, but it was downregulated by relaxin. Another polypeptide that is expressed in leiomyomas and myometrium is parathyroid hormone-related peptide with elevated levels reported in leiomyomas compared to myometrium, particularly during the proliferative phase of the menstrual cycle (175). TGF-ß1 has also been shown to induce the production of parathyroid hormone-related peptide (178), which is considered to be important in cellular calcium flux and in tissue remodeling (6). These data suggest that the interaction between relaxin, parathyroid hormone-related peptide, and TGF-ß1 results in modulation of ECM turnover, which is essential for structural modification of myometrial cells and leiomyomas during growth and regression.

PROSPECTIVE

Although many leiomyomas are asymptomatic and <1% become malignant, the presence of these tumors causes substantial morbidity, usually in the form of chronic pelvic pain and abnormal uterine bleeding. Because of their sensitivity to ovarian steroid actions the current medical interventions to relieve the symptoms and/or regress their growth center around the use of progestin, GnRHa, or antiprogestin therapies. These therapies are expensive and associated with various side effects, and many affected patients end up requiring a hysterectomy after conservative medical therapy that is either poorly tolerated or ineffective. Hysterectomies are among the most common operations performed in the United States of which a third are due to leiomyomas. It is perhaps paradoxical that so little is known about the biology of a tumor that is associated with such high cost and morbidity.

What initiates the conversion of normal myometrial smooth muscle cells into leiomyomas is unknown. A combination of mitotic activity, cellular hypertrophy, and ECM accumulation contributes to leiomyoma growth, but the relative contribution of these is poorly defined. Our knowledge regarding the contribution of ECM components in leiomyomas is limited to only a few studies, and is nonexistent on cellular hypertrophy. In addition to ovarian steroid action, it is clear that various autocrine and paracrine growth factors may influence leiomyoma growth. Our current understanding of cytokine expression in leiomyomas is limited, but it should not be surprising to find the expression of many cytokines in these tumors. Whether any of these growth factors and cytokines participate in the initial conversion of myometrial smooth muscle cells into leiomyoma is difficult to establish, however, it is certain that they are involved in leiomyoma growth. These growth factors and cytokines are critical in cellular transformation, movement, growth, differentiation, metabolic homeostasis, cellular hypertrophy, and expression of various components of ECM and adhesion molecules in various normal and tumor cells. Among these growth factors so far examined, the level of their expression in leiomyomas is not explicitly different from those in adjacent myometrium, which is a quiescent tissue. This difference may lie in their intracellular signaling pathways, which are commonly shared to promote various cellular activities. However, how this signaling leads to cell proliferation versus cell differentiation in tumors such as leiomyomas is not known. Therefore, to elucidate the role of growth factors and cytokines in leiomyoma it is essential to understand the molecular and cell biology surrounding changes in normal myometrium during the menstrual cycle.

The mechanism of RU-486 therapy-induced uterine blood flow and uterine/leiomyomas volume reduction requires investigation at the molecular level. From an endocrinologic standpoint, the reduction in uterine blood flow and volume cannot be explained by decreased levels of ovarian estrogens as seen with GnRHa therapy, because the hormonal milieu to which the uterus is exposed when a low dose of RU-486 is used is of unopposed estrogen, which argues against a hypoestrogenic effect of RU-486. It is of major interest to define the effects of antiprogestin in vivo on the expression of growth factors and cytokines in leiomyomas and in vitro on their isolated cell types. In this regard lessons learned from the effects of progestins and antiprogestins in breast and other estrogen-sensitive tumors may be applied to studies of leiomyoma. Furthermore, the potential direct action of GnRHa in leiomyomas should be further explored, in particular the effect of growth factors and cytokine expression. Because of leiomyoma's fibrotic nature it is essential to examine further the effect of antiprogestin and antiestrogen on ECM turnover, which is critical in leiomyoma growth and regression and is regulated by a balance between ECM deposition and differential expression of MMPs and TIMPs. Thus the expression, interaction, and cross-talk between their signaling pathways may collectively determine the importance of growth factors and cytokines in leiomyoma growth.

REFERENCES

1. Wilcox LS, Koonin LM, Pokras R, et al. Hysterectomy in the United States, 1988–1990. Obstet Gynecol 1994;83:549–555.

2. Buttram VC, Reiter RC. Uterine leiomyomata: Etiology, symptomatology and management. Fertil Steril 1981;36:433–445.

3. Vollenhoven BJ, Lawrence AS, Healy DL. Uterine fibroids: a clinical review. Br J Obstet Gynecol 1990;97:258–298.

4. Scully RE. Pathology of leiomyomas. Semin Reprod Endocrinol 1992;10:325–331

5. Cramer SF, Patel A. The frequency of uterine leiomyomas. Am J Clin Pathol 1990;94:435–438.

6. Anderson J. Growth factors and cytokines in uterine leiomyomas. Semin Reprod Endocrinol 1996;14:269–282.

7. Rotmensch J, Bosnyak S, Montag A. Malignant transition of uterine leiomyomata. Int Gynecol Obstet 1992;42:47–49.

8. Pandis N, Heim S, Bardi G, et al. Chromosome analysis of 96 uterine leiomyomas. Cancer Genet Cytogenet 1991;55:11–18.

9. McKusick VA. Mendelian inheritance. In: Man: Catalogs of Autosomal Recessive and X-linked Phenotypes. 9th ed. Baltimore: The Johns Hopkins University Press, 1990.

10. Meloni AM, Surti U, Contento AM, et al. Uterine leiomyomas: Cytogenetic and histologic profile. Obstet Gynecol 1992;80:209–217.

11. Nibert M, Heim S. Uterine leiomyoma cytogenetics. Genes Chromosomes Cancer 1990;2:3–13.

12. Han K, Lee W, Harris CP, et al. Comparison of chromosome aberrations in leiomyoma and leiomyosarcoma using FISH on archival tissues. Cancer Genet Cytogenet 1994;74:19–24.

13. Rein MS, Barbieri RL, Friedman AJ. Progesterone: a critical role in the pathogenesis of uterine myomas. Am J Obstet Gynecol 1995;172:14–18.

14. Chrapusta S, Sieinski W, Konopka B, et al. Estrogen and progestin receptor levels in uterine leiomyomata: relation to the tumor histology and the phase of menstrual cycle. Eur J Gynecol Oncol 1990;11:381–387.

15. Chrapusta S, Konopka B, Paszko Z, et al. Immunoreactive and estrogen-binding estrogen receptors, and progestin receptor levels in uterine leiomyomata and their parental myometrium. Eur J Gynecol Oncol 1990;11:275–281.

16. Nardelli GB, Mega M, Bertasi M, et al. Estradiol and progesterone binding in uterine leiomyomata and pregnant myometrium. Clin Exp Obstet Gynecol 1987;14:155–160.

17. Brandon DD, Erickson TE, Keenan EJ, et al. Estrogen receptor gene expression in human uterine leiomyomata. Clin Endocrinol 1995;80:1876–1881.

18. Howe SR, Gottardis MM, Everitt JI, et al. Estrogen stimulation and tamoxifen inhibition of leiomyoma cell growth in vitro and in vivo. Endocrinology 1994;136:4996–5003.

19. Howe SR, Gottardis MM, Everitt JI, et al. Rodent model of reproductive tract leiomyomata. Establishment and characterization of tumor-derived cell lines. Am J Pathol 1995;146:1568–1579.

20. Gibson JP, Sells DM, Cheng HC, et al. Induction of uterine leiomyomas in mice by medroxalol and prevention by propranolol. Toxicol Pathol 1987;4:468–473.

21. Porter KB, Tsibris JC, Nicosia SV, et al. Estrogen-induced guinea pig model for uterine leiomyomas: do the ovaries protect? Biol Reprod 1995;52:824–832.

22. Romagnolo B, Molina T, Leroy G, et al. Estradiol-dependent uterine leiomyomas in transgenic mice. J Clin Invest 1996;98:777–784.

23. Bulum SE, Simpson ER, Word RA, et al. Expression of the CYP19 gene and its products aromatase cytochrome P450 in human uterine leiomyoma tissues and cells in culture. J Clin Endocrinol Metab 1994;78:736–743.

24. Brandon DD, Bethers CL, Strawn ET, et al. Progesterone receptor messenger ribonucleic acid and protein are overexpressed in human uterine leiomyomas. Am Obstet Gynecol 1993;169:78–85.

25. Stewart EA, Austin DJ, Jain P, et al. RU486 suppresses prolactin production in explant cultures of leiomyoma and myometrium. Fertil Steril 1996;65:1119–1124.

26. Fujimoto J, Ichigo S, Hori M, et al. Expression of progesterone receptor form A and B mRNAs in gynecologic malignant tumors. Tumor Biol 1995;16:254–260.

27. Vegeto E, Shahbaz MM, Wen DX-G, et al. Human progesterone receptor A form is a cell- and promoter-specific repressor of progesterone receptor B function. Mol Endocrinol 1993;7:1244–1255.

28. Carr BR, Marshburn PB, Weatherall PT, et al. An evaluation of the effect of gonadotropin-releasing hormone analogs and medroxyprogesterone acetate on uterine leiomyomata volume by magnetic resonance imaging: a prospective, randomized, double blind, placebo-controlled, crossover trial. J Clin Endocrinol Metab 1993;76:1217–1223.

29. Harrison-Woolrych M, Robinson R. Fibroid growth in response to high-dose progestogen. Fertil Steril 1995;64:191–192.

30. Zhao K, Kuperman L, Geimonen E, et al. Progestin represses human connexin 43 gene expression similarly in primary cultures of myometrial and uterine leiomyomas. Biol Reprod 1996;54:607–615.

31. Andersen J, DyReyes V, Barbieri RL, et al. Leiomyoma primary cultures have elevated transcriptional response to estrogen compared to autologous myometrial cultures. Soc Gynecol Invest 1995;2:542–551.

32. Rutgers JL, Spong CY, Sinow R, et al. Leuprolide acetate treatment and myoma arterial size. Obstet Gynecol 1995;86:386–388.

33. Friedman AJ. Treatment of uterine myomas with GnRH agonists. Semin Reprod Endocrinol 1993;11:154–161.

34. Rein MS, Friedman AJ, Stuart JM, et al. Fibroid and myometrial steroid receptors in women treated with gonadotropin-releasing hormone agonist leuprolide acetate. Fertil Steril 1990;53:1018–1023.

35. Pasqualini JR, Cornier E, Grenier J, et al. Effect of Decapeptyl, an agonistic analog of gonadotropin-releasing hormone on estrogens, estrogen sulfates, and progesterone receptors in leiomyoma and myometrium. Fertil Steril 1990;53:1012–1017.

36. Lumsden MA, West CP, Hawkins RA, et al. The binding of steroids to myometrium and leiomyomata (fibroids) in women treated with the gonadotrophin-releasing hormone agonist Zoladex (ICI 118630). J Endocrinol 1989;121:389–396.

37. Friedman AJ, Daly M, Juneau-Norcross M, et al. A Prospective, randomized trial of gonadotropin-releasing hormone agonist plus estrogen-progestin or progestin "add-back" regimens for women with leiomyomata uteri. J Clin Endocrinol Metab 1993;76:1439–1445.

38. Reinsch RC, Murphy AA, Morales AJ, et al. The effects of RU486 and leuprolide acetate on uterine artery blood flow in the fibroid uterus: A Prospective, randomized study. Am J Obstet Gynecol 1994;170:1623–1628.

39. Murphy AA, Morales AJ, Kettel LM, et al. Regression of uterine leiomyomata to the antiprogesterone RU486: Dose-response effect. Fertil Steril 1995;64:187–190.

40. Horwitz KB, Tung L, Takimoto GS. Novel mechanisms of antiprogestin action. J Steroid Biochem Mol Biol 1995;53: 9–17.

41. Wiznitzer A, Marbach M, Hazum E, et al. Gonadotropin-releasing hormone specific binding sites in uterine leiomyomata. Biochem Biophys Res Commun 1988;152:1326–1331.

42. Emons G, Schroder B, Ortmann O, et al. High affinity binding and direct antiproliferative effects of luteinizing hormone-releasing hormone analogs in human endometrial cancer cell lines. J Clin Endocrinol Metab 1993;77:1458–1464.

43. Fiorelli G, De Bellis A, Longo A, et al. Insulin-like growth factor-I receptors in human hyperplastic prostate tissue: Characterization, tissue localization, and their modulation by chronic treatment with a gonadotropin-releasing hormone analog. J Clin Endocrinol Metab 1991;72:740–746.

44. Emanuele NV, Emanuele MA, Tentler J, et al. Rat spleen lymphocytes contain an immunoactive and bioactive luteinizing hormone-releasing hormone. Endocrinology 1990;126:2482–2486.

45. Pati D, Habibi HR. Inhibition of human hepatocarcinoma cell proliferation by mammalian and fish gonadotropin-releasing hormones. Endocrinology 1995;136:75–84.

46. Thompson MA, Adelson MD, Kaufman LM. Lupron retards proliferation of ovarian epithelial tumor cells cultured in serum-free medium. J Clin Endocrinol Metab 1991;72:1036–1041.

47. Kleinman D, Roberts CT Jr, LeRoith D, et al. Regulation of endometrial cancer cell growth by insulin-like growth factors and the luteinizing hormone-releasing hormone antagonist SB-75. Regul Pept 1993;48:91–98.

48. Gorden JD, Polan ML. The use of GnRH agonists in breast and gynecologic cancers. Semin Reprod Endocrinol 1993;11:187–194.

49. Harris N, Dutlow C, Eidne E, et al. Gonadotropin-releasing hormone gene expression in MDA-MB-231 and ZR-75-1 breast carcinoma cell lines. Cancer Research 1991;51:2577–2581.

50. Minaretzis D, Jakubowski M, Mortola JF, et al. Gonadotropin-releasing hormone receptor gene expression in human ovary and granulosa-lutein cells. J Clin Endocrinol Metab 1995;80:430–434.

51. Fraser HM, Bramley TA, Miller WR, et al. Extra pituitary actions of LHRH analoguses in tissues of human female and investigation of the existence and function of LHRH-like peptides. Prog Clin Biol Res 1986;22:29–54.

52. Kendall JZ, Mathias JR, Van Hook JW. Leuprolide acetate stimulates smooth muscle of human reproductive tract. Fertil Steril 1991;56:993–995.

53. Chegini N, Rong H, Dou Q, et al. The direct action of gonadotropin-releasing hormone analogues on myometrial smooth muscle cells and their interaction with ovarian steroids. J Clin Endocrinol Metabol 1996;81:3215–3221.

54. Hartz PH. Proliferation of muscle cells in the myometrium of the nonpregnant uterus. Arch Pathol 1945;39:323.

55. Kawaguchi K, Fujii S, Konishi I, et al. Ultrastructural study of cultured smooth muscle cells from uterine leiomyoma and myometrium under the influence of sex steroids. Gynecol Oncol 1985;21:32–41.

56. Kawaguchi K, Fujii S, Konishi I, et al. Mitotic activity in uterine leiomyomas during the menstrual cycle. Am J Obstet Gynecol 1989;160:637–641.

57. Cramer SF, Robertson AL, Ziats NP, et al. Growth potential of human uterine leiomyomas: some in vitro observations and their implications. Obstet Gynecol 1985;66:36–41.

58. Cramer SF, Meyer JS, Kraner JF, et al. Metastasizing leiomyomata of the uterus- S phase fraction, estrogen receptor, and ultrastructure. Cancer 1980;45:932–937.

59. Tiltman A. The effect of progestins on the mitotic activity of uterine fibromyomas. Int Gynecol Pathol 1985;4:89–96.

60. Rossi MJ, Chegini N, Masterson BJ. Presence of epidermal growth factor, platelet-derived growth factor and their receptors in human myometrial tissue and smooth muscle cells:Their action in smooth muscle cells *in vitro*. Endocrinology 1992;130:1716–1727.

61. Tang X-M, Rossi MJ, Masterson BJ, et al. Insulin-like growth factor I (IGF-I), IGF-I receptors and IGF binding proteins 1-4 in human uterine tissue: tissue localization and IGF-I action in endometrial stromal and myometrial smooth muscle cells *in vitro*. Biol Reprod 1994;50:1113–1125.

62. Chen L, Lindner HR, Lancet M. Mitogenic action of oestradiol-17ß on human myometrial and endometrial cells in long-term tissue cultures. J Endocrinol 1973;59:87–97.

63. Upadhyaya NB, Doody MC, Googe PB. Histological changes in leiomyomata treated with leuprolide acetate. Fertil Steril 1990;54:811–814.

64. Honore LH. Menorrhagia, diffuse myometrial hypertrophy, and the intrauterine contraceptive device: A report of fourteen cases. Acta Obstet Gynecol Scand 1979;58:283–285.

65. Puistola U, Ristili L, Ristili J, et al. Collagen metabolism in gynecologic patients: changes in the concentration of the aminoterminal propeptide of type III procollagen in serum. Am J Obstet Gynecol 1990;163:1276–1281.

66. Stewart EA, Friedman AJ, Peck K, et al. Relative overexpression of collagen type I and collagen type III messenger ribonucleic acids by uterine leiomyomas during the proliferative phase of the menstrual cycle. J Clin Endocrinol Metab 1994;79:900–906.

67. Engel J. Common structural motifs in proteins of the extracellular matrix. Curr Opin Cell Biol 1991;3:779–785.

68. Fukai N, Apte SS, Olsen BR. Nonfibrillar collagens: In; Extracellular matrix components. Ruoslahti E, Engvall, E., eds., San Diego, CA: Academic Press, 1994:3–28.

69. Hay ED. Collagen and other matrix glycoproteins in embryogenesis. In: Hay ED, ed. Cell Biology of the Extracellular Matrix. New York: Plenum Press, 1991:419–462.

70. Lin CQ, Bissell MJ. Multi-faceted regulation of cell differentiation by extracellular matrix, FASEB J. 1993;7:737–743.

71. Juliano RI, Haskill S. Signal transduction from the extracellular matrix. J Cell Biol 1992;120:577–589.

72. Taylor CV, Letarte M, Lye SJ. The expression of integrins and cadherins in normal human uterus and uterine leiomyomas. Am J Obstet Gynecol 1996;175:411–419.

73. Hynes RO. Fibronectins. New York: Springer-Verlag, 1990.

74. Brown LF, Dubin D, Lavigne L, et al. Macrophages and fibroblasts express "embryonic" fibronectins during cutaneous wound healing. Am J Pathol 1993;142:793–801.

75. McDonald JA, Quade BJ, Broekelmann TJ, et al. Fibronectin's cell-adhesive domain and an amino-terminal matrix assembly domain participate in the assembly into fibroblast pericellular matrix. J Biol Chem 1987;262:2957–2967.

76. Mosher DE, Sottile J, Wu C, et al. Assembly of extracellular matrix. Curr Opin Cell Biol 1992;4:810–818.

77. Somers CE, Mosher DF. Protein kinase C modulation of fibronectin matrix assembly, J Biol Chem 1993;268:22277–22280.

78. Werb Z, Tremble P, Damsky CH. Regulation of extracellular matrix degradation by cell—extracellular matrix interactions. Cell Differ Dev 1990;32:299–306.

79. Zhang Z, Morla AO, Vuori K, et al. The αvß1 integrin functions as a fibronectin receptor but does not support fibronectin matrix assembly and cell migration on fibronectin. J Cell Biol 1993;122:235–242.

80. Xu J, Clark RAF. Extracellular matrix alters PDGF regulation of fibroblast integrins. J Cell Biol 1996;132:239–249.

81. Werb Z, Tremble PM, Behrendtsen O, et al. Signal transduction through the fibronectin receptor induces collagenase and stromelysin gene expression, J Cell Biol 1989;109:877–889.

82. Huhtala P, Humphries MJ, McCarthy, et al. 1995, α4ß1 and α5ß1 play differential roles in metalloproteinase induction. J Cell Biol 1995;129:867–879.

83. Wight TN, Heinegard D K, Hascall VC. Proteoglycans: structure and function. In: Hay ED, ed. Cell Biology of Extracellular Matrix. New York: Plenum Press, 1991:45–78.

84. Yamagata M, Saga S, Kato M, et al. Selective distributions of proteoglycans and their ligands in pericellular matrix of cultured fibroblasts. Implications for their roles in cell-substratum adhesion, J Cell Sci 1993;106:55–65.

85. Toole BP. Protoglycans and hyaluronan in morphogenesis and differentiation. In: Hay, ED, ed., Cell Biology of the Extracellular Matrix. New York: Plenum Press, 305–341.

86. Yamaguchi T, Mann DM, Ruoslahti E. Negative regulation of transforming growth factors by the proteoglycan decorin, Nature 1990;346:281–284.

87. Castellot JJ, Addonizio ML, Rosenberg R, et al. Vascular endothelial cells produce a heparin-like inhibitor of smooth muscle growth. J Cell Biol 1981;90:372–379.

88. Guimond S, Maccarana M, Olwin BB, et al. Activating and inhibitory heparin sequences for FGF-2 (basic FGF): Distinct requirements for FGF-1, FGF-2 and FGF-4. J Biol Chem 1993;268:23906–23914.

89. Yayon A, Klagsbrun M, Esko JD, et al. Cell surface, heparin-like molecules are required for binding of basic fibroblast growth factor to its high affinity receptor, Cell 1991;64:841–848.

90. Reich-Slotky R, Bonneh-Barkay D, Shaoul E, et al. Differential effect of cell-associated heparan sulfates on the binding of keratinocyte growth factor (KGF) and acidic fibroblast growth factor to the KGH receptor. J Biol Chem 1994;269:32279–32285.

91. Gitay-Goren H, Soker S, Viodavsky I, et al. The binding of vascular endothelial growth factor to its receptors is dependent on cell surface-associated heparin-like molecules. J Biol Chem 1992;267:6093–6098.

92. McCaffrey TA, Falconed DJ, Dud B. Transforming growth factor-ß1 is a heparin-binding protein: Identification of putative heparin-binding regions and isolation of heparins with varying affinity for TGF-ß1. J Cell Physiol 1992;152:430–440.

93. Roberts AR. Transforming growth factor ß: activity and efficacy in animal models of wound healing. Wound Rep Reg 1995;3:408–418.

94. Westermark B. The molecular and cellular biology of platelet-derived growth factor. Acta Endocrinol (Copenh) 1990;123:131–142.

95. Jones J, Clemmons D. Insulin-like growth factors and their binding proteins, biological actions. Endocrine Rev 1994;16:3–34.

96. Baserga R. Growth in cell size and DNA synthesis. Exp Cell Res 1984;151:1–5.

97. Geisterfer A, Peach MJ, Owens GK. Angiotensin II induces hypertrophy, not hyperplasia of cultured rat aortic smooth muscle cells. Circ Res 1988;62:749–756.

98. Turner JD, Rotwein P, Novakofski J, et al. Induction of mRNA for IGF-I and II during hormone stimulation of muscle hypertrophy. Am J Physiol 1988;255:513–517.

99. Owens GK, Geisterfer AAT, Yang YW-H, et al. Transforming growth factor-ß-induced growth inhibition and cellular hypertrophy in cultured vascular smooth muscle cells. J Cell Biol 1988;107:771–780.

100. Harrison-Woolrych ML, Charnock-Jones DS, Smith SK. Quantification of messenger ribonucleic acid for epidermal growth factor in human myometrium and leiomyomata using reverse transcription polymerase chain reaction. J Clin Endocrinol Metab 1994;78:1179–1184.

101. Mangrulkar RS, Ono M, Ishikawa M, et al. Isolation and characterization of heparin-binding growth factors in human leiomyomas and normal myometrium. Biol Reprod 1995;53:636–646.

102. Yeh J, Rein M, Nowak R. Presence of messenger ribonucleic acid for EGF and EGF receptor demonstrable in monolayer cell cultures of myometrial and leiomyomata. Fertil Steril 1991;56:997–1000.

103. Chegini N, Rao ChV, Wakim N, et al. Binding of ^{125}I-epidermal growth factor in human uterus. Cell Tissue Res 1986;246:543–548.

104. Hoffmann GE, Rao ChV, Barrows GH, et al. Binding sites for epidermal growth factor in human uterine tissues and leiomyomas. J Clin Endocrinol Metab 1984;58:880–884.

105. Tommola P, Pekonen F, Rutanen EM. Binding of epidermal growth factor and insulin-like growth factor I in human myometrium and leiomyomata. Obstet Gynecol 1989;74:658–662.

106. Lumdsden MA, West CP, Bramley TA, et al. The binding of epidermal growth factor to the human uterus and leiomyomata in women rendered hypoestrogenic by continuous administration of an LhRH agonist. Br J Obstet Gynecol 1988;95:1299–1306.

107. Boehm KD, Daimon M, Gorodeski IF, et al. Expression of the insulin-like and platelet-derived growth factor genes in human uterine tissues. Mol Reprod Dev 1990;27:93–101.

108. Terracio L, Ronnstrand L, Tingstrom A, et al. Induction of platelet-derived growth factor receptor expression in smooth muscle cells and fibroblasts upon tissue culturing. J Cell Biol 1988;107:1947–1957.

109. Giudice LC, Irwin JC, Dsupin BA, et al. Insulin-like growth factor (IGF), IGF binding protein (IGFBP), and IGF receptor gene expression and IGFBP synthesis in human uterine leiomyomata. Human Reprod 1993;8:1796–1806.

110. Vollenhoven Bj, Herrington AC, Healy DL. Messenger ribonucleic acid expression of the insulin-like growth factors and their binding proteins in uterine fibroids and myometrium. J Clin Endocrinol Metab 1993;76:1106–1110.

111. Gloudemans T, Prinsen I, Van Unnik JA, et al. Insulin-like growth factor gene expression in human smooth muscle tumors. Cancer Res 1990;50:6689–6695.

112. Hoppener JW, Mosselman S, Roholl PJ, et al. Expression of insulin-like growth factor-I and -II genes in human smooth muscle tumors. EMBO J 1988;7:1379–1385.

113. Rein MS, Friedman AJ, Pandian MR, et al. The secretion of insulin-like growth factors I and II by explant cultures of fibroids and myometrium from women treated with a gonadotropin-releasing hormone agonist. Obstet Gynecol 1990;76:388–394.

114. Chandrasekhar Y, Heimer J, Osuamkpe C, et al. Insulin-like growth factor I and II binding in human myometrium and leiomyomas. Am J Obstet Gynecol 1992;166:64–69.

115. Fayed YM, Tsibsis JCM, Langenberg PW, et al. Human uterine leiomyoma cells: binding and growth responses to EGF, platelet-derived growth factor, and insulin. Lab Invest 1989;60:30–37.

116. Strawn EY Jr, Novy MJ, Burry KA, et al. Insulin-like growth factor I promotes leiomyoma cell growth in vitro. Am J Obstet Gynecol 1995;172:1837–1844.

117. Chegini N, Zhao Y, Williams RS, et al. Human uterine tissue throughout the menstrual cycle expresses TGF-ß1, TGF-ß2, TGF-ß3 and TGF-ß type II receptor mRNAs and proteins and contain ^{125}I-TGF-ß1 binding sites. Endocrinology 1994;135:439–449.

118. Vollenhoven BJ, Herington AC, Healy DL. Epidermal growth factor and transforming growth factor-beta in uterine fibroids and myometrium. Gynecol Obstet Invest 1995;40:120–124.

119. Dou Q, Zhao Y, Tarnuzzer WR, et al. Suppression of TGF-ßs and TGF-ß receptors mRNA and protein expression in leiomyomata in women receiving gonadotropin releasing hormone agonist therapy. J Clin Endocrinol Metabol 1996;81:3222–3230.

120. Tang X-M, Dou Q, Zhao Y, et al. The expression of transforming growth factor-ß (TGF-ßs) and TGF-ß receptors mRNA and protein and the effect of TGF-ßs on human myometrial smooth muscle cells *in vitro*. Mol Human Reprod 1997;3:233–240.

121. Yates RA, Nanney LB, Gates RE et al. Epidermal growth factor and related growth factors. Int J Dermatol 1991;30:687–694.

122. Klagsbrun M. The fibroblast growth factor family: structural and biological properties. Prog Growth Factor Res 1990;1:207–235

123. Higashiyama S, Abraham JA, Klagsbrun M. Heparin-binding EGF-like growth factor synthesis by smooth muscle cells. Horm Res 1994;42:9–13.

124. Massague J. The transfórming growth factor-ß family. Ann Rev Cell Biol 1990;6:597–641.

125. Border WA, Noble NA. Transforming growth factor ß in tissue fibrosis. New Engl J Med 1994;331:1286–1292.

126. Massague J. Receptors for the TGF-ß family. Cell 1992;69:1067–1070.

127. Lin HY, Wang XF, Ng-Eaton E, et al. Expression cloning of the TGF-ß type II receptor, a functional transmembrane serine/threonine kinase. Cell 1992;68:775–785

128. Ebner R, Chen R, Shum L, et al. Cloning of a type I TGF-ß receptor and its effect on TGF-ß binding to the type II receptor. Science 1993;260:1344–1347.

129. Bassing CH, Yingling JM, Howe DJ, et al. A transforming growth factor ß type I receptor that signals to activate gene expression. Science 1994;263:87–89.

130. ten Dijke P, Yamashita H, Ichijo H, et al. Characterization of type I receptors for transforming growth factor-ß and activin. Science 1994;264:101–104.

131. Wrana JL, Attisano L, Wieser R, et al. Mechanism of activation of the TGF-ß receptor. Nature 1994;370:341–347.

132. Chegini N. The role of growth factors in peritoneal healing. Transforming growth factor ß (TGF-ß). Eur J Surg 1997; (Suppl. 577):163:17–23.

133. Matrisian LM. Matrix metalloproteinases gene expression. In: Greenwald RA, Goublm LM, eds. Inhibition of matrix metalloproteinases: therapeutic potential. Ann NY Acad Sci 1994;732:42–50.

134. Overall CM. Regulation of tissue inhibitor of matrix metalloproteins expression. In: Greenwald RA, Goublm LM, eds. Inhibition of matrix metalloproteinases: Therapeutic potential. Ann NY Acad Sci 1994;732:51–64.

135. Hulboy DL, Rudolph LA, Matrisian LM. Matrix metalloproteinases as mediators of reproductive function. Mol Human Reprod 1997;3:27–45.

136. Tang XM, Ghahary A, Chegini N. The interaction between transforming growth factor ß and relaxin leads to modulation of matrix and matrix metalloproteinases expression in human uterus. J Soc Gynecol Invest 1996;3: Abstract No. 205.

137. Dou Q, Tarnuzzer WR, Williams RS, et al. Differential expression of matrix metalloproteinases and their tissue inhibitors in leiomyomas: A mechanism for gonadotropin releasing hormone agonist-induced tumor regression. Mol Human Reprod 1997;3:1005–1014.

138. Rodgers WH, Matrisian L, Guidice LC, et al. Pattern of matrix metalloproteinase expression in cycling endometrium imply differential functions and regulation by steroid hormones. J Clin Invest 1994;94:946–953.

139. Sato T, Ito A, Mori Y, et al. Hormonal regulation of collagenolysis in uterine cervical fibroblasts. Biochem J 1991;275:645–650.

140. Appling WD, O'Brien WR, Johnston DA, et al. Synergistic enhancement of type I and III collagen production in cultured fibroblasts by transforming growth factor beta and ascorbate. FEBS Lett. 1989;250:541–544.

141. Fine A, Goldstein RH. The effect of transforming growth factor beta on cell proliferation and collagen formation by lung fibroblast. J Biol Chem 1987;262:3897–3902.

142. Fine A, Poliks CF, Smith BD, et al. The accumulation of type I collagen mRNAs in human embryonic lung fibroblast stimulated by transforming growth factor beta. Connect Tissue Res 1990;24:237–247.

143. Raghow R, Postlethwaite AE, Keskioj, et al. Transforming growth factor ß increases the steady state levels of type I procollagen and fibronectin messenger RNAs postranscriptionally in cultured human dermal fibroblasts. J Clin Invest 1987;79:1285–1288.

144. Inagaki Y, Truter S, Ramirez F. Transforming growth factor-beta stimulates alpha 2 (I) collagen gene expression through a cis-acting element that contains an Sp1-binding site. J Biol Chem 1994;269:14828–14834.

145. Rossi P, Krsenty G, Roberts AB, et al. A nuclear factor I binding site mediates the transcriptional activation of type I collagen promoter by transforming growth factor ß. Cell 1988;52:405–414.

146. Circolo A, Welgus HG, Pierce GF, et al. Differential regulation of the expression of proteinases/antiproteinases in fibroblasts. Effects of interleukin-1 and platelet-derived growth factor. J Biol Chem 1991;266:12283–12288.

147. Ito A, Goshowaki H, Sato T, et al. Human recombinant interleukin 1α-mediated stimulation of procollagenase production and suppression of biosynthesis of tissue inhibitor of metalloproteinases in rabbit uterine cervical fibroblasts. FEBS Lett 1988;234:326–330.

148. Unemori EN, Ehsani N, Wang M, et al. Interleukin-1 and transforming growth factor-alpha: synergistic stimulation of metalloproteinases, PGE2, and proliferation in human fibroblasts. Exp Cell Res 1994;210:166–171.

149. Falcone DJ, McCaffrey TA, Haimovitz FA, et al. Macrophage and foam cell release of matrix bound growth factors. Role of plasminogen activation. J Biol Chem 1993;268:11951–11958.

150. Falcone DJ, McCaffrey TA, Haimovitz-Friedman A, et al. Transforming growth factor-beta 1 stimulates macrophage urokinase expression and release of matrix-bound basic fibroblast growth factor. J Cell Physiol 1993;155:595–605.

151. Ito A, Sato T, Iga T, et al. Tumor necrosis factor bifunctionally regulates matrix metalloproteinases and tissue inhibitor of metalloproteinases (TIMP) production by human fibroblasts. FEBS Lett 1990;269:93–95.

152. Mendoza AE, Young R, Orkin SH, et al. Increased PDGF A-chain expression in human uterine smooth muscle cells during the physiologic hypertrophy of pregnancy. Proc Natl Acad Sci USA 1990;87:2177–2181.

153. Raines EW, Dower SK, Ross R. Interleukin-1 mitogenic activity for fibroblasts and smooth muscle cells is due to PDGF-AA. Science 1989;243:393–396.

154. Shaw RJ, Benedict SH, Clark RAF, et al. Pathogenesis of pulmonary fibrosis in interstitial lung disease: Alveolar macrophage PDGF (B) gene activation an up-regulation by interferon gamma. Am Rev Respir Dis 1991;143:167–173.

155. Vollenhoven BJ, Herington AC, Healy DL. Messenger RNA encoding the insulin-like growth factors and their binding proteins, in women with fibroids, pretreated with luteinizing hormone-releasing hormone agonists. Human Reprod 1994;9:214–219.

156. Johnson LK, Baxter JD, Vlodausky I, et al. Epidermal growth factor and expression of specific genes: effect on cultured rat pituitary cells are dissociable from the mitogenic response. Proc Natl Acad Sci USA 1980;77:394–398.

157. Schonbrunn A, Krasnoff M, Westenclorf JM, et al. Epidermal growth factor and thyrotropin-releasing hormone act similarly on a clonal pituitary cell strain. J Cell Biol 1980;85:786–797.

158. Polet H. Epidermal growth factor stimulates DNA synthesis while inhibiting cell multiplication of A-431 carcinoma cells. Exp Cell Res 1990;186:390–393.

159. Gill GN, Lazer CS. Increased phosphotyrosine content and inhibition of proliferation in EGF-treated A431 cells. Nature 1981;293:305–307.

160. King ICL, Sartorelli AC. The relationship between epidermal growth factor receptors and the terminal differentiation of A431 carcinoma cells. Biochem Biophys Res Commun 1986;140:837–843.

161. Fisher DA, Lakshmanan J. Metabolism and effects of epidermal growth factor and related growth factors in mammals. Endocrine Rev 1990;11:418–442.

162. Chinkers M, McKanna JA, Cohen S. Rapid rounding of human epidermoid carcinoma cell A-431 induced by epidermal growth factor. J Cell Biol 1981;88:422–429.

163. Haigler HT, McKanna JA, Cohen S. Rapid stimulation of pinocytosis in human carcinoma cell A-431 by epidermal growth factor. J Cell Biol 1979;83:82–90.

164. Chegini N, Rong H, Zhao Y, et al. Gonadotropin hormone releasing hormone agonist (GnRHa) suppresses the expression of mRNA and proteins for growth factors and their receptors in uterine leiomyomata. Society for Gynecologic Investigation 41st Annual Meeting. 1994: Abstract No. P260.

165. Koji T, Chedid M, Rubin JS, et al. Progesterone-dependent expression of keratinocyte growth factor mRNA in stromal cells of the primate endometrium: keratinocyte growth factor as a progestomedin. J Cell Biol 1994;125:393–401

166. Pekonen F, Nyman T, Rutanen EM. Differential expression of keratinocyte growth factor and its receptor in the human uterus. Mol Cell Endocrinol 1993;95:43–49.

167. Rauk PN, Suriti S, Roberst JM, et al. Mitogenic effect of basic fibroblast growth factor and estradiol on cultured human myometrial and leiomyoma cells. Am J Obstet Gynecol 1995:173:571–577.

168. Charnock-Jones DS, Sharkey AM, Rajput-Williams J, et al. Identification and localization of alternately spliced mRNAs for vascular endothelial growth factor in human uterus and estrogen regulation in endometrial carcinoma cell lines. Biol Reprod 1993;48:1120–1128.

169. Sournia A, Koutsilieris M. Purification and partial sequencing of the major mitogen for human uterine smooth muscle like cells in leiomyoma extracts. J Clin Invest 1995;96:751–758.

170. Stewart EA, Jain P, Penglase MD, et al. The myometrium of postmenopausal women produces prolactin in response to human chorionic gonadotropin and α subunit in vitro. Fertil Steril 1995;64:972–976.

171. Daly DC, Walters CA, Prior JC, et al. Prolactin production from proliferative phase leiomyoma. Am J Obstet Gynecol 1984;148:1059–1063.

172. Rein MS, Friedman Aj, Heffner Lj. Decreased prolactin secretion by explant cultures of fibroids from women treated with a gonadotropin-releasing hormone agonist. Clin Endocrinol 1990;70:1554–1558.

173. Sharara FT, Nieman LK. Growth hormone receptor messenger ribonucleic acid expression in leiomyoma and surrounding myometrium. Am J Obstet Gynecol 1995;172:814–819.

174. Bryant-Greenwood GD. The human relaxins: Consensus and dissent. Mol Cell Endocrinol 1995;79:C125–C132.

175. Weir EC, Goad DI, Daifotis AG, et al. Relative overexpression of the parathyroid hormone-related peptide gene in human leiomyomas. J Clin Endocrinol Metabol 1994;78:784–789.

176. Singh M, Zuo J, Li X, et al. Decreased expression of functional human chorionic gonadotropin/luteinizing hormone receptor gene in human uterine leiomyomas. Biol Reprod 1995;53:591–597.

177. Rossi MJ, Pawlina W, Larkin LH, et al. Presence of relaxin binding sites in human myometrial smooth muscle cells and its inhibitory effect on EGF action in culture. Biol Reprod 1991;44 (Suppl. 1):Abstract No. 184.

178. Casey H, Mibe M, MacDonald PC. Transforming growth factor-beta 1 stimulation of parathyroid hormone-related protein expression in human uterine cells in culture: mRNA levels and protein secretion. J Clin Endocrinol Metab 1992:74:950–952.

7

CYTOKINES IN EARLY PREGNANCY SUCCESS AND FAILURE

Joseph A. Hill

Brigham and Women's Hospital, Harvard Medical School, Boston, Massachusetts

The primary function of the immune system is to differentiate between self and non-self, and to destroy nonself tissues and organisms. Immune responses are either innate or acquired, depending on the prior exposure to antigen, acquired specificity of response, and immunologic memory. Innate immunity is rapid and relatively non-specific, such as occurs in inflammation. An inflammatory response is mediated by cytokines and other soluble factors secreted by natural killer (NK) cells, macrophages, lymphocytes, mast cells, basophils, platelets, fibroblasts, and even endothelial and mucosal epithelial cells. The innate immune response is similar in intensity despite repeated antigen exposures, for it does not possess memory, unlike acquired immunity. Acquired immunity is both time dependent and specific following antigen recognition by antigen processing cells such as macrophages leading to activation and differentiation of specific T and B lymphocytes.

Antigen processing cells present antigen to immune cells in association with surface protein molecules called major histocompatibility (MHC) determinants, grouped

Cytokines in Human Reproduction, Edited by Joseph A. Hill
ISBN 0-471-35242-X   Copyright © 2000 Wiley-Liss, Inc.

as either MHC class I (HLA-A, B, C) or MHC class II (HLA-DR, DP, DQ) molecules. Class I determinants are expressed on nearly all nucleated cells and normally bind peptides from endogenously processed antigens. Class II determinants are expressed primarily on antigen processing cells where they bind peptides from exogenously derived antigens.

T cells recognize antigenic peptides in association with cell surface HLA molecules that have genetically defined tissue type differences between individuals. NK cells do not need MHC molecules for antigen recognition but can mediate cell lysis directly through their secreted cytokines or indirectly through activation of acquired T cell mediated immunity. Acquired immunity can also be initiated by antigen presentation to T cells through T cell receptor coupling to Class II MHC determinants. Cytotoxic T lymphocyte responses occur through T cell recognition of antigen peptides in association with self Class I MHC molecules.

Upon activation, antigen processing cells secrete pro-inflammatory cytokines such as interleukin (IL)-12. IL-12 is a key cytokine in immune regulation promoting both NK cell and cytotoxic T-lymphocyte activity. IL-12 also modulates IgA synthesis and induces T cell commitment from the T helper O (ThO) to Th1 phenotype characterized by interferon gamma (IFN-γ) secretion. IFN-γ secretion by Th1 cells mediates both cellular immunity and organ-specific autoimmunity.

Acquired immunity is often mediated by a dichotomous T cell cytokine response dominated by either Th1 or Th2 cytokines. Th1 cytokines include IL-2, IL-12, IFN-γ, tumor necrosis factor (TNF) β and perhaps TNF-α. Th2 cytokines include IL-4, IL-5, IL-6, IL-10, and perhaps IL-13. Th1 cytokines generally result in cellular immunity, whereas Th2 cytokines activate B cells, causing their differentiation into antibody secreting plasma cells. Acquired immunity does not depend upon either a Th1 or Th2 cytokine response, but may include components of both in a Th3 response dominated by both IFN-γ and IL-4. The outcome of an immune response dominated by either cellular versus antibody mediated immunity is best predicted by the IL-4 to IFN-γ ratio. An inflammatory response may be determined by the ratio of Th2 inhibiting cytokines to Th1 activating cytokines. Loss of self-tolerance leading to inflammatory autoimmunity may result owing to deficient IL-4 production. Uncontrolled immunity is normally prevented by the elimination of antigen, stimulation of T suppressor cells, antibody feedback mechanisms, and cytokine regulation. Immunologic tolerance is fundamental to the immune system with loss culminating in autoimmunity and autoimmune disease. Cytokines may also affect tolerance through upregulation or induction of expression of MHC molecules and through autoregulatory feedback stimulation and inhibition.

Suppressor cells are thought to be stimulated by some antigens. These cells function by nonspecific mechanisms such as through secretion of IFN-γ, which can inhibit B lymphocyte proliferation; production of transforming growth factors (TGF-β), which can inhibit T and B cell proliferation or in some cases increase their proliferation; and inhibit IL-2 production, and absorption of growth factors and cytolysis of specific T helper and B cells expressing antigens in association with MHC determinants. T suppressor cells may also nonspecifically downregulate specific immune responses through IL-2 activation of macrophage TNF production, leading to immune cell destruction through apoptosis.

Antibodies specifically neutralize antigens through the formation of antigen-antibody complexes or by binding to antigenic determinants, blocking their access to specific membrane immunoglobulin on B cell derived plasma cells. Cytokine cascades may also be initiated by antigen-antibody complexes.

Autoantibody production occurs in normal individuals. These autoantibodies are often transient and of low level. Autobodies can be upregulated during an immune response to foreign antigens, but these are generally low affinity IgM and neither are generated with T cell help nor lead to tissue injury. Pathological autoimmunity may occur if high titer, high affinity autoantibodies are produced with assistance provided by autoreactive T cells.

THE DECIDUA

The endometrium cyclically prepares to receive a fertilized egg in a process known as the menstrual cycle. The endometrium is an immunologically dynamic tissue containing a myriad of immune and inflammatory cells capable of activation and cytokine secretion (1–10) as is endometrial epithelium (8, 10) as discussed in Chapters 5 and 8.

Following ovulation, the endometrium decidualizes under the influence of progesterone secreted by the corpus luteum. At the time of implantation (approximately 7–9 days postovulation) the endometrial leukocyte population is made up predominantly of large granulated lymphocytes expressing the NK cell phenotypic marker CD56 followed closely by macrophages and CD3 T-lymphocytes, of which CD8 suppressor T cells predominate (11–13).

In early pregnancy CD56 positive, large-granulated lymphocytes predominate (12, 14–16). The few T lymphocytes that are present do not express the IL-2 receptor (17). These cells have been described to be the source of several cytokines (18), such as TGF-β (19), granulocyte colony stimulating factor (G-CSF), and macrophage CSF (CSF, 20). These factors have been proposed to contribute to successful human pregnancy just as it has in murine gestation (21) in a process referred to as immunotrophism (21–22). However, these cells are also capable of secreting TNF-α (23) and, at term, IFN-γ (24). TNF and INF-γ have been postulated to have immunodystropic effects leading to pregnancy loss if secreted in high levels (25).

IMMUNOSUPPRESSION

Immunologically, the conceptus is a hemiallograft and thus should be rejected unless immunoregulatory mechanisms intervene to protect the allogenic pregnancy. One such mechanism may be that placental syncytiotrophoblast at the maternal fetal interface does not express the classic major histocompatibility complex (MHC) class I and class II molecules (26) except for HLA-C, HLA-E and HLA-G (27–28). The precise function(s) of these molecules is unknown, although one function of HLA-G may be to regulate NK activity within the uterus (29). Syncytiotrophoblast also expresses complement regulatory proteins that can bind complement and thus prevent complement mediated attack (30). IFN-γ and TNF have been reported to induce MHC expression in trophoblast (31, 32), which has been proposed to be a mechanism of immunologic reproductive failure (33). However, data derived from in vivo studies of spontaneously aborted trophoblast indicate that this potential mechanism is unlikely to be responsible for recurrent pregnancy loss in women (34).

There is evidence that immunosuppression occurs in pregnancy. Antibody dependent cellular cytotoxicity (ADCC) and NK cell activity are diminished in pregnant women compared to women who are not pregnant (35). Although diminished NK cell activity occurs in pregnancy, neither the number nor the percentage of NK cells in the peripheral circulation are associated with NK activity (36) and thus cannot be used to predict pregnancy outcome (37, 38). The potential immunosuppressive factors produced during pregnancy include progesterone, pregnancy-associated alpha 2-glycoprotein, alpha-fetoprotein, transforming growth factor-beta (TGF-β), and T-helper (Th)2 cytokines. The Fas ligand-Fas receptor system may also be involved in immunomodulation (Reviewed in 39). There is also evidence that immunosuppression is necessary for pregnancy as suggested by the finding that loss of response to recall antigens is associated with successful pregnancy (40).

Further evidence that immunomodulation occurs during pregnancy comes from observations in women and in animal models. In women with rheumatoid arthritis, disease status improves generally during pregnancy (41); women with systemic lupus erythematosus, disease often is exacerbated or remains unchanged (42). One potential mechanism responsible for these observations is downregulation of TNF-α (43) and IL-2 (44) which correlates with clinical improvement in rheumatoid arthritis (41) and exacerbation of systemic lupus erythematosus (45), respectively.

IMMUNOTROPISM VERSUS IMMUNODYSTROPISM

The absolute need for an intact maternal immune system during pregnancy appears unlikely, for successful breeding occurs in immune deficient mice (46–48). However, cytokine mediated reproductive failure may still occur. In animal models, downregulation of Th1 type cytokines in favor of Th2 type cytokines has been demonstrated in normal pregnant mice (49) prompting the hypothesis that successful pregnancy is a Th2 phenomenon (50). The administration of Th1 cytokines to pregnant mice has also been observed to lead to fetal demise (51). Several of the Th1 cytokines, including IFN-γ and TNF, have been shown to have direct toxic effects on many reproductive processes including embryo development (52), implantation events (53), and trophoblast growth (54) in vitro. One potential mechanism whereby IFN-γ may mediate embryotoxicity is by inhibiting transmembrane mobility of cytoskeletal proteins (55). TNF may also accelerate apoptosis (56). In abortion prone mice the expression of mRNA for IL-2, IFN-γ, and TNF-α were reported to be quantitatively higher in the placentae of mice undergoing resorption compared to placentae from normal murine pregnancies (57). Levels of IL-2 and IFN-γ were also increased in supernatants of mixed lymphocytes and placental cells from this same animal model of spontaneous abortion (58).

The first studies suggesting a Th1-Th2 paradigm in recurrent pregnancy loss in women demonstrated in vitro that peripheral blood mononuclear cells from many women with unexplained recurrent pregnancy loss were more likely to proliferate (59) and secrete embryotoxic and trophoblast-toxic cytokines such as IFN-γ than cells from fertile controls or from women with other explanations for their pregnancy losses (60). Of 244 women with unexplained recurrent spontaneous abortion, 160 responded to trophoblast antigens in vitro by producing embryotoxicity in a murine culture system and by secreting high levels of IFN-γ, TNF-α, and TGF-β as measured by ELISA, but very low levels of IL-4 and IL-10 in trophoblast activated peripheral blood mononuclear cell culture supernatants. Conversely, women without a history of recurrent pregnancy loss responded with IL-10 and, to a much lower extent, IL-4 (61). These data prompted the hypothesis that as in mice, Th2 type of immunity may be the natural response to trophoblast; Th1 type immunity may be aberrant and may potentially play a role in the reproductive difficulty of women exhibiting such a response (61). More recent data from our laboratory suggest that this paradigm may not be as simplistic as we originally proposed, for we have been unable to substantiate consistently that peripheral blood mononuclear cells cultured with trophoblast from women with successful pregnancy histories have a predominant Th2 response. Women both with and without recurrent pregnancy loss may make IL-10 and IFN-γ but Th1 type immunity still predominates in some women with reproductive difficulty (62). IL-12, which favors Th1 immunity (63), may also be involved in these women (64). Our most recent data parallel a recent study identifying Th1 and Th2 cytokines in human late-gestation decidual tissues where unlike in mice, late gestation human decidual tissue does not preferentially express a Th2 type cytokine profile (65).

We have also been unable to confirm a report that peripheral serum levels of TNF and IL-2 (66) or any Th1 or Th2 cytokine or the soluble intracellular adhesion molecule ICAM-1 is predictive of pregnancy outcome (67). One potential reason for this discrepancy may be that in our study, serum samples were obtained upon documenting fetal cardiac activity and later correlated with subsequent pregnancy outcome, whereas in the study reporting that TNF and IL-2 were associated with pregnancy loss the investigators did not state whether the fetus was alive or dead at the time of obtaining the serum. This is potentially important because in cases of a missed abortion where the fetus has already died, it may not be surprising to find elevations in inflammatory cytokines. Similarly, assessment of embryotoxicity of maternal serum in murine culture systems is also not scientifically valid unless heat inactivation to destroy complement and preabsorption with murine splenocytes to remove heterophilic antimurine antibodies is first accomplished. Particular attention to serum collection tubes is also important because the rubber tops of vacutainer serum collection tubes are embryotoxic (68).

CONCLUSIONS

Data to date although tantalizing does not prove definitively that Th1 immunity to trophoblast causes human reproductive failure. At best our data imply a very strong association with recurrent pregnancy loss. A definitive answer must await the outcome of experiments performed in the decidua of early human pregnancy in which comparisons are made between euploid and aneuploid spontaneous losses and elective pregnancy terminations. Such studies are currently being performed in our laboratory.

REFERENCES

1. Kazza BA. Specific endometrial granular cells: A semiquantitative study. Eur J Obstet Gynecol 1972;3:77–84.

2. Morris H, Edwards J, Tiltman A, et al. Endometrial lymphoid tissue: an immunohistologic study. J Clin Pathol 1985;38:644–652.

3. Kamat BR, Isaccson PG. The immuno cytochemical distribution of leukocytic subpopulations in human endometrium. Am J Pathol 1987;127:66–73.

4. Marshall RJ, Jones DB. An immunohistochemical study of lymphoid tissue in human endometrium. Int Gynecol Pathol 1988;7:225–235.

5. King A, Wellins V, Gardner L, Loke YW. Immunocytochemical characterization of the unusual large granular lymphocytes in human endometrium throughout the menstrual cycle. Human Immunol 1989;24:195–205.

6. Tabibzadeh SS. Evidence of T cell activation and potential cytokine action in human endometrium. J Clin Endocrinol Metab 1990;71:645–649.

7. Starkey PM, Glover LM, Rees MCP. Variation during the menstrual cycle of immune cell populations in human endometrium. Eur J Obstet Gynecol Reprod Biol 1991;39:203–207.

8. Kauma SW, Aukerman SC, Eiserman D, et al. Colony stimulating factor-1 and c-fms expression in human endometrial tissues and placenta during the menstrual cycle and early pregnancy. J Clin Endocrinol Metab 1991;73:746–751.

9. Bulmer JN, Marrison L, Longfellow M, Kitson A, Pace D. Granulated lymphocytes in human endometrium: histochemical and immunohistochemical studies. Human Reprod 1991;6:791–798.

10. Tabibzadeh SS, Sun XZ. Cytokine expression in human endometrium through the menstrual cycle. Human Reprod 1992;7:1214–1221.

11. Kientxeris LD, Bulmer JN, Warren A, Morrison L, Li TC, Cooke ID. Endometrial lymphoid tissue in the timed endometrial biopsy: morphometric and immunohistochemical aspects. Am J Obstet Gynecol 1992; 167:667–674.

12. King A, Loke YW, Chaouat G. NK cells and reproduction. Immunology Today 1997;18:64–66.

13. Vassiliadou N, Bulmer JN. Quantitative analysis of T lymphocyte subsets in pregnant and nonpregnancy human endometrium. Biol Reprod 1996;55:1017–1022.

14. Bulmer JN, Sutherland CA. Immunohistological characterization of lymphoid cell populations in the early human placental bed. Immunology 1984;152:349–357.

15. Starkey PM, Sargent IL, Redman CWG. Cell populations in human early pregnancy decidua: characterization of large granular lymphocytes by flow cytometry. Immunology 1988;65:129–134.

16. Vince GS, Starkey PM, Jackson MC, Sargent LL, Rednian CWG. Flow cytometric characterization of cell populations in human pregnancy decidua and isolation of decidual macrophages. J Immunol Methods 1990;132:181–189.

17. Bulmer JN, Johnson PM. The T-lymphocyte population in first-trimester human decidua does not express the interleukin-2 receptor. Immunology 1986;58:685–687.

18. Jokhi PP, King A, Sharkey AM, Smith SH, Loke YW. Screening for cytokine messenger ribonucleic acids in purified human decidual lymphocyte populations by the reverse-transcriptase polymerase chain reaction. J Immunol 1994;153:4427–4435.

19. Clark DA, Vince G, Flanders KC, Horte H, Starkey P. CD56+ lymphoid cells in human first trimester pregnancy decidua as a source of noel transforming growth factor-β-2-related immunosuppressive factors. Human Reprod 1994;19:2270–2277.

20. Shorter SC, Vine GS, Starkey PM. Production of granulocyte colony stimulating factor at the maternal-fetal interface in human pregnancy. Immunology 1992;75:468–474.

21. Athanassakis I, Bleakley CR, Paetkau V, Gilbert C, Barr PJ, Wegmann TG. The immuno-stimulatory effect of T cells and the T cell lymphokines on murine fetally-derived placental cells. J Immunol 1987;130:37.

22. Wegmann TG, Athanassakis I, Gilbert L, Branch D, Dy M, Menu E, Chaouat G. The role of M-CSF and GM-CSF in fostering placental growth and fetal survival. Transpl Proc 1989;21:566.

23. Vince G, Shorter S, Starkey P, Humphreys J, Clover L, Wilkins T, Sargent I, Redman C. Localization of tumor necrosis factor production in cells at the materno/fetal interface in human pregnancy. Clin Exp Immunol 1992;88:174–180.

24. Jones CA, Finlay-Jones II, Hart PH. Type 1 and Type 2 cytokines in human late gestation decidual tissue. Biol Reprod 1997;57:303–311.

25. Hill JA, Anderson DJ. Cell-mediated immune mechanisms in recurrent spontaneous abortion. In: Talwar GP ed. Contraceptive Research for Today and the Nineties. New York: Springer Verlag, 1988:171–180.

26. Faulk WP, Emple A. Distributing beta 2 microglublin and HLA in chorimic villi of human placentae. Nature 1976;262:799–802.

27. Ellis SA, Sergeant IL, Redman CW, McMichael AT. Evidence for a novel aHLA antigen found on human extravillous trophoblast and a choriocarcinoma cells line. Immunology 1986;59:595–601.

28. Kovats S, Main EK, Librach C, Stubblebine M, Fisher SJ, DeMars R. A class I antigen, HLA-G expressed in human trophoblasts. Science 1990;248:220–233.

29. Pasnany L, Mandelboim O, Vales-Gomez M, David DM, Gomez HT, Strominger JL. Protection form natural killer cell-mediated lysis by HLA-G expression in target cells. Science 1996;274:792–295.

30. Purcell DF, McKenzie IF, Lublin DM, et al. The human cell-surface glycoproteins HuLy-m5, membrane co-factor protein (MCP) of the complement system, and trophoblast leucocyte-common (TLX) antigen, are CD46. Immunology 1990;70:155–161.

31. Anderson DJ, Berkowitz RS. Gamma-interferon enhances expression of class I MHC antigens in the early HLA(+) human choriocarcinoma cell line BeWo but does not induce MHC expression in the HLA(–) choriocarcinoma cell line JAR. J Immunol 1985;135:2498–2502.

32. Feinman MA, Kliman JH, Main EK. HLA antigen expression and induction by gamma interferon in cultural human trophoblast. Am J Obstet Gynecol 1987;157:1429–1434.

33. Hunt JS, Hsi BL. Evasive strategies of trophoblast cells: selective expression of membrane antigens. Am J Reprod Immunol 1990;23:57–63.

34. Hill JA, Melling GC, Johnson PM. Immunohistochemical studies of human utero-placental tissues from first trimester spontaneous abortion. Am J Obstet Gynecol 1995;173:90–96.

35. Hill JA, Hsia S, Doran DW, Bryans CI, Jr. Natural killer cell activity and antibody dependent cell-mediated cytotoxicity in Preeclampsia. J Reprod Immunol 1986;9:205–212.

36. Hill JA. Natural killer cells in endometriosis. Fertil Steril 1993;60:928–929.

37. Hill JA, Canning C, Collins H, Ritz J. Peripheral blood T-cell and NK cell immunophenotypes are not clinically useful in predicting pregnancy outcome in women with recurrent spontaneous abortion. Fertil Steril 1996; ASRM Abstract: 565.

38. Dudley DJ, Green W, Silver RM, Branch DW, Scott JR. White blood cell markers do not identify a unique subset of women with unexplained recurrent pregnancy loss. J Soc Gynecol Invest 1997;4:185A.

39. Ashkenazi A, Dixit VM. Death receptors: signaling and modulation. Science 1998;281:1305–1308.

40. Bermas BL, Hill JA. Proliferative responses to recall antigens are associated with pregnancy outcome in women with a history of recurrent spontaneous abortion. J Clin Invest 1997;100:1330–1334.

41. Klipple GL, Cecere FA. Rheumatoid arthritis and pregnancy. Rheum Dis Clin N Am 1989;15:213–239.

42. Petri M, Howard D, Repke J. Frequency of lupus flare in pregnancy. The Hopkins Lupus Pregnancy Center experience. Arthritis Rheum 1991;34:1538–1545.

43. Rankin EC, Choy EH, Kassimos D, Kingsley GH, Supwith AM, Isenberg DA, Panayi GS. The therapeutic effects of an engineered human anti-tumor necrosis factor alpha antibody (CDP571) in rheumatoid arthritis. Br J Rheumatol 1995;34:334–342.

44. Stallmach T, Hebisch G, Joller-Jemelka HI, Orban P, Schuffer J, Engelmann H. Cytokine production and visualized effects in the feto-maternal unit: quantitative and topographic data on cytokines during intrauterine disease. Lab Invest 1995;73:384–392.

45. Bermas BL, Petri M. Goldman D, Mittleman K, Miller MW, Stacks NI, Via CS, Shearer GM. T-helper cell dysfunction in systemic lupus erythematosis (SLE): relation to disease activity. J Clin Immunol 1994;14:169–177.

46. Croy BA, Chapeau CJ. Evaluation of the pregnancy immunotrophism hypothesis by assessment of the reproductive performance of young adult mice of genotype scid/scid, bg/bg. J Reprod Fert 1990;88:231–239.

47. Pfeffer K, Mak TW. Lymphocyte antogeny and activation in gene targeted mutant mice. Ann Rev Immunol 1994;12:367–411.

48. Guimond MJ, Luross JA, Wang B, Terhost C, Daniel S, Crowy BA. Absence of natural killer cells during murine pregnancy is associated with reproductive compromise in TgE26 mice. Biol Reprod 1997;56:169–179.

49. Lin H, Mosmann TR, Guilbert L, Tuntipopipat S, Wegmann TG. Synthesis of T helper 2-type cytokines at the materno-fetal interface. J Immunol 1993;151:4562–4573.

50. Wegmann TG, Lin H, Guilbert L, Mosman TR. Bidirectional cytokine interactions in the maternal-fetal relationship. Is successful pregnancy a Th2 phenomena? Immunol Today 1993;14:353–356.

51. Chaouat G, Menu E, Clark D, Dy M, Minkowski M, Wegmann TG. Control of fetal survival in CBAx DBA/2 mice in lymphokine therapy. J Reprod Fertil 1990;89:447–458.

52. Hill JA, Haimovici F, Anderson DJ. Products of activated lymphocytes and macrophages inhibit mouse embryo development in vitro. J Immunol 1987;132:2250–2254.

53. Haimovici F, Hill JA, Anderson DJ. The effects of soluble products of activated lymphocytes and macrophages on blastocyst implantation events in vitro. Biol Reprod 1991;44:69–75.

54. Berkowitz RS, Hill JA, Kurtz CB, Anderson DJ. Effects of products of activated leukocytes (lymphokines and monokines) on the growth of malignant trophoblast cells in vitro. Am J Obstet Gynecol 1988;158:199–203.

55. Polgar K, Yacono P, Golan D, Hill JA. Immune interferon gamma inhibits transitional mobility of a plasma membrane protein in preimplantation stage mouse embryos. A T helper 1 mechanisms for immunologic reproductive failure. Am J Obstet Gynecol 1996;174:282–287.

56. Beutler B, Von Haffel C. Unraveling function in the TNF ligand and receptor families. Science 1994;264:667–668.

57. Tangri S, Raghupathy R. Expression of cytokines in placenta of mice undergoing immunologically mediated spontaneous fetal resorptions. Biol Reprod 1993;49:850–856.

58. Tangri S, Wegmann TG, Raghupathy R. Meternal anti-placental reactivity in natural immunologically-mediated fetal resorptions. J Immunol 1994:152:4903–4911.

59. Yamada H, Polgar K, Hill JA. Cell-mediated immunity to trophoblast antigens in women with recurrent spontaneous abortion. Am J Obstet Gynecol 1994;170:1339–1344.

60. Hill JA, Polgar K, Harlow BL, Anderson DJ. Evidence of embryo and trophoblast toxic cellular immune response(s) in women with recurrent spontaneous abortion. Am J Obstet Gynecol 1992;166:1044–1052.

61. Hill JA, Polgar K, Anderson DJ. Th1 type immunity to trophoblast antigens in women with recurrent spontaneous abortion. JAMA 1995;273:1933–1936.

62. Choi BC, Hill JA. Th1 (IFN-γ), Th2 (IL-10) and TGF-β1 secretion in response to trophoblast and progesterone in women with unexplained recurrent pregnancy loss and for the controls. American Society of Reproductive Medicine 53rd Annual Meeting 1997, S17.

63. Trinchieri G, Interleukin-12 and its role in the generation of Th1 cells. Immunol Today 1993;14:335–338.

64. Hill JA, Xiao L, Choi BC. IL-12 and IL-15 secretion in response to trophoblast in women with and without evidence of Th1 associated recurrent abortion and fertile controls. American Society of Reproductive Medicine 53rd Annual Meeting 1997, S16.

65. Jones CA, Finlay-Jones JJ, Hart PH. Type 1 and Type 2 cytokines in human late-gestation and decidual tissue. Biol Reprod 1997;57:303–3 11.

66. Mallman P, Mallman R, Krebs D. Determination of tumor necrosis factor alpha and interleukin 2 in women with idiopathic recurrent miscarriage. Arch Gynecol Obstet 1991;249:73–78.

67. Schust DJ, Hill JA. Correlation of serum cytokine and adhesion molecule determinations with pregnancy outcome. J Soc Gynecol Invest 1996;3:259–261.

68. Haimovic, F, Hill JA, Anderson DJ. Variables affecting toxicity of human sera in mouse embryo cultures. J In Vitro Fertil Embryo Transfer 1988;5:202–206.

8

CYTOKINES IN PRETERM AND TERM PARTURITION

Donald J. Dudley

University of Texas San Antonio School of Medicine, San Antonio, Texas

Little progress has been made in the treatment and prevention of preterm labor and delivery in the United States over the past 20 years (1, 2). One reason for the lack of progress in preventing and treating preterm labor is a poor understanding of the pathophysiology of this condition. One important concept that has been elucidated in the course of studies over the past several years is that preterm labor is a heterogeneous syndrome with many possible causes (3). As a result of these insights, different immune mechanisms have been postulated to contribute to a significant proportion of preterm labor. The purpose of this chapter is to review the immunobiologic mechanisms that may mediate both normal and abnormal parturition.

INNATE VERSUS ADAPTIVE IMMUNITY

Immune responses generally are divided into two types of responses, innate and adaptive (4). Innate immune responses are directed against foreign antigens in nonspecific fashion, have no memory component, and are mediated by immune effector cells such as macrophages and neutrophils. Adaptive immune responses are usually directed

Cytokines in Human Reproduction, Edited by Joseph A. Hill
ISBN 0-471-35242-X   Copyright © 2000 Wiley-Liss, Inc.

against specific antigen after intricate antigen processing and presentation by antigen presenting cells such as macrophages and dendritic cells. These processed antigens are recognized by T cells bearing specific receptors for antigen, resulting in T cell proliferation with consequent cytotoxicity and/or antibody production. Unlike innate responses, adaptive responses are characterized by memory of the antigen leading to secondary immune responses.

A key mediator of any immune response is the production and activity of cytokines. Cytokines are proteins that can be produced by any cell after damage, but usually are messengers from one immune effector cell to other immune effector cells, resulting in changes in cellular activity. During pregnancy, the most likely immune response is at a primitive immunologic level (5), and normal adaptive mechanisms leading to cytotoxicity are attenuated (6, 7). However, aberrations in normal adaptive immunity may play a part in abnormal pregnancy, such as recurrent pregnancy loss (8) and preeclampsia (9). This chapter focuses on cytokine immunobiology during innate immune responses and addresses the possible role of cytokines in normal and abnormal parturition.

BASIC CONCEPTS OF CYTOKINE BIOLOGY

There have been more than 50 different proteins that can be classified as cytokines. The nomenclature for these proteins presents the novice with a confusing morass of names such as interleukin, tumor necrosis factor, and interferon, among others. Currently, the naming of a cytokine requires that the amino acid sequence be known and the gene for the protein cloned prior to name designation. There are currently 18 interleukins (IL-1 through IL-18), two TNFs, three interferons, and numerous chemokines. A detailed review of each cytokine is beyond the scope of this chapter, but excellent reviews have been published recently for each of these cytokines (see bibliography).

Cytokines in Innate Immune Responses

In innate inflammatory responses, there are generally four activities: initiation, immune effector cell attraction, immunomodulation, and inhibition/resolution (Fig. 8.1). After an inflammatory stimulus, damaged cells usually promptly produce interleukin-1 (IL-1) (10) and tumor necrosis factor-α (TNF-α) (11). These two cytokines are encoded by different genes on different chromosomes yet have similar activities. They act as endogenous pyrogens, activate endothelial cells, mediate shock responses, stimulate fibroblast proliferation, trigger the acute phase response (perhaps via IL-6), and promote the gene for prostaglandin H synthase 2 (or cyclooxygenase II), leading to increased prostaglandin production. These cytokines thus are key to the initiation of the inflammatory response.

One key role of IL-1 and TNF-α is the stimulation of chemokine (or *chemo*attractant cyto*kine*) production. The inflammatory stimulus itself can also elicit the production of these so-called, 10 to 20 kDa "small cytokines." In general, chemokines are classed into two broad families, termed the C-X-C chemokines and C-C chemokines,

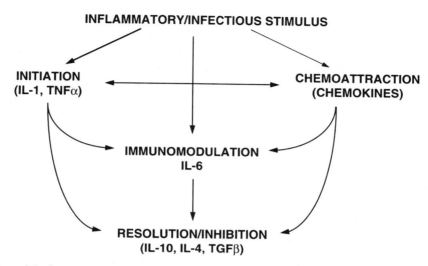

Figure 8.1. General concept of inflammation. After an infectious stimulus, initiation and chemoattration occur followed by immunomodulation. The inflammatory process then is inhibited and resolves. Each of these steps is mediated by different cytokines as noted.

based upon cysteine moieties in a conserved amino acid sequence of the proteins (12). C-X-C chemokines (or α chemokines) include IL-8, growth-related oncogenes (GROα, GROß, GROγ), IP-10, and ENA-78, among many others. This family of chemokines generally act to attract and activate neutrophils. The C-C chemokines (or ß chemokines) include macrophage inflammatory protein-1α (MIP-1α) and MIP-1ß, monocyte chemotactic protein-1 (MCP-1), MCP-2, MCP-3, and RANTES (regulated on activation normal T cell expressed and secreted), among others. C-C chemokines generally attract and activate monocytes, macrophages, and T cells. Although the differences between subfamilies in general hold true, some chemokines can influence many different types of immune effector cells, including neutrophils, monocytes, mast cells, T cells, and many other cell types. Chemokines act by establishing a concentration gradient from the site of inflammation upon which different immune effector cells migrate. As the cells migrate into the area, they become activated against antigen in either nonspecific or specific fashion depending upon the lineage of the cell. Chemokines generally are produced early in inflammatory responses, soon after IL-1 and TNF-α.

After the first few hours of an inflammatory stimulus, immunomodulatory cytokines such as IL-6 are expressed (13). IL-6 has many different functions depending on the context of the site of action and the cells being signaled by the cytokine. IL-6 can act as a growth factor, stimulates B cells to become high antibody-producing plasma cells, activates T cells, and is a critical mediator of the acute phase response by the liver. Other cytokines in the same class as IL-6 include leukemia inhibitory factor (LIF), oncostatin-M (OSM), and IL-11. They utilize the gp130 subunit in their receptors, matched with other specific subunits for each cytokine (see below). The precise role of these cytokines in the inflammatory response is not entirely clear, although it is felt that they act in an immunomodulatory fashion by maintaining the immune response to an eliciting antigen without promoting adjacent tissue damage.

Occurring late in the inflammatory process, IL-10 (14), IL-4 (15), and TGF-ß (16) species are produced and act to inhibit cytokine synthesis and thus are the "braking system" for the inflammatory process. IL-10 was originally termed "cytokine synthesis inhibitory factor" and is produced by monocytes, macrophages, and T cells after stimuli such as lipopolysaccharide (LPS) and other specific antigens. IL-4 similarly acts as an "anti-inflammatory" cytokine and regulates inflammatory responses, differentiates B cell and T cells, and serves as a growth factor for mast cells. TGFß comes in several different isoforms, the best described being TGFß1, TGFß2, and TGFß3, with similar biologic properties. TGFß isoforms have a key role in tissue remodeling after injury, and induce fibrosis in damaged tissues. Overexpression of TGFß appears to be one key pathophysiological feature of glomerulonephritis (17).

Normal inflammatory responses, as carefully scripted by regulatory factors, result in destruction of the invading stimulus while maintaining normal tissue architecture and function. Recent investigations have shown that, when the normal processes regulating the inflammatory response are disturbed, pathological injury to the host results. Perhaps this is best exemplified by the current theories regarding the pathophysiology of septic shock, in which an abnormally regulated inflammatory response to a stimulus results in overproduction of cytokines such as IL-1 and TNF-α (18). This then leads to the characteristic clinical spectrum of sepsis as marked by hypotension and organ dysfunction. Better understanding of the factors regulating cytokine production during inflammatory responses is needed to better define pathological processes and develop improved immunotherapeutic agents.

Cytokine Receptors

Although studies regarding the regulation of cytokine production by cells are needed, similar studies to understand the factors that regulate cytokine receptor expression are essential. Cytokines effect their actions on target cells only if these cells bear specific cytokine receptors. In general, cytokine receptors are dimers or trimers of membrane-bound subunits which, when bound, change conformation and trigger a signal via the intracellular component of the receptor. Then, through a variety of intracellular signaling mechanisms (often coupled with G proteins), cellular activity is altered after translocation of the signal into the cell nucleus and binding to the appropriate gene promoter(s).

Cytokine receptors tend to have similar structure and function. For example, there are three members of the IL-1 receptor family, IL-1RI, IL-1RII, and T1/ST2/Fit-1 (10). The extracellular domains of these receptors share significant homology with three immunoglobulin-like domains, but their intracellular structures are quite different. Most IL-1 mediated activities are translated through IL-1RI, but the definitive signal transduction mechanisms utilized by this receptor have yet to be fully characterized. Notably, the cytosolic portion of IL-1RII is truncated, such that this receptor acts as a "decoy" receptor and no intracellular signal is transmitted after binding IL-1.

Additionally, IL-1α and IL-1ß appear to bind to different and distinct peptide sequences on the same receptor. Like IL-1, TNF-α utilizes several dimeric receptors. The TNF-α receptor family includes two primary types, the 55 kDa and 75 kDa receptors, which mediate intracellular signals via several novel intracellular proteins called TRAFs (TNF receptor associated factors) as well as several other proteins that appear to transmit death signals to the cell nucleus (e.g., fas) (11).

A complicated family of receptors binds to IL-6 and related proteins. These receptors all contain gp130, along with one or two other monomers that confer specificity for each cytokine (14). The IL-6 receptor has one IL-6 binding receptor that pairs with a gp130/gp130 homodimer, whereas LIF binds to the LIF receptor and one gp130 monomer. OSM binds to either LIF/gp130 or OMR/gp130, making dimers, and IL-11 binds to a specific receptor that binds to a homodimer of gp130, similar to IL-6. Thus these cytokines all require gp130 for normal function and transmission of intracellular signals, all utilizing the JAK-STAT signal transmitting system.

Among the two chemokine families, chemokine-receptor interactions are varied, being either relatively exclusive or more indiscriminate (12). The CC-CKR-1 receptor binds most C-C chemokines, but few of the C-X-C chemokines, whereas the CXC-CKR-1 receptor binds most C-X-C chemokines but none of the other family. Of these two receptor types, there are at least four subtypes of CXC-CKR and five subtypes of CC-CKR. Chemokine receptor expression appears to play a key role in the pathogenesis of HIV infection leading to AIDS. HIV utilizes chemokine receptors for entry into macrophages and T cells, and occupation of the receptors with their specific chemokine prevents cellular infection.

Although a receptor for IL-10 has been detected, it is unclear if IL-10 receptors fall into families such as described above (14). IL-4 and related cytokines bind with high affinity to hematopoietin receptors but, unlike other members of the family that bind to heterodimers, IL-4 binds to a single hematopoietin-binding domain (15). There have been at least two TGF-ß receptors identified, and a recently described receptor named endoglin binds to TGF-ß1 and TGF-ß3, but not TGF-ß2 (16). Endoglin is highly expressed on endothelial cells and binds with TGF-ß1 and TGF-ß3 with high affinity. Thus receptor availability for any cytokine is critical for each specific cytokine to exert its action on the target cells.

Key Characteristics of Cytokines

Notably, several cytokines are described in each type of immune response, highlighting important characteristics of cytokines. First, there is great *redundancy* in cytokines, such that several cytokines may have similar function. An excellent example is provided by IL-1 and TNF-α, where cytokines coded by different genes on different chromosomes have remarkably similar effects. Another important characteristic of cytokines is *pleiotropy*, or multiple activities for one protein. An excellent example of this characteristic is IL-6, in that this cytokine has multiple and varied activities depending upon the experimental conditions employed. The nature of cytokines thus clouds the certainty for the specific role for each cytokine in any one condition. Although transgenic technology has helped to elucidate some roles for cytokines in mice, these experiments often result in prompting more questions rather than providing definitive answers. Lastly, cytokines can have *different effects at differing concentrations*. An excellent example in animal reproductive biology is the role of TNF-α during pregnancy, where physiological TNF-α appears to play an important role in early embryonic development (19), but can be embryolethal at high concentrations later in pregnancy (20).

Clearly, a detailed understanding of the regulation of cytokine production by immune effector cells and other cells not classically considered immune effectors is critical to understanding the role of cytokines in normal physiological processes and pathophysiological conditions.

SOME PRECAUTIONARY NOTES

The remainder of this chapter will addresses the potential role(s) of cytokines in preterm labor and normal labor at term. In the following discussions, there are references to the detection of cytokines in the amniotic fluid and serum of pregnant women during normal and preterm labor. One must be extremely cautious in interpreting the meaning of cytokines detected in body fluids, particularly with regard to inferring causative pathophysiology for these different conditions.

In an insightful review, Whiteside (21) notes that cytokine concentrations in body fluids are subject to a number of potentially confounding variables. For example, many ELISA kits for cytokines detect only monomers of the protein, whereas cytokines often tend to form multimers and would thus escape detection. Also, some cytokines are bound to carrier proteins and may escape detection, but some of the same cytokine may be free, thus leading to spurious results. Thus there may be nonspecific and specific binding proteins that could interfere with detection. Additionally, several cytokines (e.g., IL-6, TNF-α) have circulating receptors that can alter assay results, and IL-1 has a circulating receptor antagonist (IL-1Ra) that must be accounted for when evaluating the effects of IL-1. Other similar proteins yet to be discovered could exist for other cytokines. Moreover, circulating antibodies specific for cytokines have been described and viruses have been reported to produce a protein similar to a TNF receptor that is detected by the assay. Also, Epstein–Barr virus produces a truncated form of IL-10 that has only some of the activity of native IL-10 but binds in assays.

Other considerations include the short half-life of cytokines in the circulation, usually less than a few minutes. Thus cytokines are rarely detected in the serum of normal healthy individuals. Excess cytokine detected in serum could suppress production of other cytokines and excessive utilization of a cytokine may make it undetectable. Some cytokines, such as TNF-α, are active in a membrane-bound form and thus would not be detected in serum and still have potent activity.

Lastly, different commercially available kits for the same cytokine in a specific sample may yield different values. There have been international standards developed for clinical use by the World Health Organization through the Biological Response Modifier Program in Frederick, Maryland (21). However, most commercially available kits for cytokine detection for research purposes do not undergo such careful scrutiny. Certainly, different antibody pairs used in these kits can have different specificities for different antigenic epitopes on the cytokine itself. These differences could account for some of the differences in cytokine levels in amniotic fluid and serum reported from different laboratories, as described below. Hence caution must be used when comparing values from different laboratories, particularly with regard to cutoff values as determined using receiver–operator curves.

THE ROLE OF CYTOKINES IN PRETERM LABOR

General Concepts

Depending upon the patient population, anywhere from 10% to 30% of instances of preterm labor may be due to intrauterine infection, often subclinical in nature (22). Only a minority of cases of preterm labor can be attributed to clinically evident intrauterine infection. Hence most cases of preterm labor due to intrauterine infection are likely the result of an inflammatory response in the gestational tissues. This inflammatory process is mediated by cytokine production and results in prostaglandin production, which plays an important role in the onset and propagation of myometrial contractility and subsequent labor and birth (23).

Inflammatory Stimuli: Bacteria as a Possible Cause of Preterm Labor

As noted above, classic inflammatory responses can be considered to consist of four different phases: initiation, attraction of immune effector cells, immunomodulation, and resolution. Obviously, inflammatory responses can be initiated by any number of potential stimuli, from foreign bodies (e.g., splinters) to specific bacterial pathogens. In preterm labor, there are a number of candidate organisms that may elicit an inflammatory response that could mediate preterm contractions (Table 8.1) (24). Among those listed, the most likely common organisms include bacterial vaginosis (BV), Group B streptococci (GBS), trichomonas, and gram-negative organisms. How these different organisms initiate the inflammatory response in maternal decidua is not clear. Figure 8.2 shows the anatomy of human gestational tissues upon which most of the following discussion is based. One possible conceptual framework for the pathogenesis of infection associated preterm labor is suggested in Figure 8.3 and is discussed in greater detail.

Some investigators have challenged the postulated role for infection in the pathogenesis of preterm labor (25). However, each of these criticisms can be addressed by a careful review of the literature and prudent interpretation of pertinent studies. First, recent studies regarding the association of BV strongly suggest that alterations of the vaginal microflora contribute to preterm birth. McGregor et al. (26) showed convincingly that, in a high-risk population for preterm birth, treatment of common genital tract infections detected at the first prenatal visit could significantly reduce the chances for preterm birth. In their population, 19% of women with BV left untreated delivered preterm, whereas 9% of women negative for BV experienced preterm birth.

Table 8.1. Organisms implicated in infection-associated preterm labor (24)

Bacteroides sp.
Chlamydia trachomatis
Coliforms
   Enterobacter sp.
   Escherichia coli
   Klebsiella pneumoniae
   Proteus mirabilis
Fusobacterium nucleatum
Gardnerella vaginalis
Hemophilus influenzae
Listeria monocytogenes
Mobiluncus sp.
Mycoplasma hominis
Neisseria gonorrheae
Staphylococcus aureus
Streptococcus agalactiae (Group B)
Streptococcus faecalis (Group D)
Treponema pallidum
Trichomonas vaginalis

If treated, however, BV positive women had the same rate of preterm birth as BV negative women. Hillier et al. (27) showed in a low-risk population that screening women at 23 to 26 weeks gestation for BV could identify a high-risk population for preterm birth, and that BV was associated with preterm birth independent of other previously described risk factors such as socioeconomic class and prior history of preterm birth. Additionally, Hauth (28) showed that, in a high-risk population for preterm birth, 49% of women with untreated BV experienced preterm birth whereas 31% of treated BV-positive women delivered preterm. He concluded that antibiotic treatment for BV significantly reduced rates of preterm birth in women with BV. These studies strongly suggest that BV is an independent risk factor for preterm birth, indicating a possible cause and effect relationship.

Although it is impossible to test this theory in women, several animal models have been developed that further support the role of infection as a cause of preterm labor. Gravett et al. (29) have pioneered the use of a primate model for infection-induced preterm labor. In their model, pregnant rhesus monkeys on day 130 of gestation (of a 167 day gestation) can be infected intraamniotically (or via other routes) resulting in preterm birth. Moreover, amniotic fluid (AF) in these monkeys displays a similar pattern of pro-inflammatory cytokines and prostaglandins as noted in women (see below). Several investigators, including Oshiro et al (30), Hirsh et al. (31), Fidel et al. (32), and Kaga et al. (33) (among others), have developed the mouse as a possible model for infection associated preterm labor. In our model, we inject pregnant mice at days 12–14 of a 19 day gestation with LPS or pro-inflammatory cytokines and have noted preterm delivery within 24 h of injection. After injection, cytokine and

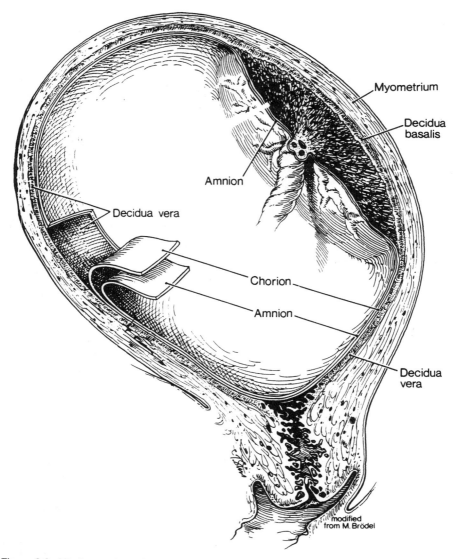

Figure 8.2. Uterine anatomy. In this cross-sectional drawing, note the close approximation of fetal membranes to vagina via the cervix. Modified from Cunningham FG, MacDonald PC, Gant N, et al (eds). Williams Obstetrics (20th ed). Stamford: Appleton & Lange, 1997:112. Reprinted with permission.

prostaglandin production by decidual explants as noted in other animal models occurs. Romero et al. (34) showed that IL-1 induces preterm delivery in mice, and their group also determined that peritoneal injection of LPS in pregnant mice at day 15 of gestation resulted in marked increases of serum and amniotic fluid concentrations of

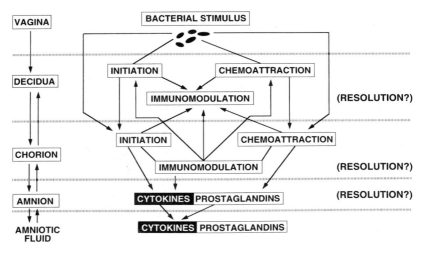

Figure 8.3. General concept of infection-associated preterm labor. In this figure, vaginal microbial flora ascend through the cervix to elicit a cytokine response from the maternal decidua. The maternal decidua and fetal chorion and amnion then transmit signals via different classes of cytokines with the ultimate result being prostaglandin production leading to uterine activity.

IL-1-α and IL-6. Also, Dombroski et al. (35) have developed an ascending infection model for preterm birth using pregnant rabbits. In this model, bacterial inoculation via the vagina results in preterm birth. Thus animal models also strongly suggest that there is a possible cause and effect relationship between infection and preterm birth.

In studies of human gestational membranes isolated from women with infection associated preterm birth, there is a strong association between infection of the chorioamnion and histological chorioamnionitis. Hillier et al. (36) showed that the recovery of any organism from the chorioamnion was strongly associated with histological chorioamnionitis with an odds ratio of 7.2. Moreover, the proportion of placentas with evidence of infection was greatest among those women delivering earliest. In a follow-up study, Hillier et al. (37) correlated AF cytokine production with histological chorioamnionitis and preterm birth. They found that elevations of amniotic fluid cytokines and prostaglandins predicted delivery at less than 34 weeks and within 7 days of amniocentesis. Romero et al. (38) showed that there was a strong association between positive AF bacterial cultures and histological chorioamnionitis as well as the severity of inflammation. Acute inflammation of the chorionic plate was the most sensitive indicator of microbial invasion of the amniotic cavity, and they concluded that the presence of acute inflammatory lesions in the chorioamnion was a marker of infection in the amniotic fluid. These in vivo studies of tissues are limited because the tissues are isolated after birth, and hence a definitive cause and effect relationship cannot be proved. Regardless, they are strong evidence that infection of the gestational tissues is associated with histological chorioamnionitis and is highly correlated with the cytokines and prostaglandins detected in the amniotic fluid of women with infection associated preterm labor.

McDonald and Casey (25) also argue that the marked differences in cytokine and prostaglandin concentrations in two different compartments of amniotic fluid indicate that infection does not play a role in preterm labor and that these substances are the result of labor rather than the cause. They suggest that the increased concentrations of these substances in the "forebag" at the cervix are greater than the "hindbag" near the uterine fundus are merely the result of the labor process. First, it is difficult to prove or disprove any hypothesis based upon amniotic fluid concentrations of cytokines and arachidonic acid metabolites. As noted above (21), one must use great caution when interpreting the data collected from the detection of substances, such as cytokines and prostaglandins, in the serum and amniotic fluid of women. Just as one cannot, using such studies, prove that a cause and effect relationship between infection and preterm birth exists, one also cannot prove that one does not exist. These substances in AF have many potential sources and possible confounding influences. Second, cytokines and prostaglandins are merely messengers produced by cells in response to a stimulus. In this regard, their argument is entirely correct in that these substances are not the cause per se of labor. An alternative interpretation is that they are mediating the inflammatory response stimulated by bacterial inoculation of the maternal and fetal tissues overlying the cervix and in the lower uterine segment. These intermediaries then transmit their messages to adjacent tissues, inducing gap junctions and promoting the final common pathway of labor.

In summary, there is strong evidence that infection of the maternal decidua and the fetal chorioamniotic membranes is causative for some cases of preterm labor. The following discussion focuses on the intermediary role of cytokines in this pathophysiological process. In this context, cytokines do not cause preterm labor but are likely key messengers relaying an inflammatory signal from the stimuli to the myometrium, resulting in uterine activity and eventual birth.

Initiation: Interleukin-1 and Tumor Necrosis Factor α

Both IL-1 and TNF-α can be found in elevated concentrations in the AF of women experiencing preterm labor. IL-1ß was found to be key component among IL-1 subtypes, and there was a strong correlation between IL-1ß and prostaglandin concentrations in one report by Romero et al. (39). In a subsequent report regarding IL-1α and IL-1ß in preterm labor (40), this group found that 100% of women with positive cultures had detectable IL-1ß, whereas half of women with negative cultures of AF had detectable IL-1ß. Also, IL-1 was found in greater AF concentrations in women with preterm PROM, preterm labor, and with positive AF cultures. Similarly, Carroll et al. (41) found elevated IL-1ß concentrations of AF taken from women with preterm PROM and early delivery.

IL-1Ra is detected in very high concentrations in AF, but in one study AF IL-1Ra was not increased in the AF of women with preterm labor despite increases in AF IL-1α and IL-1ß found in these same samples (42). Notably, this same group later found that IL-1Ra was indeed significantly increased in fetal serum and AF in the presence of microbial invasion (43). Potential sources of IL-1Ra from human gestational tissues include amnion, chorion, and decidua, but the decidua appears to be the primary source (44). IL-1Ra significantly inhibited PGE2 production by cultured human amnion cells and chorion cells (42), but IL-1Ra was found to have a partial agonist effect on human decidual cell PGE2 production. Two groups have shown that IL-1Ra stimulates PGE2 production by decidual cells (45, 46), the first such finding for this receptor antagonist. Thus the role of IL-1Ra in human parturition is not clear.

TNF-α is also elevated in the amniotic fluid of women with infection associated preterm labor. AF TNF-α concentrations are highest in women with preterm PROM, preterm labor, and positive AF bacterial cultures, whereas TNF-α was detectable in only 10% of women with negative AF cultures experiencing preterm labor (47). Additionally, Kupferminc et al. (48) showed that soluble TNF receptors p55 and p75 are physiological constituents of maternal plasma and amniotic fluid in the second trimester, and concentrations increase into the third trimester, but TNF-α is elevated in the maternal plasma but not amniotic fluid in the second trimester. Laham et al. (49) further showed that maternal TNF-α concentrations did not change with pregnancy or labor, but that AF TNF-α concentrations increased over the course of pregnancy and in association with preterm labor. In an interesting study evaluating TNF-α in the lower genital tract, Inglis et al. (50) found that the presence of TNF-α in cervical secretions was predictive of subsequent preterm delivery at a rate similar to fetal fibronectin, with an odds ratio of 6.2.

Maternal decidua is one potential source for TNF-α. Casey et al. (51) showed that cultured decidual cells and decidual explants produced TNF-α after stimulation with LPS. Vince et al. (52) also found that term decidual explants produced TNF-α after stimulation with LPS. TNF-α in the first trimester was primarily localized to the decidual macrophages, but in the third trimester both decidual and chorionic villous trophoblast contained TNF-α mRNA. Fortunato et al. (53) also found that explants of human fetal membranes produced TNF-α after stimulation with LPS and that non-stimulated explants of amniochorion contained TNF-α in amnion and chorion, as well as TNF-α p55 receptor, although they do not specify the number of samples used. Dudley et al. (54) found TNF-α mRNA expressed in only one-third of gestational membranes isolated from more than 50 women experiencing a variety of clinical scenarios, including normal term labor, preterm labor and delivery, and infection associated preterm labor and delivery. Austgulen et al. (55) found abundant expression of TNF receptors p55 and p75 in human placenta, and in particular the p55 receptor was found in villous syncytiotrophoblasts and decidual cells. These receptors likely mediate the cytotoxic effects of TNF-α on human placental trophoblasts noted by Yui et al. (56), suggesting that TNF-α may have an apoptotic role in placenta. Also, TNF-α has been reported to stimulate metalloproteinases by human chorionic cells and thus may contribute to collagenase remodeling of the uterine cervix (57).

Along with TNF-α, decidua can produce IL-1, as shown by Romero and colleagues (58). In these experiments, decidual explants produced IL-1 in response to LPS. Baergan et al. (59) found IL-1 using immunocytohistological techniques in the amnion, trophoblast, and decidua from all placentas evaluated. Using placental cell cultures, Steinborn et al. (60) found increased IL-1ß production women delivering preterm compared to women delivering at term not in labor. Dudley et al. (54) found that IL-1ß mRNA is distributed throughout the decidua, chorion, and amnion of women after preterm and term labor, regardless of being associated with clinically evident infection.

One note of caution is needed regarding the use of dispersed cell monolayers as opposed to explant cultures. Lonsdale et al. (61) found that the dispersion of decidual cells into monolayer cultures resulted in significant production of inflammatory cytokines, 10- to 300-fold greater than produced by explants. Their data indicate that it is difficult to infer many conclusions regarding in vivo pathophysiology utilizing dispersed cells. However, studies of the regulation of cytokine production using monolayer cell cultures can still provide valuable data as to the regulatory influences that can modify cytokine production by these cells. In a separate compelling study from the same group (62), it was found that intact membranes from term pregnancies did not allow the passage of a significant proportion of cytokines from one side to the other (generally less than 15%). However, this study did not address membranes from preterm deliveries or from membranes with inflammation.

Animal models similarly show a possible role for IL-1 and TNF-α in preterm delivery. Romero et al. showed that IL-1 stimulated preterm delivery in mice (34) and that this effect was abrogated with the IL-1 receptor antagonist (63). In a separate study, injection of pregnant rats with TNF-α, IL-1, and LPS caused fetal deaths and resorptions associated with necrosis (64). Silver et al. (65) showed that LPS-induced fetal death in mice is likely due to a maternal response to LPS rather than a direct toxic effect of the LPS, mostly mediated by TNF-α. Treatment with IL-1Ra and soluble TNF receptor/Fc fusion protein did not prevent preterm birth after LPS administration to pregnant mice (66). Baggia et al. (67) showed that IL-1ß infusion in the amniotic cavity of rhesus monkeys resulted in intra-amniotic production of TNF-α and prostaglandins with resultant uterine activity, suggesting that IL-1ß and TNF-α may act synergistically to elicit uterine contractions. In this same model, intraamniotic infection with GBS induces significant amounts of AF IL-1Ra (68). In the rabbit model of preterm labor, intracervical inoculation of *E. coli* is associated with increased AF concentrations of TNF-α, IL-1, and prostaglandins (69). These animal studies indicate that IL-1 and TNF-α mediate the pathophysiological events leading to pregnancy loss associated with LPS, IL-1, or TNF-α administration.

In summary, there are compelling data from human and animal studies to indicate that a critical component of the inflammatory response in gestational tissues to bacterial stimuli is the production of IL-1 and TNF-α, and that these pro-inflammatory cytokines are important signals to the innate immune response to become activated and amplified. Moreover, these cytokines themselves appear to have toxic properties against maternal and fetal tissues at the high concentrations noted in these pathological conditions. Hence the maternal response appears to be key component of the pathophysiology of infection associated preterm labor.

Chemoattraction: Chemokines

Chemokines have elevated AF and serum concentrations in women experiencing preterm labor. IL-8, previously known as neutrophil attractant/activating peptide-1, has perhaps been the most extensively studied chemokine in pregnancy. Romero et al.

(70) first reported elevations of IL-8 in AF of women with preterm labor, and they found the highest concentrations of IL-8 in the AF of women with microbial invasion of the amniotic cavity. In a follow-up study from their previous work evaluating leukotactic factors in AF, Chernouny et al. (71) also found that IL-8 was elevated in the AF of women with histological chorioamnionitis and preterm labor. Further, they found that AF IL-8 was a more sensitive indicator of histological chorioamnionitis and preterm delivery than AF culture. Puchner et al. (72) found AF IL-8 concentrations highest in women with clinically evident intrauterine infection, and only rarely were IL-8 concentrations elevated in women with no evidence of infection. Albert et al. (73) found that AF IL-8 concentrations could predict responsiveness to tocolytic therapy, and that IL-8 concentrations of greater than 15 ng/mL were associated with inevitable labor and delivery. Conversely, Laham et al. (74) reported that AF IL-8 concentrations were not elevated in women with preterm labor, but that they were elevated in term labor. However, there is considerable overlap of values in their data. Another C-X-C chemokine, GROα, has been reported to be elevated in AF of women with intra-amniotic infection (75).

In cord serum, IL-8 concentrations had more sensitivity and specificity than did other conventional markers of infection such as C-reactive protein, in the early detection of chorioamnionitis (76). However, in maternal plasma Laham et al. (74) found no increase in IL-8 concentrations with labor or intrauterine infection.

Representing the C-C chemokines, MIP-1α is also increased in the AF of women with infection associated preterm labor. Romero et al. (77) reported that MIP-1α concentrations were elevated in the AF of women with microbial invasion of the AF, both in term and preterm labor. Also, MIP-1α concentrations correlated well with AF IL-8 and white blood cell count. Dudley et al. (78) also reported elevated concentrations of MIP-1α in the AF of women with preterm labor and clinically evident intrauterine infection. Moreover, there were elevations of AF MIP-1α with normal term labor and a significant correlation between AF MIP-1α concentrations and cervical dilation in women with term labor.

Potential sources of the chemokines noted in these AF samples include maternal decidua and fetal chorion and amnion. Kelly et al. (79) first reported that choriodecidual cells in culture produced IL-8, and that this IL-8 production was inhibited by progesterone at 1 μmol/L. The uterine cervix has also been found to produce relatively large amounts of IL-8 in vitro and thus may be another source for the IL-8 found in amniotic fluid (80). Dudley et al. (81) found that cultured decidual cells and chorion cells produced IL-8 in a concentration-dependent fashion after incubation with IL-1ß, TNF-α, and LPS. Additionally, Trautman et al. (82) found that amnion cells similarly produced significant quantities of IL-8 after incubation with these same substances, and Fortunato et al. (53) found that amniochorion produced IL-8. Dudley et al. (54) found that IL-8 mRNA was expressed throughout the decidua, chorion, and amnion in all patients tested after labor, regardless of whether the labor was term, preterm, or associated with clinically evident intrauterine infection.

Placental explants obtained from different clinical scenarios were compared by Shimoya et al. (83) with regard to IL-8 production. They found that the presence or absence of labor did not affect IL-8 production, but that placentas with histological chorioamnionitis had significantly higher IL-8 production that those without chorioamnionitis. Histological analysis revealed that IL-8 was produced by trophoblast cells and macrophage-like cells. Similarly, Saito et al. (84) showed that IL-8 immunolocalized to cytotrophoblast, syncytiotrophoblast, Hofbauer cells, decidual stromal cells and lymphocytes, and endometrial gland cells. Notably, Reisenberger et al. (85) showed that the placenta is relatively impermeable to transfer or diffusion of IL-8, and they conclude that this finding may account for the differences in serum and AF IL-8 concentrations.

Dudley et al. (86) reported that human decidual cells produced MIP-1α in response to IL-1, TNF-α, IL-4, and LPS. Moreover, they have reported that cultured human decidual cells (87) and chorion cells (88) produce MIP-1α in response to heat-killed GBS and to purified bacterial virulence factors such as lipoteichoic acid and sialic acid. Hence decidual cells and chorion cells are potential sources for chemokines noted in infection associated preterm labor.

In rabbits, IL-8 is cross-reactive with human IL-8, whereas no homologue for IL-8 has been described for the mouse. Using reagents for human IL-8, Ito et al. (89) found that IL-8 production by fibroblast isolated from the rabbit cervix was inhibited by physiological concentrations of progesterone, similar to reports of Barclay et al. (80). El Maradney et al. (90) found that human IL-8 induced cervical ripening in nonpregnant and pregnant rabbits, and this cervical ripening was associated with a significant neutrophilic infiltrate. Although it is difficult to reconcile rabbit studies with human IL-8, these studies provide compelling evidence for a potential role of IL-8 in parturition, particularly with regard to cervical remodeling.

In summary, chemokines are found to be markedly elevated in the AF of women with infection-associated preterm labor and human gestational tissues are one potential source for these chemokines. Given the regulation of chemokine production by IL-1ß and TNF-α, it seems likely that chemoattraction into gestational tissues with resultant chorioamnionitis is intimately associated with the production of IL-1ß and TNF-α. Moreover, there is evidence that bacterial stimuli will induce chemokine production directly from these cells. Chemokines therefore likely play a key role in amplifying the inflammatory response in these tissues.

Immunomodulation: IL-6

Perhaps the best studied of all cytokines during pregnancy is IL-6. IL-6 has been found to be elevated in the amniotic fluid of women with preterm labor and infection associated preterm labor in numerous studies. Romero et al. (91) in the first report of elevated concentrations of AF IL-6 also found that decidual explants produced IL-6 in response to LPS. In subsequent studies by this group, IL-6 has been found to be among the most sensitive and specific indicators of infection associated preterm labor. In consecutive studies, they found that IL-6 was a better indicator of microbial invasion of the amniotic cavity, amniocentesis-to-delivery interval, and neonatal complications than gram stain, glucose concentration, and white blood cell count in women with both preterm labor with intact membranes (92) and preterm PROM (93). They proposed a cutoff of 11.2 ng/mL IL-6 in AF based upon re-

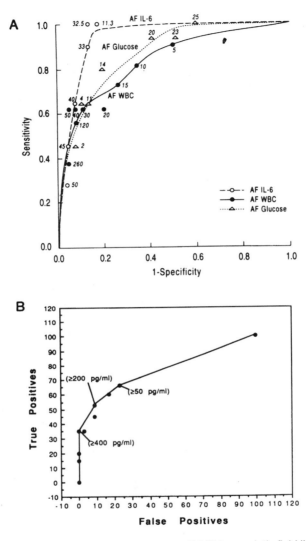

Figure 8.4. Comparison of receiver–operator curves (ROC) for amniotic fluid IL-6. Panel A represents one ROC from one study in which the discriminatory value for amniotic fluid IL-6 is 11.3 ng/mL, whereas the ROC depicted in panel B shows a discriminatory value for IL-6 to be 200 pg/mL. The lower panel shows a third discriminatory value for IL-6 of 6.17 ng/mL. These figures show that different studies with different assays will yield different discriminatory values for this cytokine. (Panel A is reprinted with permission from Romero R, et al., Am J Obstet Gynecol 1993;169:805–816. © 1993 Mosby-Year Book, Inc. Panel B is reprinted with permission from Dudley BJ, et al., Br J Obstet Gynecol 1994;101:592–597. © 1994 Royal College of Obstetricians and Gynecologists. Panel C is reprinted by permission from Coultrip LL, et al., Am J Obstet Gynecol 1994;171:901–911. © 1994 Mosby-Year Book, Inc.).

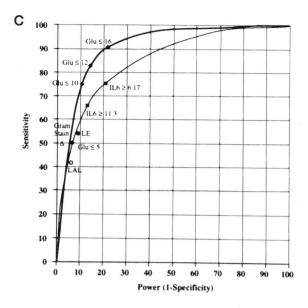

ceiver–operator curves (see Fig. 8.4). In a follow-up study, Romero et al. (94) found that AF IL-6 was a sensitive and rapid test for the detection of microbial invasion of the amniotic cavity and suggested that the test may be useful in identifying women at risk for preterm birth and neonates at increased risk for morbidity and mortality. Also, Yoon et al. (95) determined that AF IL-6 was a sensitive test for the prospective diagnosis of histological chorioamnionitis, but that the best discriminatory value was 17 ng/mL. Moreover, AF IL-6 was more sensitive for predicting infectious morbidity than AF culture.

Saito et al. (96) also found that AF obtained from women with infection associated preterm labor had 20- to 30-fold higher concentrations than did women with no evidence of infection. Greig et al. (97) reported that AF IL-6 concentrations correlated well with the presence of histological chorioamnionitis and positive AF cultures in women with preterm labor and intact membranes. They found evidence for a discriminatory value of 600 pg/mL with 100% sensitivity and 89% specificity, with a positive predictive value of 85%. Contrary to the findings of Romero et al. (92) Coultrip et al. (98) found that AF glucose concentrations were slightly more specific and sensitive then AF IL-6 determinations in women with preterm labor (Fig. 8.4). Moreover, they found that a discriminatory value of 6.17 ng/mL was more predictive of preterm delivery. Lastly, Andrews et al. (99) confirmed these studies and found that AF IL-6 concentrations were higher and inversely proportional to gestational age in women with intact membranes and reflected chorioamnion colonization even when AF cultures were negative.

Similarly, Dudley et al. (100) found that AF IL-6 concentrations were increased in women with preterm labor, and that IL-6 was predictive of preterm birth regardless of infectious morbidity (Fig. 8.4). However, we found a different discriminatory value for IL-6 in the prediction of preterm birth at 200 pg/mL. The discrepancy in the suggested discriminatory values between the three groups depicted in Figure 8.4 likely is the result of the use of different assays and indicates the need for universal agreement on assays and standards before widespread clinical application of this test.

In the only study regarding other immunomodulatory cytokines during preterm labor, Waring et al. (101) reported that AF LIF concentrations were also elevated in women with preterm labor associated with intra-amniotic infection. They also found that human gestational tissue explants produced LIF in response to LPS, IL-1ß, and TNF-α. Little work has been done regarding the possible contribution of oncostatin M and IL-11 to the pathophysiology of preterm labor.

Serum IL-6 concentrations have also been found to be elevated in women with preterm PROM and preterm labor. Murtha et al. (102) found that serum IL-6 concentrations were much greater in women with preterm PROM, particularly if they delivered within 24 h of sampling, and that these values correlated well with both clinical and histological chorioamnionitis. Laham et al. (103) similarly found that plasma IL-6 concentrations were elevated in women with preterm labor, but were not elevated in women at term in normal labor. Conversely, Lencki et al. (104) found no correlation of serum IL-6 concentrations with clinical chorioamnionitis, although umbilical cord blood IL-6 concentrations were elevated in this setting. Moreover, Yoon et al. (105) found that umbilical cord plasma IL-6 concentrations were highly correlated with the occurrence of periventricular leukomalacia (PVL) in neonates. Their findings supported the hypothesis that cytokines may mediate brain injury resulting in PVL and that intrauterine infection may play an important role in the pathophysiology of white matter damage. Further, they suggest that strategies to prevent PVL should commence prior to birth.

As noted above, IL-6 has been shown to be produced by decidual explants (91). Dudley et al. (106) showed that production of IL-6 by cultured monolayers of human decidual cells was regulated by IL-1ß, TNF-α, and LPS. Similar findings were made for cultured monolayers of human chorion cells (107). Matsuzaki et al. (108) found that explants of placentas obtained from women with clinical chorioamnionitis produced more IL-6 than placental explants from women at term, both in labor and not in labor. Additionally, Pasetto et al. (109) used decidual explants and fetal membrane explants to show that IL-6 was produced by these tissues but there was no difference between women in labor and women having cesarean section. Saito et al. (96) showed that IL-6 was immunolocalized to syncytiotrophoblast, cytotrophoblast, Hofbauer cells, decidual stromal cells, and maternal macrophages. Utilizing decidual stromal cell cultures, Montes et al. (110) showed that secretion of decidual cell IL-6 production was inhibited by progesterone at concentrations of 100 nmol/L.

Menon et al. (111) isolated mRNA from amniochorionic membranes of women with and without intrauterine infection and found that amnion and chorion from women with infection expressed both mRNA and protein for IL-6. Dudley et al. (54) isolated mRNA from the gestational tissues from over 50 women experiencing normal term labor, preterm labor, and preterm labor associated with intrauterine infection and showed that IL-6 mRNA was expressed throughout decidua, chorion, and amnion in similar patterns in all women after labor regardless of the presence of infection. In a recent publication, Laham et al. (112) showed that IL-6 is a physiological constituent of amniotic fluid and that IL-6 production by human gestational tissues is differentially regulated by LPS and the spontaneous onset of labor. In this study, they found that IL-6 production by explant cultures of membranes and placenta could be detected after labor, and that LPS stimulated significant production of IL-6 by placental and choriodecidual explants but not by explants of amnion.

Besides the potential clinical value of AF IL-6 determinations, studies have shown that determination of IL-6 in vaginal secretions may also have clinical applicability. Lockwood et al. (113) found that IL-6 in cervical secretions was associated with preterm delivery. In this study, an IL-6 level in cervical secretions of greater than 250 pg/mL was an independent predictor of preterm delivery. However, IL-6 concentration in cervical secretions, although specific, was not a particularly sensitive indicator of women with preterm deliveries and did not correlate with maternal intrauterine infection. In a confirmatory study, Rizzo et al. (114) showed that IL-6 at a concentration of greater than 410 pg/mL had a sensitivity of 67% and a specificity of 91%, similar to that of Lockwood's study. They also found no correlations between cervical IL-6 concentrations, the occurrence of bacterial vaginosis, and other cervical pathogens. Cervical concentrations of IL-6 correlated well with the presence of chorioamnionitis even in the absence of positive amniotic fluid cultures.

It is interesting to note that, although IL-6 is among the most extensively studied cytokines in preterm labor, the role that IL-6 plays in intrauterine infection and preterm labor remains to be elucidated. Mitchell et al. (115) showed that IL-6 stimulated PGE_2 production by amnion cells and decidual cells, but only at high concentrations. IL-6 plays a key endocrine role by activating the acute phase response and thus is likely an important mediator of the systemic response to intrauterine infection. However, this has not been definitively shown in either human or animal models. We have found that murine decidual explants produce increased amounts of IL-6 after administration of LPS (116), but could not establish a role for IL-6. Regardless, IL-6 determinations in amniotic fluid, serum, and/or cervical secretions appear to have the best potential for clinical utility among all the cytokines studied thus far.

Resolution and Inhibition: IL-10, IL-4, and TGF-ß

Studies regarding the role of immunosuppressive cytokines in preterm labor are still in their infancy. IL-10 is a key cytokine synthesis inhibitor, yet little is know about IL-10 during pregnancy. Heyborne et al. (117) found that IL-10 concentrations in the AF of women taken at the time of genetic amniocentesis in the early second trimester could predict the occurrence of small-for-gestational age (SGA) infants. They found that IL-10 concentrations were elevated in the AF of pregnancies destined to become SGA and speculated that this reflected a generalized or dysregulated immune activation during pregnancy. Conversely, Spong et al (118) could not confirm these findings in their patient population. In the setting of preterm labor, Greig et al. (119) reported that AF concentrations of IL-10 were elevated in women with clinically evident chorioamnionitis, a finding that Dudley et al. (120) were unable to confirm.

Regarding the potential sources of IL-10 from gestational tissues, Cadet et al. (121) first reported that IL-10 was expressed in placenta and placental bed. Roth et al. (122) also reported that human placental cytotrophoblasts from all stages of pregnancy produced IL-10 and they were able to detect IL-10 in placenta and placental bed. Based on these findings, both groups suggested that IL-10 may be important in maintaining maternal tolerance of the allogeneic fetus. Similarly, Trautman et al. (123) have detected IL-10 in trophoblasts, but can find little IL-10 production by chorion cells and amnion cells in culture. We found that cultured human decidual cells secreted modest amounts of IL-10 after stimulation with IL-1ß and LPS. Speculating that fetal membranes may be deficient in the ability to make IL-10, further studies of chorion cells showed that these cells were able to make small amounts of IL-10 in response to LPS (124). Also, IL-10 was expressed in most human gestational tissues after labor, suggesting that an inflammatory infiltrate may contribute to the IL-10 mRNA detected in these samples. Regarding the possible role for IL-10 in infection-associated preterm labor, Fortunato et al. (125) found that IL-10 transcriptionally regulated IL-6 production by human amniochorionic membrane explants. These studies, though provocative, indicate that the role, regulation, and effects of IL-10 during infection associated preterm labor have yet to be elucidated.

Similarly, little is known about the activities of IL-4. Dudley et al. (126) found significant elevations of IL-4 in the amniotic fluid of women with clinically evident intrauterine infection. However, IL-4 has yet to be shown to be produced by human gestational tissues, although IL-4 receptor is present in early pregnancy decidua (127). IL-4 has an interesting paradoxical behavior in human gestational tissues. In monocytes, IL-4 inhibits cyclooxygenase activity and decreases prostaglandin production, suggesting that this is one mechanism by which IL-4 exerts antiinflammatory effects (128). However, in human amnion cells (129), chorion cells, and decidual cells (130), IL-4 enhances prostaglandin production. In a subsequent and confirmatory study, Spaziani et al. (131) found that IL-4 induced cyclooxygenase-II enzyme and PGE_2 production by cultured amnion cells. However, Pasetto et al. (109) found that explants of decidua and fetal membranes obtained from term vaginal deliveries and cesarean deliveries produced no IL-4.

Although TGFß appears to have a key role in the maintenance of pregnancy, TGFß has only rarely been studied for its possible role in infection associated preterm labor. Bry and Hallman (132) found that TGFß inhibited IL-1 and TNF-α stimulated PGE2 production by amnion cells, and they speculated that TGFß may have an important inhibitory role in the pathogenesis of preterm labor. In a subsequent study, they also found that TGF-ß2 prevented preterm birth using a rabbit model of cytokine induced preterm birth and this was associated with decreased AF PGE_2 concentrations (133).

The paucity of studies regarding the resolution and inhibitory phase of inflammation during preterm labor leads to no definitive conclusions. The published studies suggest that these normally inhibitory influences may be abrogated or perhaps paradoxically switched to contribute to uterine activity (e.g., via PGE_2 induced myometrial activity). Much more research is needed to ascertain further the roles of these inhibitory substances during preterm labor.

AN INTRAUTERINE INFLAMMATORY RESPONSE SYNDROME?

Recently, the concept of a systemic inflammatory response syndrome to account for cases of sepsis where no focus of infection is evident has been suggested (Table 8.2) (18). In this emerging paradigm, patients who develop evidence of early sepsis but with no identified causative organism have SIRS, whereas patients with a known source of infection have sepsis. Patients with severe organ dysfunction have multiple organ dysfunction syndrome (MODS) and a high mortality rate. One extension of this hypothesis applicable to preterm labor is to consider the inflammation in maternal decidua to be a local inflammatory response syndrome, or intrauterine inflammatory response syndrome (IUIRS). When an organism is identified as a likely cause of the infection (e.g., positive amniotic fluid cultures, positive vaginal cultures), then the diagnosis of intrauterine infection would be made (Table 8.3).

Table 8.2. ACCP/SCCM classification of sepsis (18)

Systemic Inflammatory Response Syndrome (SIRS)

No documented infection
Two or more of the following conditions:
   Temperature > 38°C or < 36°C
   Pulse > 90 beats per minute
   Respiratory rate > 20 breaths per minute or $PaCO_2$ < 32 mm Hg
   White blood cell count > 12, 000/mm^3, < 4,000/mm^3, or > 10% immature (band) forms

Sepsis

Culture-proven or documented infection, with two or more of the following conditions:
   Temperature > 38°C or < 36°C
   Pulse > 90 beats per minute
   Respiratory rate > 20 breaths per minute or $PaCO_2$ < 32 mm Hg
   White blood cell count > 12, 000/mm3, < 4,000/mm3, or > 10% immature (band) forms

Severe Sepsis

Sepsis associated with:
   Organ dysfunction
   Hypoperfusion as manifested by lactic acidosis, oliguria, or an acute alteration in mental status
   Hypotension (systolic blood pressure < 90 mm Hg or a reduction of [2] 40 mm Hg from baseline in the absence of other causes of hypotension

Septic Shock

Sepsis-induced hypotension despite adequate fluid resuscitation along with hypoperfusion (lactic acid)

Multiple Organ Dysfunction Syndrome (MODS)

Presence of altered organ function in an acutely ill patient such that homeostasis cannot be maintained without intervention

---

Table 8.3. Proposed classification for intrauterine inflammatory response syndrome[a]

Intrauterine Inflammatory Response Syndrome (IUIRS)

No documented infection
Preterm labor with documented cervical change
Clinical signs of intrauterine infection (two or more of the following):
    Temperature > 38°C
    Uterine tenderness
    White blood cell count > 20,000/mm^3
    Foul-smelling vaginal discharge
Amniotic fluid glucose < 15 mg/dL
Increased amniotic fluid cytokine concentrations (e.g., IL-6 > 11.3 ng/mL)

Intrauterine Infection

Documented infection with positive amniotic fluid bacterial cultures or vaginal cultures
Meets criteria for IUIRS (as noted above)

[a] For sepsis, severe sepsis, septic shock, and multiple organ dysfunction syndrome (MODS), see table 8.2.

Chorioamnionitis would thus be limited to a pathological diagnosis and not imply any causative organism.

As SIRS is thought to be the result of an abnormally regulated inflammatory response to a bacterial insult affecting the entire organism, so IUIRS would be the result of an abnormally regulated cytokine response to the inflammatory stimuli affecting gestational tissues (Fig. 8.5). Given the close apposition of gestational tissues to the microbial flora of the vagina, it seems likely that these tissues are often exposed to in-

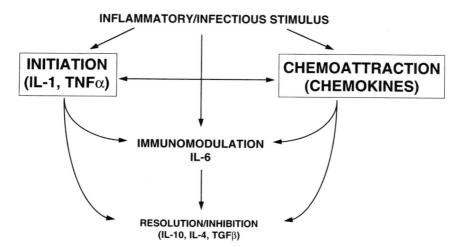

Figure 8.5. General concept for intrauterine inflammatory response syndrome. In this figure, the initiation and chemoattraction phases are enlarged to depict the possible enhanced roles of these phases, whereas the resolution phase is diminished.

flammatory stimuli throughout pregnancy. Yet most pregnancies continue without complications of preterm labor. However, one hypothesis to account for preterm labor is that in some women the normal milieu of pregnancy regulating cytokine production becomes disturbed, thus allowing for either the diminution in the amounts and/or effects of immunosuppressive substances such as IL-10. Alternatively, the promotion of the pro-inflammatory response could overwhelm the inhibitory effects of IL-10. This dysregulated condition thus would lead to overproduction of IL-1, TNF-α, and chemokines as reflected by increased concentrations of pro-inflammatory cytokines in the amniotic fluid and serum. The ultimate response is uterine activity leading to expulsion of the fetus and ultimate resolution of the inflammation after birth.

THE ROLE OF CYTOKINES IN NORMAL PARTURITION

Evidence is emerging that cytokines may also play an intermediary role in the propagation of normal labor at term in the absence of obvious infection. However, caution must be exercised in interpreting these studies because cytokine release by gestational tissues in this setting may reflect a secondary inflammatory response occurring as labor progresses, suggesting that cytokines may have little or no role in this physiological process.

Several investigators have found that cytokines are increased in the AF in women during normal labor at term. AF concentrations of IL-1ß (40), TNF-α (47), IL-6 (100), IL-8 (96), and MIP-1α (78) have all been found to be increased by a number of investigators. We have shown that IL-6 and MIP-1α concentrations increased in AF obtained after inserting a needle into the forebag of women during labor, and that these concentrations correlated with cervical dilation. Similarly, plasma concentrations of TNF-α, IL-1, IL-6, and IL-8 are increased in women during normal term labor (134), leading these investigators to speculate that these cytokines may play a role in normal labor.

Cultured monolayers of decidual cells and chorion cells obtained from normal term pregnancies produce cytokines such as IL-6 (106, 107), IL-8 (81), and MIP-1α (86) readily after stimulation with IL-1ß, TNF-α, and LPS. Explants derived from term decidua produce most every cytokine described in this chapter. Moreover, these studies often described significant basal production of these cytokines without stimulation. Thus gestational tissues obtained from term pregnancies have the potential to produce inflammatory cytokines both constitutively and after inflammatory stimulation with pro-inflammatory cytokines such as IL-1ß and bacterial products such as LPS and lipoteichoic acid.

In vivo studies also support a potential role for cytokines in normal labor (52, 53, 59, 84, 96). Several studies have shown that mRNA for IL-1ß, TNF-α, IL-6, and IL-8 can be detected in gestational membranes obtained from women after labor. Dudley et al. (54) showed that IL-1ß, IL-6, and IL-8 mRNA was readily detected from decidua, chorion, and amnion after labor, and that the pattern of cytokine mRNA expression was similar in all women after labor, regardless of whether this occurred at term, preterm, or associated with intrauterine infection. Notably, TNF-α mRNA was not often detected, suggesting either less of a role for TNF-α or more rapid degradation of the mRNA in this setting. Osmers et al. (135) found that IL-8 was expressed in increasing amounts in gestational tissues prior to the onset of labor at term, and they suggested that IL-8 expression in these tissues may be critical to the process leading to cervical maturation in preparation for labor (Fig. 8.6). Mechanical stretching of the fetal membranes results in increased IL-8 production and collagenase activity (136), and progesterone has been found to inhibit IL-8 production by cultured decidual cells and chorion cells (137). IL-8 and other chemokines may serve to attract monocytes, macrophages, neutrophils, and other immune effector cells into the cervix and lower uterine segment. These chemokines may activate these cells to release collagenases and metalloproteinases, which then could remodel the cervical stroma prior

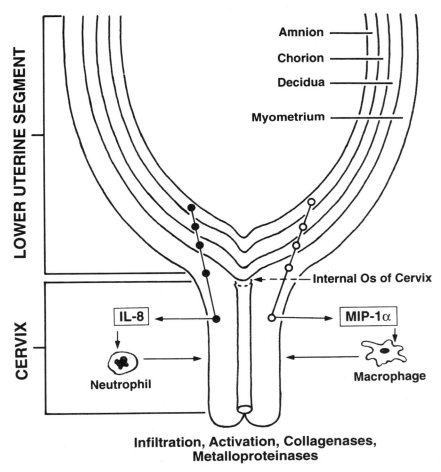

Figure 8.6. The potential role of chemokines in cervical maturation. This figure depicts the possible sources of chemokines from cells in gestational and maternal tissues and the possible effects of the chemokines on cervical status.

to and with the onset of labor (138, 139). Functional or absolute decrease in circulating progesterone may be one regulatory influence that mediates this mechanism.

CONCLUSION

Although much has been learned regarding the production and regulation of inflammatory cytokines during pregnancy, the precise role of these proteins in the physiology of labor and the pathophysiology of preterm labor remains obscure. Further research into the expression and regulation of cytokine receptors in gestational tissues and myometrium is needed, as are studies regarding the potential role for immunosuppressive cytokines in normal and abnormal pregnancies. Additionally, studies regarding bacterial attachment and the signal transduction mechanisms leading to pro-inflammatory cytokine and chemokine gene activation in gestational tissues are critically needed. Such studies could potentially lead to novel and effective immunotherapeutic agents against the inciting event rather than the final common pathway of uterine activity and thus be more effective than currently used tocolytic agents.

REFERENCES

1. Creasy RK. Preterm birth prevention: Where are we? Am J Obstet Gynecol 1993;168:1223–1230.
2. Leveno KJ, Little BB, Cunningham FG. The national impact of ritodrine hydrochloride for inhibition of preterm labor. Obstet Gynecol 1990;76:12–15.
3. Romero R, Mazor M, Munoz H, et al. The preterm labor delivery syndrome. Ann NY Acad Sci 1994:414–429.
4. Dudley DJ, Weidmeier S. The ontogeny of the immune response: perinatal perspectives. Semin Perinatol 1991;15:184–195.
5. King A, Loke YW. On the nature and function of human uterine granular lymphocytes. Immunol Today 1991;12:432–435.
6. Dudley DJ, Chen CL, Mitchell MD, et al. Adaptive immune responses during murine pregnancy: pregnancy-induced regulation of lymphokine production by activated T lymphocytes. Am J Obstet Gynecol 1993;168:1155–1163.
7. Lin H, Mosmann TR, Guilbert L, et al. Synthesis of T helper 2-type cytokines at the maternal fetal interface. J Immunol 1993;151:4562–4573.
8. Hill JA, Polger K, Anderson DJ. T-helper 1-type immunity to trophoblast in women with recurrent spontaneous abortion. JAMA 1995;273:1933–1936.
9. Dudley DJ, Hunter C, Mitchell MD, et al. Interleukin-12 concentrations are elevated in the serum of women with severe preeclampsia. J Reprod Immunol 1996;31:97–108.
10. Dinarello CA. The interleukin-1 family: 10 years of discovery. FASEB J 1994;8:1314–1325.
11. Bazzoni F, Beutler B. The tumor necrosis family ligand and receptor families. New Eng J Med 1996;334:1717–1725.
12. Adams DH, Lloyd AR. Chemokines: leucocyte recruitment and activation cytokines. Lancet 1997;349:490–495.

13. Kishimoto T, Akira S, Narazaki M, et al. Interleukin-6 family of cytokines and gp130. Blood 1995;86:1243–1254.

14. Moore KW, Ho ASY, Xu-Amano J. Molecular biology of interleukin-10 and its receptor. In: de Vries JE, de Waal Malefyt R, eds. Interleukin-10. Austin: REG Landes Co., 1995:1–10.

15. Boulay JL, Paul WE. The interleukin-4-related lymphokines and their binding to hematopoietin receptors. J Biol Chem 1992;267:20525–20528.

16. Sporn MB, Roberts AB. Transforming growth factor-ß: recent progress and new challenges. J Cell Biol 1992;119:1017–1021.

17. Border WA, Noble NA. Transforming growth factor ß in tissue fibrosis. New Engl J Med 1994;331:1286–1292.

18. Bone RC, Balk RA, Cerra RF, et al: Definitions for sepsis and organ failure and guidelines for the use of innovative therapies in sepsis. Chest 1992;101:1644–1655.

19. Hunt JS, Chen HL, Miller L. Tumor necrosis factors: pivotal components of pregnancy. Biol Reprod 1996;54:554–562.

20. Gendron RL, Nestel FP, Lapp WS, et al. Lipopolysaccharide-induced fetal resorption in mice is associated with intrauterine production of tumor necrosis factor-alpha. J Reprod Fertil 1990;90:395–402.

21. Whiteside TL. Cytokine measurements and interpretation of cytokine assays in human disease. J Clin Immunol 1994;14:327–339.

22. Gomez R, Ghezzi F, Romero R, et al. Premature labor and intra-amniotic infection: clinical aspects and role of the cyotkines in diagnosis and pathophysiology. Clin Perinatol 1995;22:281–342.

23. Mitchell MD, Romero RJ, Edwin SS, Trautman MS. Prostaglandins and parturition. In Progress in Perinatal Physiology. Reprod Fertil Develop 1995;7:469–477.

24. Dudley DJ, Trautman MS. Infection, inflammation, and contractions: the role of cytokines in the pathophysiology of preterm labor. Semin Reprod Endocrinol 1994;12:263–272.

25. MacDonald PC, Casey ML. Preterm Birth. Sci Am Sci Med 1996;3:42–51.

26. McGregor JA, French JI, Parker R, et al. Prevention of premature birth by screening and treatment for common genital tract infections: results of a prospective controlled evaluation. Am J Obstet Gynecol 1995;173:157–167.

27. Hillier SL, Nugent RP, Eschenbach DA, et al. Association between bacterial vaginosis and preterm delivery of a low-birth-weight infant. New Engl J Med 1995;333:1737–1742.

28. Hauth JC. Reduced incidence of preterm delivery with metronidazole and erythromycin in women with bacterial vaginosis. New Engl J Med 1995;333:1732–1736.

29. Gravett MG, Witkin SS, Haluska GJ, et al. An experimental model for intraamniotic infection and preterm labor in rhesus monkeys. Am J Obstet Gynecol 1994;171:1660–1667.

30. Oshiro B, Silver RM, Dudley DJ, et al. The mouse as an investigational model for preterm labor. Sem Reprod Endocrinol 1994;12:240–245.

31. Hirsch E, Saotome I, Hirsch D. A model of intrauterine infection and preterm delivery in mice. Am J Obstet Gynecol 1995;172:1598–1603.

32. Fidel PL, Romero R, Wolf N, et al. Systemic and local cytokine profiles in endotoxin-induced preterm parturition in mice. Am J Obstet Gynecol 1994;170:1467–1475.

33. Kaga N, Katsuki Y, Obata M, et al. Repeated administration of low-dose lipopolysaccharide induces preterm delivery in mice: a model for human preterm parturition and for as-

sessment of the therapeutic ability of drugs against preterm delivery. Am J Obstet Gynecol 1996;174:754–759.

34. Romero R, Mazor M, Tartakovsky B. Systemic administration of interleukin-1 induces preterm parturition in mice. Am J Obstet Gynecol 1991;165:969–971.

35. Dombroski RA, Woodard DS, Harper MJ, et al. A rabbit model for bacteria-induced preterm pregnancy loss. Am J Obstet Gynecol 1990;163:1938–1943.

36. Hillier SL, Martius J, Krohn M, et al. A case-control study of chorioamniotic infection and histologic chorioamnionitis in prematurity. New Engl J Med 1988;319:972–978.

37. Hillier SL, Witkin SS, Krohn MA, et al. The relationship of amniotic fluid cytokines and preterm delivery, amniotic fluid infection, histologic chorioamnionitis, and chorioamnion infection. Obstet Gynecol 1993;81:941–948.

38. Romero R, Salafia CM, Athanassiadis AP, et al. The relationship between acute inflammatory lesions of the preterm placenta and amniotic fluid microbiology. Am J Obstet Gynecol 1992;166:1382–1388.

39. Romero R, Brody DT, Oyarzun E, et al. Infection and labor. III. Interleukin-1: a signal for the onset of labor. Am J Obstet Gynecol 1989;160:1117–1123.

40. Romero R, Mazor M, Brandt F, et al. Interleukin-1α and interleukin-1ß in preterm and term human parturition. Am J Reprod Immunol 1992;27:117–123.

41. Carroll SG, Abbas A, Ville Y, et al. Concentration of fetal plasma and amniotic fluid interleukin-1 in pregnancies complicated by preterm prelabour amniorrhexis. J Clin Pathol 1995;48:368–371.

42. Romero R, Sepulveda W, Mazor M, et al. The natural interleukin-1 receptor antagonist in term and preterm parturition. Am J Obstet Gynecol 1992;167:863–872.

43. Romero R, Gomez R, Galasso M, et al. The natural interleukin-1 receptor antagonist in the fetal, maternal, and amniotic fluid compartments: the effect of gestational age, fetal gender, and intrauterine infection. Am J Obstet Gynecol 1994;171:912–921.

44. Fidel PL , Romero R, Ramirez M, et al. Interleukin-1 receptor antagonist (IL-1Ra) production by human amnion, chorion, and decidua. Am J Reprod Immunol 1994;32: 1–7.

45. Mitchell MD, Silver RM, Edwin SS, et al. Potential agonist action of the interleukin-1 receptor antagonist protein: implications for treatment of women. J Clin Endocrinol Metab 1993;73:1386–1388.

46. Cole OF, Sullivan MHF, Elder MG. The interleukin-1 receptor antagonist is a partial agonist of prostaglandin biosynthesis by human decidual cells. Prostaglandins 1993;46:493–498.

47. Romero R, Mazor M, Sepulveda W, et al. Tumor necrosis factor in preterm and term labor. Am J Obstet Gynecol 1992;166:1576–1587.

48. Kupferminc MJ, Peaceman A, Aderka D, et al. Soluble tumor necrosis factor receptors in maternal plasma and second-trimester amniotic fluid. Am J Obstet Gynecol 1995;173:900–905.

49. Laham N, Brennecke SP, Bendtzen K, et al. Tumour necrosis factor a during human pregnancy and labour: maternal plasma and amniotic fluid concentrations and release from intrauterine tissues. Eur J Endocrinol 1994;131:607–614.

50. Inglis SR, Jeremias BA, Kuno K, et al. Detection of tumor necrosis factor-α, interleukin-6, and fetal fibronectin in the lower genital tract during pregnancy: relation to outcome. Am J Obstet Gynecol 1994;171:5–10.

51. Casey ML, Cox SM, Beutler B, et al. Cachectin/tumor necrosis factor-a formation in the human decidua: potential role of cytokines in infection-induced preterm labor. J Clin Invest 1989;83:430–436.

52. Vince G, Shorter S, Starkey P, et al. Localization of tumour necrosis factor production in cells at the materno/fetal interface in human pregnancy. Clin Exp Immunol 1992;88:174–180.

53. Fortunato SJ, Menon RP, Swan KF, et al. Inflammatory cytokine (interleukins 1, 6, and 8 and tumor necrosis factor-α) release from cultured human fetal membranes in response to endotoxic lipopolysaccharide mirrors amniotic fluid concentrations. Am J Obstet Gynecol 1996;174:1855–1862.

54. Dudley DJ, Collmer D, Mitchell MD, et al. Detection of inflammatory cytokine mRNA in human gestational tissues utilizing polymerase chain reaction: implications for term and preterm labor. J Soc Gynecol Invest 1996;3:328–335.

55. Austgulen R, Espevik T, Mecsei R, et al. Expression of receptors for tumor necrosis factor in human placenta at term. Acta Obstet Gynecol Scand 1992;71:417–424.

56. Yui J, Garcia-Lloret M, Wegmann TG, et al. Cytotoxicity of tumour necrosis factor-alpha and gamma-interferon against primary human placental trophoblasts. Placenta 1994;15:819–835.

57. So T, Ito A, Sato T, et al. Tumor necrosis factor-a stimulates the biosynthesis of matrix metalloproteinases and plasminogen activator in cultured human chorionic cells. Biol Reprod 1992;46:772–778.

58. Romero R, Wu YK, Brody DT, et al. Human decidua: a source of interleukin-1. Obstet Gynecol 1989;73:31–34.

59. Baergen R, Benirschke K, Ulich TR. Cytokine expression in the placenta: the role interleukin 1 and interleukin 1 receptor antagonist expression in chorioamnionitis and parturition. Arch Pathol Lab Med 1994;118:52–55.

60. Steinborn A, Gunes H, Roddiger S, et al. Elevated placental cytokine release, a process associated with preterm labor in the absence of intrauterine infection. Obstet Gynecol 1996;88:534–539.

61. Lonsdale LB, Elder MG, Sullivan MHF. A comparison of cytokine and hormone production by decidual cells and tissue explants. J Endocrinol 1996;151:309–313.

62. Kent ASH, Sullivan MHF, Elder MG. Transfers of cytokines through human fetal membranes. J Reprod Fertil 1994;100:81–84.

63. Romero R, Tartakovsky B. The natural interleukin-1 receptor antagonist prevents interleukin-1-induced preterm delivery in mice. Am J Obstet Gynecol 1992;167:1041–1045.

64. Silen ML, Firpo A, Morgello S, et al. Interleukin-1α and tumor necrosis factor a cause placental injury in the rat. Am J Pathol 1989;135:239–244.

65. Silver RM, Lohner WS, Daynes RA, et al. Lipopolysaccharide-induced fetal death: the role of tumor necrosis factor alpha. Biol Reprod 1994;50:1108–1112.

66. Fidel PL, Romero R, Cutright J, et al. Treatment with the interleukin-1 receptor antagonist and soluble tumor necrosis factor receptor Fc fusion protein does not prevent endotoxin-induced preterm parturition in mice. J Soc Gynecol Invest 1997;4:22–26.

67. Baggia S, Gravett MG, Witkin SS, et al. Interleukin-1ß intra-amniotic infusion induces tumor necrosis factor-α, prostaglandin production, and preterm contractions in pregnant rhesus monkeys. J Soc Gynecol Invest 1996;3:121–126.

68. Witkin SS, Gravett MG, Haluska GJ, et al. Induction of interleukin-1 receptor antagonist in rhesus monkeys after intraamniotic infection with group B streptococci or interleukin-1 infusion. Am J Obstet Gynecol 1994;171:1668–1672.

69. McDuffie RS, Sherman MP, Gibbs RS. Amniotic fluid tumor necrosis factor-a and interleukin-1 in a rabbit model of bacterially induced preterm pregnancy loss. Am J Obstet Gynecol 1992;167:1583–1588.

70. Romero R, Ceska M, Avila C, et al. Neutrophil atrractant/activating peptide-1/interleukin-8 in term and preterm parturition. Am J Obstet Gynecol 1991;655:813–820.

71. Cherouny PH, Pankuch GA, Romero R, et al. Neutrophil atrractant/activating peptide-1/interleukin-8: association with histologic chorioamnionitis, preterm delivery, and bioactive amniotic fluid leukoattractants. Am J Obstet Gynecol 1993;169:1299–1303.

72. Puchner T, Egarter C, Wimmer C, et al. Amniotic fluid interleukin-8 as a marker of intra-amniotic infection. Arch Gynecol Obstet 1993;253:9–14.

73. Allbert JR, Naef RW, Perry KG, et al. Amniotic fluid interleukin-6 and interleukin-8 levels predict the success of tocolysis in patients with preterm labor. J Soc Gynecol Invest 1:264–268.

74. Laham N, Rice GE, Bishop GJ, et al. Interleukin 8 concentrations in amniotic fluid and peripheral venous plasma during human pregnancy and parturition. Acta Endocrinol 1993;129:220–224.

75. Cohen J, Ghezzi F, Romero R, et al. GROα in the fetomaternal and amniotic fluid compartments during pregnancy and parturition. Am J Reprod Immunol 1996;35:23–29.

76. Shimoya K, Matsuzaki N, Taniguchi T, et al. Interleukin-8 in cord sera: a sensitive and specific marker for the detection of preterm chorioamnionitis. J Infect Dis 1992;165:957–960.

77. Romero R, Gomez R, Galasso M, et al. Macrophage inflammatory protein-1α in term and preterm parturition: effect of microbial invasion of the amniotic cavity. Am J Reprod Immunol 1994;32:108–113.

78. Dudley DJ, Hunter C, Mitchell MD, et al. Elevations of amniotic fluid macrophage inflammatory protein-1α concentrations in women during term and preterm labor. Obstet Gynecol 1996;87:94–98.

79. Kelly RW, Leask R, Calder AA. Choriodecidual production of interleukin-8 and mechanism of parturition. Lancet 1992;339:776–777.

80. Barclay CG, Brennand JE, Kelly RW, et al. Interleukin-8 production by the human cervix. Am J Obstet Gynecol 1993;169:625–632.

81. Dudley DJ, Trautman MS, Mitchell MD. Inflammatory mediators regulate IL-8 production by cultured gestational tissues: evidence for a cytokine network at the chorio-decidual interface. J Clin Endocrinol Metab 1993;76:404–410.

82. Trautman MS, Dudley DJ, Edwin SS, et al. Amnion cell biosynthesis of interleukin-8: regulation by inflammatory cytokines. J Cell Physiol 1992;153:38–43.

83. Shimoya K, Matsuzaki N, Taniguchi T, et al. Human placenta constitutively produces interleukin-8 during pregnancy and enhances its production in intrauterine infection. Biol Reprod 1992;47:220–226.

84. Saito S, Kasahara T, Sakakura S, et al. Detection and localization of interleukin-8 mRNA and protein in human placenta and decidual tissues. J Reprod Immunol 1994;27:161–172.

85. Reisenberger K, Egarter C, Vogl S, et al. The transfer of interleukin-8 across the human placenta perfused in vitro. Obstet Gynecol 1996;87:613–616.

86. Dudley DJ, Spencer S, Edwin S, et al. Regulation of human decidual cell macrophage inflammatory protein-1α (MIP-1α) by inflammatory cytokines. Am J Reprod Immunol 1995;34:231–235.

87. Dudley DJ, Edwin SS, Van Wagoner J, et al. Regulation of decidual cell chemokine production by Group B Streptococci and purified bacterial cell wall components. Am J Obstet Gynecol 1997;177:666–672.

88. Dudley DJ, Edwin SS, Dangerfield A, et al. Regulation of cultured human chorion cell chemokine production by group B streptococci and purified bacterial products. Am J Reprod Immunol 1996;36:264–268.

89. Ito A, Imada K, Sato T, et al. Suppression of interleukin 8 production by progesterone in rabbit uterine cervix. Biochem J 1994;301:183–186.

90. El Maradny E, Kanayama N, Halim A, et al. Interleukin-8 induces cervical ripening in rabbits. Am J Obstet Gynecol 1994;171:77–83.

91. Romero R, Avila C, Santhanam U, et al. Amniotic fluid interleukin-6 in preterm labor: association with infection. J Clin Invest 1990;85:1392–1400.

92. Romero R, Yoon BH, Mazor M, et al. The diagnostic and prognostic value of amniotic fluid white blood cell count, glucose, interleukin-6, and Gram stain in patients with preterm labor and intact membranes. Am J Obstet Gynecol 1993;169:805–816.

93. Romero R, Yoon BH, Mazor M, et al. A comparative study of the diagnostic performance of amniotic fluid glucose, white blood cell count, interleukin-6, and Gram stain in the detection of microbial invasion in patients with preterm premature rupture of membranes. Am J Obstet Gynecol 1993;169:839–851.

94. Romero R, Yoon BH, Kenney JS, et al. Amniotic fluid interleukin-6 determinations are of diagnostic and prognostic value in preterm labor. Am J Reprod Immunol 1993;30:167–183.

95. Yoon BH, Romero R, Kim CJ, et al. Amniotic fluid interleukin-6: a sensitive test for antenatal diagnosis of acute inflammatory lesions of preterm placenta and prediction of perinatal morbidity. Am J Obstet Gynecol 1995;172:960–970.

96. Saito S, Kasahara T, Kato Y, et al. Elevation of amniotic fluid interleukin 6 (IL-6), IL-8, and granulocyte colony stimulating factor (G-CSF) in term and preterm parturition. Cytokine 1993;5:81–88.

97. Greig PC, Ernest JM, Teot L, et al. Amniotic fluid interleukin-6 levels correlate with histologic chorioamnionitis and amniotic fluid cultures in patients in premature labor with intact membranes. Am J Obstet Gynecol 1993;169:1035–1044.

98. Coultrip LL, Lien JM, Gomez R, et al. The value of amniotic fluid interleukin-6 determinations in patients with preterm labor and intact membranes in the detection of microbial invasion of the amniotic cavity. Am J Obstet Gynecol 1994;171:901–911.

99. Andrews WW, Hauth JC, Goldenburg RL, et al. Amniotic fluid interleukin-6: correlation with upper genital tract microbial colonization and gestational age in women delivered after spontaneous labor versus indicated delivery. Am J Obstet Gynecol 1995;173:606–612.

100. Dudley DJ, Hunter C, Mitchell MD, et al. Clinical value of amniotic fluid interleukin-6 determinations in the management of preterm labor. Br J Obstet Gynecol 1994;101:592–597.

101. Waring PM, Romero R, Laham N, et al. Leukemia inhibitory factor: association with intra-amniotic infection. Am J Obset Gynecol 1994;171:1335–1341.

102. Murtha AP, Greig PC, Jimmerson CE, et al. Maternal serum interleukin-6 concentrations in patients with preterm premature rupture of membranes and evidence of infection. Am J Obstet Gynecol 1996;175:966–969.

103. Laham N, Rice GE, Bishop GJ, et al. Elevated plasma interleukin 6: a biochemical marker of human preterm labor. Gynecol Obstet Invest 1993;36:145–147.

104. Lencki SG, Maciulla MB, Eglinton GS. Maternal and umbilical cord serum interleukin levels in preterm labor with clinical chorioamnionitis. Am J Obstet Gynecol 1994;170:1345–1351.

105. Yoon BH, Romero R, Yang SH, et al. Interleukin-6 concentrations in umbilical cord plasma are elevated in neonates with white matter lesions associated with periventricular leukomalacia. Am J Obstet Gynecol 1996;174:1433–1440.

106. Dudley DJ, Trautman M, Araneo BA, Edwin SE, Mitchell MD. Decidual cell biosynthesis of interleukin-6: Regulation by inflammatory cytokines. J Clin Endocrinol Metab 1992;74:884–889.

107. Dudley DJ, Lundin-Schiller S, Edwin SS, et al. Biosynthesis of interleukin-6 by cultured human chorion laeve cells: regulation by cytokines. J Clin Endocrinol Metab 1992;75:1081–1086.

108. Matsuzaki N, Taniguchi T, Shimoya K, et al. Placental interleukin-6 production is enhanced in intrauterine infection but not in labor. Am J Obstet Gynecol 1993;168:94–97.

109. Pasetto N, Piccione e, Zicari A, et al. Cytokine production by human fetal membranes and uterine decidua at term gestation in relation to labour. Placenta 1993;14:361–364.

110. Montes MJ, Tortosa CG, Borja C, et al. Constitutive secretion of interleukin-6 by human decidual stromal cells in culture. Regulatory effect of progesterone. Am J Reprod Immunol 1995;34:188–194.

111. Menon R, Swan KF, Lyden TW, et al. Expression of inflammatory cytokines (interleukin-1ß and interleukin-6) in amniochorionic membranes. Am J Obstet Gynecol 1995;172:493–500.

112. Laham N, Brennecke SP, Bendtzen K, et al. Differential release of interleukin-6 from human gestational tissues in association with labour and in vitro endotoxin treatment. J Endocrinol 1996;149:431–439.

113. Lockwood CJ, Ghidini A, Wein R, et al. Increased interleukin-6 concentrations in cervical secretions are associated with preterm delivery. Am J Obstet Gynecol 1994;171:1097–1102.

114. Rizzo G, Capponi A, Rinaldo D, et al. Interleukin-6 concentrations in cervical secretions identify microbial invasion of the amniotic cavity in patients with preterm labor and intact membranes. Am J Obstet Gynecol 1996;175:812–817.

115. Mitchell MD, Dudley DJ, Edwin SE, et al. Interleukin-6 stimulates prostaglandin production by human amnion and decidual cells. Eur J Pharmacol 1991;192:189–191.

116. Dudley DJ, Chen CL, Branch DW, et al. A murine model for preterm labor: inflammatory mediators regulate the production of prostaglandin E$_2$ and interleukin-6 by murine decidua. Biol Reprod 1993;48:33–39.

117. Heyborne KD, McGregor JA, Henry G, et al. Interleukin-10 in amniotic fluid at midtrimester: immune activation and suppression in relation to fetal growth. Am J Obstet Gynecol 1994;171:55–59.

118. Spong CY, Sherer DM, Ghidini A, et al. Second-trimester amniotic fluid or maternal serum interleukin-10 levels and small for gestational age neonates. Obstet Gynecol 1996;88: 24–28.

119. Greig PC, Herbert WNP, Robinette BL, et al. Amniotic fluid interleukin-10 concentrations increase through pregnancy and are elevated in patients with preterm labor associated with intrauterine infection. Am J Obstet Gynecol 1995;173:1223–1227.

120. Dudley DJ, Hunter C, Mitchell MD, et al. Amniotic fluid interleukin-10 (IL-10) concentrations during pregnancy and with labor. J Reprod Immunol 1997;33:147–156.

121. Cadet P, Rady PL, Tyring SK, et al. Interleukin-10 messenger ribonucleic acid in human placenta: implications of a role for interleukin-10 in fetal allograft protection. Am J Obstet Gynecol 1995;173:25–29.

122. Roth I, Corry DB, Locksley RM, et al. Human placental cytotrophoblasts produce the immunosuppressive cytokine interleukin 10. J Exp Med 1996;184:539–548.

123. Trautman MS, Collmer D, Edwin SS, et al. Expression of interleukin-10 in human gestational tissues. J Soc Gynecol Invest 1997;4:247–253.

124. Dudley DJ, Dangerfield A, Jackson K, et al. Production of interleukin-10 (IL-10) by human decidual cells and chorion cells in response to lipopolysaccharide (abstract 308). J Soc Gynecol Invest 1997;4:156A.

125. Fortunato SJ, Menon R, Swan KF, et al. Interleukin-10 inhibition of interleukin-6 in human chorioamnionic membrane: transcriptional regulation. Am J Obstet Gynecol 1996;175:1057–1065.

126. Dudley DJ, Hunter C, Varner MW, et al. Elevation of amniotic fluid interleukin-4 concentrations in women with preterm labor and chorioamnionitis. Am J Perinatol 1996;13:443–447.

127. Starkey PM. Expression of cells of early human pregnancy decidua, of the p75, IL-2 and p145, IL-4 receptor proteins. Immunology 1991;73:64–70.

128. Hart PH, Vitty GF, Burgess DR, et al. Potential anti-inflammatory effects of interleukin-4: suppression of human monocyte tumor necrosis factor α, interleukin 1 and prostaglandin E_2. Proc Natl Acad Sci (USA) 1989;86:3803–3807.

129. Adamson S, Edwin SS, LaMarche S, et al. Actions of interleukin-4 on prostaglandin biosynthesis by human amnion cells. Prostagl Leuko EFA 1994;50:133–135.

130. Adamson S, Edwin SS, LaMarche S, et al. Actions of interleukin-4 on prostaglandin biosynthesis at the chorion-decidual interface. Am J Obstet Gynecol 1993;169:1442–1447.

131. Spaziani EP, Lantz ME, Benoit RR, et al. The induction of cyclooxygenase-2 (COX-2) in intact human amnion tissue by interleukin-4. Prostaglandins 1996;51:215–223.

132. Bry K, Hallman M. Transforming growth factor-ß opposes the stimulatory effects of interleukin-1 and tumor necrosis factor on amnion cell prostaglandin E_2 production: implication for preterm labor. Am J Obstet Gynecol 1992;167:222–226.

133. Bry K, Hallman M. Transforming growth factor-ß2 prevents preterm delivery induced by interleukin-1a and tumor necrosis factor-a in the rabbit. Am J Obstet Gynecol 1993;168:1318–1322.

134. Opsjon SL, Wathen NC, Tingulstad S, et al. Tumor necrosis factor, interleukin-1 and interleukin-6 in normal human pregnancy. Am J Obstet Gynecol 1993;169:397–404.

135. Osmers RGW, Blaser J, Kuhn W, et al. Interleukin-8 synthesis and the onset of labor. Obstet Gynecol 1995;86:223–229.

136. El Maradny E, Kanayama N, Halim A, et al. Stretching of fetal membranes increases the concentration of interleukin-8 and collagenase activity. Am J Obstet Gynecol 1996;174:843–849.

137. Kelly RW, Illingworth P, Baldie G, et al. Progesterone control of interleukin-8 production in endometrium and chorio-decidual cells underlies the role of the neutrophil in menstruation and parturition. Human Reprod 1994;9:253–258.

138. Granstrom LM, Ekman GE, Malmstrom A, et al. Serum collagenases levels in relation to the state of the human cervix during pregnancy and labor. Am J Obstet Gynecol 1992;167:1284–1288.

139. Rechberger T, Woessner JF. Collagenase, its inhibitors, and decorin in the lower uterine segment in pregnant women. Am J Obstet Gynecol 1993;168:1598–1603.

9

CYTOKINE NETWORKS IN THE HUMAN PLACENTA

Joan S. Hunt

University of Kansas Medical Center, Kansas City, Kansas

The placenta is responsible for establishing and maintaining uninterrupted communication between the mother and the fetus during pregnancy. In this temporary organ, a wide range of nutrients is transported from the maternal to the fetal blood circulation and gases are exchanged (1). In addition, the placenta and associated fetal membranes produce steroid and polypeptide hormones required for the maintenance of pregnancy and fetal development (2).

Synthesis and secretion of the inter- and intracellular communication molecules called cytokines are vital, newly recognized secretory activities of the placenta (3–7). Cytokines are comparatively small polypeptides, averaging 15 to 30 kDa in molecular weight, and are short-lived but powerful modulators of autocrine and paracrine cell function. These molecules bind to specific receptors, transduce intracellular signals, and profoundly alter gene expression.

Organizing placental cytokines into defined categories, which would be helpful in predicting their functions, is a difficult and controversial task (8, 9). Designations of pro-inflammatory and anti-inflammatory have often been used to refer to the cytokines produced as the inflammatory response waxes and wanes. We use these terms here for convenience while recognizing that other well described aspects of the inflammatory

Cytokines in Human Reproduction, Edited by Joseph A. Hill
ISBN 0-471-35242-X   Copyright © 2000 Wiley-Liss, Inc.

response may or may not accompany their production during pregnancy. In mice, a simple and therefore attractive system is used, that is, Th1 type (pro-inflammatory) and Th2 type (anti-inflammatory). However, human cytokines do not fall readily into these categories, and furthermore, using these terms might give the mistaken impression that T helper cells are the main sources of cytokines, which is not the case in the placenta.

An emerging concept in reproduction is that many types of cells in pregnant uteri and placentas are capable of contributing cytokines that were first identified as products of activated leukocytes. This is clearly the case in human placentas, where trophoblast as well as stromal cells produce pro- and anti-inflammatory cytokines and transcription and translation follow highly predictable cell-specific and stage-specific temporal patterns. Readers interested in the development of this field are referred to previous reviews (3, 6). Here the focus is on recent observations and presentation of new ideas and evidence for functions of these potent molecules in human placentas. Cytokines in experimental animals with hemochorial placentation are also mentioned as needed to expand a viewpoint or idea.

PLACENTAL MORPHOLOGY AND CELLULAR COMPONENTS

Human fetuses develop from the inner cell mass of the implanted blastocyst within a shell of trophectoderm derived trophoblastic cells. The anatomic arrangements of the embryo and its associated membranes, which contain both trophoblast and inner cell mass derived mesenchymal cells, are illustrated in Figure 9.1 (10). Cytokine effects

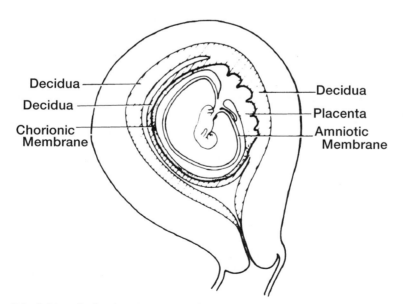

Figure 9.1. Schematic drawing showing anatomic arrangements of the human decidua, placenta, extraplacental membranes (chorionic membrane, amniotic membrane), and embryo (center) during the first trimester of pregnancy. Reprinted by permission of the American Association of Immunologists (10).

are invariably concentration-dependent, so it is important to be familiar with the anatomic features and cellular components of the placenta and its membranes in order to predict the potential autocrine, paracrine, and juxtacrine functions of these powerful, short-lived molecules.

Trophoblast Cell Subpopulations

Implantation in humans and mice is slightly different although both species show an adhesion phase and a penetration phase (Fig. 9.2) (11). Following implantation there is an initial wave of syncytiotrophoblast invasion, and this is followed by cytotrophoblastic cell invasion (Fig. 9.3) (12, 13). Trophoblast invasion is a complicated process involving breakdown of matrix, proliferation, and migration (14, 15). Cytotrophoblastic cells erupt from some of the placental villi in columns as their tips contact decidua, then fan out to form the cytotrophoblastic shell. Cells in columns undergo predictable changes in expression of integrins, which bind extracellular matrix components such as laminin and fibronectin, and those that facilitate cell–cell binding (ICAMs). Cytotrophoblast cells termed interstitial cells march through the decidualized endometrial stroma toward the uterine spiral arteries, where they replace the endothelial cells and assume the designation of endovascular cytotrophoblast cells. Extravillous cytotrophoblastic cells make up the only subpopulation that is in direct contact with decidual cells.

Many placental villi do not attach to the decidua. In these floating villi the layer of trophoblast cells facing the mother is syncytialized, having formed from underly-

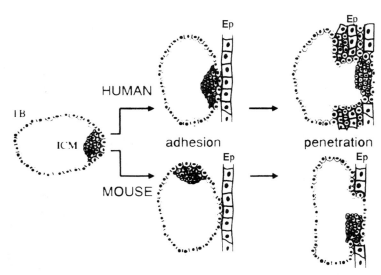

Figure 9.2. Implantation in the human and mouse species. Penetration in humans involves infiltration of the uterine epithelial cells by trophoblast. Ep, uterine luminal epithelial cells; TB, trophoblast cells; ICM, inner cell mass. Reprinted by permission of J.B. Lippincott Publishing Company (11).

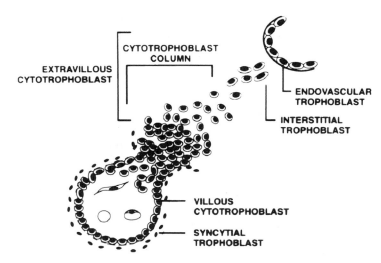

Figure 9.3. Schematic illustration of trophoblast subpopulations in first trimester placentas. A villus composed of an outer layer of syncytialized trophoblast and an inner layer of cytotrophoblast cells is shown in cross section. Cytotrophoblast cells form a column that attaches to and invades maternal decidua. Individual cells (interstitial trophoblast) intermingle with decidual cells, and some cells (endovascular trophoblast) replace the endothelial cells of the spiral arteries. Reprinted by permission of R.G. Landes Publishing Company (12).

ing cytotrophoblastic cells. Syncytiotrophoblast is the only subpopulation continuously exposed to maternal blood.

As pregnancy progresses, trophoblast migration is halted and the villi regress to form the defined placenta and extraplacental membranes (Fig. 9.1). Extravillous cytotrophoblastic cells that are continuous with the placenta make up the chorion membrane, which is directly apposed to maternal decidua. Stroma containing fetal fibroblasts and macrophages is associated with the fetal side of the chorion membrane but there are no fetal capillaries. The amnion membrane, a single layer of epithelial cells, encases the amniotic fluid and embryo throughout pregnancy.

Cellular Components of Placental Villous Mesenchyme

Villous cytotrophoblast and syncytiotrophoblast are separated from the placental villous mesenchyme by a thick basement membrane. The major populations of cells found in the stroma, which is derived from the inner cell mass and is contiguous with the umbilical cord, are undifferentiated fibroblastic type cells, fetal placental macrophages (also known as Hofbauer cells), endothelial cells lining fetal capillaries, and blood cells.

Hematopoietic cells that can be identified by immunohistology in early human placental villous mesenchyme are mainly macrophages, and these remain the predominant leukocyte population in late gestation placentas (16). Macrophages are also the major leukocyte population in the stroma of the extracellular membranes (17).

Flow cytometry experiments on cells harvested from washed term placentas, which included both stromal cells and fetal blood cells but not maternal leukocytes, show that placentas specifically select certain leukocytes (18). CD3neg16+56+57+ natural killer cells are five- to sixfold more common and CD8+ cytotoxic/suppressor T cells are significantly elevated in placentas as compared to cord blood. CD14+ macrophages are present in approximately the same proportions whereas antigen-specific CD4+ helper type T lymphocytes are threefold less common in placentas than in cord blood.

PRO-INFLAMMATORY CYTOKINES IN PLACENTAS: SYNTHESIS AND POTENTIAL FUNCTIONS

Inflammation associated cytokines are usually considered to include tumor necrosis factors (TNF-α, TNF-ß), interferon-γ (IFN-γ), interleukin-2 (IL-2), and interleukin-1β (IL-1ß). Interleukin-6 is listed among the pro-inflammatory cytokines because of being synthesized early but has transitional properties associated with an anti-inflammatory state. Growth factors such as colony stimulating factor-1 (CSF-1, M-CSF), granulocyte macrophage colony stimulating factor (GM-CSF), granulocyte colony stimulating factor (G-CSF), and insulin, which promote proliferation and differentiation of cells, are also considered functionally pro-inflammatory but are not discussed here.

Pro-inflammatory cytokines are most prominent at the beginning and end of pregnancy. For example, TNF-α and IL-1ß are high in the supernatant culture media of first trimester decidua and these cytokines as well as IL-6 increase dramatically in human placentas and amniotic fluid with the onset of labor (19–21). This may be due to the "inflammatory" nature of the implantation and parturition processes where hematopoietic cells, whose cytokine genes are highly sensitive to inducing factors, appear to be the major contributors. Although the same cytokines may be synthesized in nonhematopoietic cells through much of pregnancy, their production is significantly lower than that of activated immune cells (22, 23).

Tumor Necrosis Factor Gene Family

TNF-α was the first member of the multigene TNF family to be identified and characterized, and LT-α (formerly known as TNF-ß) was the second (24–28). These two genes are located within the class III region of the human, mouse, and rat major histocompatibility complexes. Additional members have now been identified by virtue of sequence similarities among their receptors. These include nerve growth factor, Fas ligand (FasL), CD40 ligand, CD27 ligand, CD30 ligand, 4-1BB ligand, and OX40 and TRAIL. Of these, the TNFα, FasL, and TRAIL genes, whose proteins mediate apoptosis, are known to be expressed in human placentas and, in the case of TNFα and FasL, specifically by trophoblast cells (29–31). TNFα and FasL have also been identified in mouse placental trophoblast cells (32, 33).

TNF-α and LT-α bind to the same two receptors, TNF-R1 and TNF-R2, both of which are present in human and mouse placentas (34, 35). Signaling involves interactions among a large number of intracellular proteins that include the TNF receptor associated factors (TRAFs) and death domain homologues (36). Similar proteins mediate signaling through the receptor for FasL, Fas (Fas-R, CD95), and TRAIL (37, 38). Fas-R and TRAIL receptors are as yet unreported in human placentas.

TNF-α. TNF-α, the flag carrier of the TNF gene family, is a potent pro-inflammatory cytokine first identified as a product of activated macrophages that is now known to be expressed in many normal tissues, including the cycling uteri and decidua of women, rats, and mice (39). Mammalian placentas may also be major sources of TNF-α; in situ hybridization and immunohistochemical experiments done in our laboratory detected TNF-α gene products in trophoblast cells at early stages of gestation and in fetal and maternal macrophages near the basal plate and chorion membrane at term (29). Haynes et al. also reported TNF-α transcripts in first trimester trophoblast cells (40). However, Wang and Walsh failed to detect TNF-α mRNA by RT-PCR and northern blotting in normal term placental villi taken distal to the basal plate (41). Thus there may be regional differences in production of TNF-α in term placentas, or perhaps TNF-α-like transcripts and proteins rather than authentic TNF-α was identified in some studies. These questions remain to be resolved.

TNF-α is a highly versatile cytokine. It is best known for its ability to mediate cell death and tissue destruction via stimulation of apoptosis (programmed cell death) through one of its receptors, TNF-R1. This could be its major function during the menstrual cycle, where gene expression is highest in the menstrual phase (42). Another role is postulated for TNF-α in human placentas; Yui et al. (43) proposed the interesting idea that TNF mediated programmed death of cytotrophoblast cells permits closer associations between placental capillaries and maternal blood as pregnancy progresses to term.

The more common role of this powerful pro-inflammatory cytokine may be to program gene expression. Despite its name, binding of TNF-α by many types of cells has no apparent effect on cell growth and may even stimulate DNA synthesis and cell proliferation. Yet many other cellular functions are affected. Of particular importance to pregnancy, there is ample evidence in humans and mice that TNF-α regulates hormone synthesis and release by trophoblast cells (39, 44). Although TNF-α has no effect on major histocompatibility antigen expression in trophoblast cells, this potent, pleiotrophic cytokine might influence both angiogenesis and tissue remodeling by controlling production of certain enzymes.

The question then arises as to what model system might be used to prove or disprove these possibilities. Fortunately, mice have the same patterns of TNF-α gene expression as women so it is appropriate to conduct experiments in this species that cannot be done on humans. Recently, we initiated studies on TNF-α/LT-α deficient (knockout) mice in collaboration with H. Bluethmann of Hoffmann-La Roche, Basel, Switzerland, and TNF-R knockout mice with J. Peschon, Immunex, Seattle, WA. The mice are fertile but are susceptible to certain diseases. Preliminary results suggest that an absence of TNF-α or its receptors results in subtle changes in certain aspects of placentas and offspring (45). These observations are in keeping with the postulate that TNF-α has a central role in the uteroplacental cytokine networks that drive pregnancy to successful completion. Yet the absence of a major influence on fertility and pregnancy indicates that other cytokines that could include IL-1 as well as other TNF gene family members with similar actions (FasL, TRAIL) compensate when TNF-α actions are interrupted.

Other TNF Gene Family Members. Vince et al. were the first to report low levels of LT-α and its mRNA in human placentas (46). More recently, low levels of LT-α, which is usually produced by activated T helper cells (Th1 type), have been reported in maternal plasma and normal term amniotic fluid (47). The cytokine may be neutralized by forming heterodimers with membrane LTß, which is present in similar amounts (47).

Experimental evidence has been presented in support of an important role for FasL in pregnancy. Runic et al. (30) have identified FasL in cytotrophoblast cells and syncyotrophoblast in human placentas by immunohistology and have proposed that the cytokine confers immune privilege in the placenta just as it does in the eye and testis. We have shown that FasL mRNA and protein are present in mouse uterus and placenta, where it is positioned to interfere with trafficking of immune cells between the mother and the fetus (33). In its absence, leukocytes flood the maternal–fetal interface. Thus we have suggested that chimerism as well as immunoprotection during pregnancy may be prevented by FasL.

The FasL/Fas-R system, which is best known for its role in programmed cell death, might also assist in organ development and tissue remodeling required during pregnancy. Suzuki et al. have identified the protein in the cervix and vagina where it appears to play a role in the dynamic estrogen driven morphological and functional changes that take place during the menstrual cycle (48). It is not inconceivable that the uterus and placenta might also make use of this powerful cytokine; unpublished immunohistochemical studies done recently in our laboratory suggest that Fas-R and FasL are co-expressed in/on mouse uterine and placental cells.

Recently, investigators uncovered TRAIL in human placentas (31). Binding of TRAIL involves several proteins that include signal transducing receptors (37, 38). Current experiments in our laboratory are addressing the expression, regulation, and function(s) of these newly identified members of the TNF ligand and receptor gene families.

Interferon-γ

Interferon-γ (IFN-γ) is a second powerful pro-inflammatory cytokine that is found in the pregnant female reproductive tract. Immunoreactive IFN-γ has been detected in several subpopulations of trophoblast cells and is found in amniotic fluid at termination (49, 50). The cytokine may be produced locally. Specific mRNA has been identified in human first trimester villous cytotrophoblast cells by in situ hybridization (40) and trophoblast cells in other species produce IFN-γ. Further molecular localization studies are indicated; human placental cells exhibit IFN-γR (51), so receptor binding of cytokine made elsewhere could account for the immunohistochemical results.

In mice, immunoreactive IFN-γ has been identified in early gestation uteroplacental units by ELISA (52). Preliminary studies suggest that the protein is present in cells surrounding the implantation site during early mouse pregnancy, is found in maternal blood spaces at midgestation, and is localized to metrial gland cells and placental cells at late stages (53). IFN-γ mRNA is present in circulating maternal leukocytes (54) but in the absence of in situ hybridization data the possibility of additional local synthesis cannot be eliminated. IFN-γ receptors (IFN-γR) are expressed by many types of mouse uterine cells during gestation whereas expression in placental cells is not initiated until approximately gestation day 12 (55, 56). Differential expression of IFN- γR mRNA is a characteristic of embryonic cells from gestation day 14 onward.

Expression patterns for the IFN-γ and IFN- γR genes in the uterus, placenta, and embryo strongly support the idea of a role for this potent cytokine in pregnancy. Three well-described functions of IFN-γ are to (1) guard against virus infections by stimulating the production of proteins conferring resistance, (2) control cell growth, and (3) stimulate display of major histocompatibility antigens. Two of these have garnered experimental support. IFN-γ reduces proliferation of human trophoblast cells and augments the apoptotic actions of TNF-α (57). It enhances the expression of major histocompatibility complex class I antigens but not class II antigens by selected subpopulations of human, mouse, and rat trophoblast cells (7, 11). The ability of IFN-γ to increase TNF-R density three- to fivefold, thereby augmenting the actions of TNF-α, as well as multiple other functions are discussed in detail by Sheehan and Schreiber (58).

Interleukin-2

Interleukin-2 (IL-2) is an autocrine growth factor produced by activated T helper cells that is required for their proliferation and clonal expansion. IL-2 mRNA has been reported in human syncytiotrophoblast (59). Recent sequencing of placental IL-2 cDNA by the same group indicates that the 5′ end is 247 bp longer than lymphocyte IL-2 and may represent an alternative splice form (60). However, efforts to identify bioactive cytokine in uteri and placentas have failed. Recently, Vince and Johnson proposed that it is the absence of IL-2 that comprises the central aspect of immunoprotection at the human maternal–fetal interface rather than a particular bias toward anti-inflammatory cytokines, as proposed by Wegmann et al. to be the case in mice (8, 61). It has been suggested that uteroplacental prostaglandin E$_2$ (PGE2) may interfere with the production of IL-2, which would disallow proliferation of maternal anti-fetal immune cells in the uterus and placenta (62).

Interleukin-1

Interleukin-1ß (IL-1ß) is a potent cytokine produced by activated macrophages that initiates immune responses by targeting to and activating T helper cells. In an early report, Flynn et al. (63) showed that human placental macrophages produce IL-1, presumably IL-1ß, which is the preferred species in monocyte/macrophages. Immunohistochemical studies in our laboratory identified IL-1ß in maternal macrophage-like cells in fibrin associated with first trimester villi and in fetal leukocytes in term placentas and membranes (64). Weak immunoreactivity was also observed in some trophoblast. Subsequently, two groups have submitted evidence for production of this cytokine by extravillous trophoblast cells. Librach et al. reported IL-ß1 synthesis by cells harvested from first trimester placentas that had been enriched for cytotrophoblasts (mainly extravillous cytotrophoblasts), and Menon et al. showed that human term chorion membrane (residual extravillous cytotrophoblast cells) contains IL-1ß mRNA as well as protein (65, 66). IL-1ß production by placental trophoblast cell subpopulations, that is, syncytiotrophoblast and villous cytotrophoblast cells, may be artifactually induced by cell harvesting procedures and in vitro culture (67).

It is not certain how IL-1ß might promote pregnancy, but one possibility is that IL-1ß produced in placental macrophages assists in host defense against microbial invaders by promoting lymphocyte proliferation (63). A second is that IL-1ß in cytotrophoblast cells, which display type I 80 kDa IL-1 receptors, stimulates autocrine circuits leading to increased production of matrix metalloproteinase-9 (MMP-9), thereby facilitating the invasive process (65). IL-1 and TNFα have many overlapping functions and a deficiency of one might be compensated by the other.

A TRANSITION CYTOKINE: INTERLEUKIN-6

Interleukin-6 (IL-6) is now regarded as a major mediator of host responses to infections and tissue damage. Its role is intermediary, and it is referred to in the scientific literature as both pro- and anti-inflammatory. This cytokine is increased by PGE2, which downregulates production of inflammation-associated cytokines (IL-2, IFN-γ) and increases anti-inflammatory cytokines (IL-4, IL-10) via autocrine/paracrine pathways (68). The PGE2/IL-6 loop may therefore constitute a transition between the pro- and anti-inflammatory phases of pregnancy.

IL-6 is clearly involved in reproduction and various phases of pregnancy. It is produced in glandular epithelial cells of the cycling uterus, particularly after stimulation with IL-1, and immunoreactive IL-6 has been reported in coelomic and amniotic fluids as well as in extracts of first trimester placental and decidual tissues (69, 70). The cytokine has been identified in the same tissues by immunohistochemistry (69). Positive signals in the immunostains were mainly limited to trophoblast, and syncytiotrophoblast exhibited the strongest reactivity. Hofbauer cells and placental endothelial cells were negative, although decidual cells and decidual macrophages were weakly positive. In situ hybridization studies to localize gene transcription to specific types of cells have not been reported. Yet it is important to map this cytokine because increased IL-6 in amniotic fluids is a comparatively reliable marker of approaching parturition.

It is not certain exactly how IL-6 might function in pregnancy and no studies in knockout mice have been reported that might be informative. Jauniaux et al. have proposed that IL-6 may function in placental remodeling as well as in hematopoiesis in early yolk sac and angiogenesis (70). In mice, IL-6 is produced in luminal epithelial cells following mating and may serve as a signal of pregnancy (71).

ANTI-INFLAMMATORY CYTOKINES IN PLACENTAS: SYNTHESIS AND POTENTIAL FUNCTIONS

Interleukin-4 (IL-4), interleukin-10 (IL-10), and transforming growth factor-ß (TGF-ß1) are among the anti-inflammatory cytokines. All these cytokines are made in human placentas. The first two are prominent in cycling uteri and levels increase with pregnancy (72). Recent preliminary studies suggest that implantation defects are associated with markedly reduced endometrial expression (73). The anti-inflammatory cytokines may be reinforced by the bioactive lipid PGE2 (68), which itself has immunosuppressive properties (62).

Interleukin-4

Interleukin-4 (IL-4) and its receptors have been localized to human term placentas, decidua, and membranes by immunohistology and radiolabel binding assays (74). Cytotrophoblast, decidual macrophages, and maternal and fetal endothelial cells expressed IL-4, whereas syncytiotrophoblast and placental macrophage immunostaining was inconsistent. Term placentas and membranes contained IL-4 mRNA. By contrast, IL-4 is not detectable in either unstimulated or enterotoxin B-stimulated human cord blood leukocytes (75). IL-4 receptors are present on both trophoblast and trophoblast cell lines (Jar, BeWo, JEG-3) (74). In mice, higher levels of IL-4 in uteroplacental tissues than in other organs have been detected, although the cellular sources of this cytokine have not been determined (52). Greater IL-4 mRNA expression in placentas than in maternal blood has been reported (52, 54).

Human placental IL-4 has been proposed to promote maturation of uteroplacental macrophages while inhibiting natural killer cell activation and to serve as a negative regulator of immune cell activity at the fetal–maternal interface (52, 74). One potential pathway of immunosuppression is via induction of inducible cyclooxygenase (COX-2) and production of PGE2 from amnion membranes (76), which could inhibit lymphocyte proliferation.

Interleukin-10

Interleukin-10 (IL-10) is a well described inhibitor of immune responses that is usually produced primarily by Th2 type lymphocytes and macrophages, but may also arise from trophoblast cells. Although IL-10 concentrations are elevated in patients with infection associated preterm labor, which is believed to be caused in large part by cytokines from activated macrophages (77, 78), Roth et al. have recently reported that cells selectively harvested from early, middle, and late stages of pregnancy that are enriched for cytotrophoblasts produce increasing amounts of IL-10 as gestation progresses to termination (79). Placental fibroblasts tested in the same experiments were nonproducers. Although the authors reached the conclusion that human cytotrophoblast cells were the major sites of synthesis of IL-10, macrophages were not specifically excluded from the cell preparations and immunostaining of trophoblast cells for IL-10 was weak, so the conclusion that cytotrophoblast cells are IL-10 contributors may yet require modification.

IL-10 is among the cytokines identified by Lin et al. at the mouse maternal–fetal interface that are proposed to convey an immunosuppressive environment to the pregnant uterus (52). This might be achieved by inhibiting adhesion of leukocytes to activated endothelial cells as shown by Krakauer (80) or by inhibiting production of pro-inflammatory cytokines such as IFN-γ, a well described activity of IL-10.

Transforming Growth Factor ß

TGF-ß1 is produced in large amounts by selectively harvested first trimester decidual cells, particularly stromal cells, large granular leukocytes (natural killer-like lymphocytes), and trophoblast cells (19). TGF-ß1 mRNA is present in first trimester syncytiotrophoblast and, at term, in syncytiotrophoblast, placental villous mesenchymal cells and the chorion membrane (81). In mice and rats, the TGF-ß1 gene is expressed in luminal epithelium and endometrial glands as well as in uterine natural killer cells and macrophages (82, 83).

TGF-ß1 is a negative modulator of synthesis of pro-inflammatory cytokines such as TNF-α by macrophages and enhances their ability to produce IL-10 (84). It is a potent inhibitor of differentiation and represses secretion of chorionic gonadotropin and placental lactogen by monolayer cultures of human term cytotrophoblast cells (85). Because levels of TGF-ß are high and its actions are invariably inhibitory, this cytokine is likely to be among the most important of modulators of immune and other types of cells at the maternal–fetal interface. As an example of this latter type of activity, TGF-ß1 produced in decidua is believed to have a critical role in limiting trophoblast invasion (86).

Other Anti-Inflammatory Substances: Bioactive Lipids

The uterus and placenta are sites of synthesis of several products of arachadonic acid metabolism. Although these are too numerous and too complex in action to discuss here in detail, any listing of anti-inflammatory substances in the uterus and placenta would be incomplete without some mention being made of these powerful mediators. It is important to recognize that prostaglandin G/H synthase is an early response gene in macrophages and that PGE2 serves as a negative feedback signal, reducing production of pro-inflammatory cytokines by hematopoietic cells (62).

Regulation of synthesis of PGE2 differs among cell lineages and is stimulated by multiple signals, as shown recently in the peri-implantation mouse uterus (87). Prostaglandin receptor genes are also differentially regulated in mouse uterus (88). In human chorion and decidual cells, PGE2 synthesis is stimulated by both IL-1β and IL-4 (89, 90), and multiple studies have shown that prostaglandins have diverse roles, being central to successful implantation but also importantly involved in parturition (89).

Hormonal Regulation of Inflammatory and Anti-Inflammatory Cytokines

Evidence is mounting in support of the idea that female sex steroid hormones supervise cytokine production in the uterus and placenta (7, 91, 92). In our own work, for example, we learned that TNF-α production in cycling uteri of women and mice is clearly regulated by estrogens and progesterone and that regulation is cell type-specific as well as concentration-dependent (42, 93). As regards estrogens, production of TNF-α/β by human helper T cells is enhanced by low doses of estradiol-17β whereas expression of the TNF-α gene in mouse uterine epithelial cells is enhanced by progesterone rather than estrogen (93, 94). Furthermore, T helper clones are suppressed for production of TNF-α/β by high doses of estrogen (93). The Th clones were also induced by estradiol to secrete higher levels of both IL-10 and IFN-γ while having no effect on secretion of IL-4 or TGF-β (94).

Overall, progesterone has profound inhibitory effects on immunological phenomena. For example, progesterone has negative effects on TNF-α transcription and translation in macrophages (Miller L, Hunt JS, unpublished data), suppresses phagocytosis by decidual stromal cells (95), promotes lymphocyte production of Th2-type anti-inflammatory cytokines in Th1 cell clones (96), and may therefore be a major regulatory force in determining balances and proportions of inflammatory and anti-inflammatory cytokines during most of pregnancy. Potential influences of placental polypeptide hormones, human choriogonadotropin and placental lactogen, have not been thoroughly investigated but should not be underestimated. Schafer et al. reported that these two hormones suppress production of IL-2 while enhancing production of TNF-α, IL-1β, and IL-6 by blood mononuclear cells (97).

Cytokines also regulate hormone production. For instance, Feinberg et al. showed that progesterone production by the choriocarcinoma cell line, JEG-3, is stimulated by IL-1α, IL-1β and TNF but not by IL-2 or IFN-γ (98). This finding not only illustrates reciprocal regulation but suggests distinct functional patterns within subgroups of pro-inflammatory cytokines.

SUMMARY

Placentas transcribe and translate essentially all of the prominent pro- and anti-inflammatory cytokines that have been reported in other systems, with the possible exception of IL-2. Even in the case of IL-2, message is present. This is not at all surprising given the dynamic changes that take place in this remarkable organ and the complex requirements of pregnancy. Placentas are also, according to Adamson, home to all of the oncogenes ever identified (99) and it is these and other transcription factors that carry out cytokine instructions in ever-fluctuating intracellular signaling pathways.

Significant progress has been made in defining the cytokine motifs that characterize successful pregnancy although much remains to be learned, particularly about newly identified cytokines such as IL-12 and IL-15. Nonetheless, certain general principles are emerging from the data collected thus far. It is clear that pro- and anti-inflammatory cytokines have specific temporal and spatial patterns and that production must be tightly regulated. At present this appears to be achieved by placental/maternal hormones, bioactive lipids, and the cytokines themselves. Although novel production by trophoblast cells has captured the interest of many investigators, placental mesenchymal cells are major players and the influences of maternal cells cannot be overlooked. Clinical and basic immunologists must now work toward effective translation of these findings into methods for identifying disorders of cytokine synthesis in women (100) and therapies for improving reproductive performance.

ACKNOWLEDGMENTS

These studies are supported by grants from the National Institutes of Health (HD24212, HD29156, HD26429), the Kansas Mental Retardation Research Center (HD02528), and the Kansas University P30 Center for Reproductive Sciences (HD33994). I am indebted to the numerous colleagues, postdoctoral fellows, students, and technical assistants who have contributed to these studies.

REFERENCES

1. Fox H. Physiology of the placenta. In: Bennington JL, ed. Pathology of the Placenta. Vol. VII, Major Problems in Pathology. London: W.B. Saunders. 1978:38–49.

2. Casey ML, MacDonald PC, Simpson ER. Endocrinological changes of pregnancy. In: Wilson JD, Foster DW, eds. Williams Textbook of Endocrinology. Philadelphia: W.B. Saunders, 1992;977–991.

3. Hunt JS. Cytokine networks in the uteroplacental unit: Macrophages as pivotal regulatory cells. J Reprod Immunol 1989;16:1–17.

4. Pollard JW, Pampfer S, Daiter E, et al. Cytokines at the maternal fetal interface: colony stimulating factor-1 as a paradigm for the maternal regulation of pregnancy. In: Strauss JF III, Lyttle CR, eds. Uterine and Embryonic Factors In Early Pregnancy. New York: Plenum Press, 1991:107–118.

5. Rappolee DA, Sturm KS, Schultz GA, et al. Expression and function of growth factor ligands and receptors in preimplantation mouse embryos. In: Schomberg DW, ed. Growth Factors in Reproduction. New York: Springer-Verlag, 1991:207–218.

6. Mitchell MD, Trautman MS, Dudley DJ. Cytokine networking in the placenta. Placenta 1993;14:249–275.

7. Hunt JS, Soares MJ. The placenta. In: Marsh JA, Kendall MD, eds. The Physiology of Immunity. Boca Raton: CRC Press, 1995:277–295.

8. Vince GS, Johnson PM. Is there a Th2 bias in human pregnancy? J Reprod Immunol 1996;32:101–104.

9. Guilbert LJ. There is a bias against type 1 (inflammatory) cytokine expression and function in pregnancy. J Reprod Immunol 1996;32:105–110.

10. Schmidt CM, Chen H-L, Chiu I, et al. Temporal and spatial expression of HLA-G mRNA in extraembryonic tissues of transgenic mice. J Immunol 1995;155:619–625.

11. Hunt JS, Roby KF. Implantation factors. Clin Obstet Gynecol 1994;37:635–645.

12. Hunt JS, Soares MJ. Features of the maternal-fetal interface. In: Hunt JS, ed. HLA and the Maternal–Fetal Relationship. Austin:Landes Pub. Co., 1996:1–26.

13. Enders AC, Welsh AO. Structural interactions of trophoblast and uterus during hemochorial placenta formation. J Exp Zool 1993;266:578–587.

14. Bischof P, Martelli M, Campana A. Controlled extracellular matrix degradation: a fundamental mechanism in the implantation process. In: Glasser SR, Mulholland J, Psychoyos A, eds. Endocrinology of Embryo–Endometrium Interactions. New York: Plenum Press, 1994:379–389.

15. Damsky CH, Schick SF, Klimanskaya I, et al. Adhesive interactions in peri-implantation morphogenesis and placentation. Reprod Toxicol 1997;11:367–375.

16. Vince GS, Johnson PM. Immunobiology of human uteroplacental macrophages—friend and foe? Placenta 1996;17:191–199.

17. Lessin DL, Hunt JS, King CR, et al. Antigen expression by cells near the maternal-fetal interface. Am J Reprod Immunol Microbiol 1988;16:1–7.

18. Roussev RG, Higgins NG, McIntyre JA. Phenotypic characterization of normal human placental mononuclear cells. J Reprod Immunol 1993;25:15–29.

19. Jokhi PP, King A, Loke YW. Cytokine production and cytokine receptor expression by cells of the human first trimester placental-uterine interface. Cytokine 1997;9:126–137.

20. Opsjon SL, Wathen NC, Tingulstad S, et al. Tumor necrosis factor, interleukin-1 and interleukin-6 in normal human pregnancy. Am J Obstet Gynecol 1993;169,397–404.

21. Steinborn A, Gunes H, Roddiger S, et al. Elevated placental cytokine release, a process associated with preterm labor in the absence of intrauterine infection. Obstet Gynecol 1996;88:534–439.

22. Libby P, Warner SJC, Galin CB. Human vascular smooth muscle cells can transcribe the tumor necrosis factor/cachectin gene and respond to inflammatory mediator. Clin Res 1987;35:297A.

23. Jaattela M. Biologic activities and mechanisms of action of tumor necrosis factor-α cachectin. Lab Invest 1991;64:724–742.

24. Beutler B, Cerami A. The biology of cachectin/TNF—a primary mediator of the host response. Ann Rev Immunol 1989;7:625–55.

25. Arai K-I, Lee F, Miyajima A, Miyatake S, Arai N, Yokota T. Cytokines: coordinators of immune and inflammatory responses. Ann Rev Biochem 1990;59:783–836.

26. Camussi G, Albano E, Tetta C, Bussolino F. The molecular action of tumor necrosis factor-α. Eur J Biochem 1991;202:3–14.

27. Bazan JF. Emerging families of cytokines and receptors. Curr Biol 1993;3:603–606.

28. Beutler B, van Huffel C. Unraveling function in the TNF ligand and receptor families. Science 1994;264:667–668.

29. Chen HL, Yang Y, Hu XL, et al. Tumor necrosis factor-alpha mRNA and protein are present in human placental and uterine cells at early and late stages of gestation. Am J Pathol 1991;139:327–335.

30. Runic R, Lockwood CJ, Ma Y, et al. Expression of Fas ligand by human cytotrophoblasts: implications in placentation and fetal survival. J Clin Endocrinol Metab 1996;81:3119–3122.

31. Wiley SR, Schooley K, Smolak PJ, et al. Identification and characterization of a new member of the TNF family that induces apoptosis. Immunity 1995;3:673–682.

32. Hunt JS, Chen HL, Hu XL, et al. Normal distribution of tumor necrosis factor-α messenger ribonucleic acid and protein in virgin and pregnant osteopetrotic (*op/op*) mice. Biol Reprod 1993;49:441–452.

33. Hunt JS, Vassmer D, Miller L, et al. Fas ligand is positioned in mouse uterus and placenta to prevent trafficking of activated leukocytes between the mother and the conceptus. J Immunol 1997;158:4122–4128.

34. Yelavarthi KK, Hunt JS. Analysis of p60 and p80 tumor necrosis factor-α mRNA and protein in human placentas. Am J Pathol 1993;143:1131–1141.

35. Roby KF, Laham N, Kroning H, et al. Expression and localization of messenger RNA for tumor necrosis factor receptor (TNF-R) I and TNF-RII in pregnant mouse uterus and placenta. Endocrine 1995;3:557–562.

36. Darnay BG, Aggarwal BB. Early events in TNF signaling: a story of associations and dissociations. J Leukocyte Biol 1997;61:559–566.

37. Chinnaiyan AM, O'Rourke K, Yu GL, et al. Signal transduction by DR3, a death domain-containing receptor related to TNF-R-1 and CD95. Science 1996;274:990–992.

38. Kitson J, Raven T, Jiang YP, et al. A death domain-containing receptor that mediates apoptosis. Nature 1996; 384:372–375.

39. Hunt JS, Chen HL, Miller L. Tumor necrosis factors: Pivotal factors in pregnancy? Biol Reprod 1997;54:554–562.

40. Haynes MK, Shepley KS, Jackson LG, et al. Cytokine production in first trimester chorionic villi: detection of mRNAs and protein products in situ. Cell Immunol 1993;151:300–308.

41. Wang Y, Walsh SW. TNFα concentrations and mRNA expression are increased in preeclamptic placentas. J Reprod Immunol 1996;32:157–170.

42. Hunt JS, Chen HL, Hu XL, et al. Tumor necrosis factor-α mRNA and protein in human endometrium. Biol Reprod 1992;47:141–147.

43. Yui J, Hemmings D, Garcia-Lloret M, et al. Expression of the human p55 and p75 tumor necrosis factor receptors in primary villous trophoblasts and their role in cytotoxic signal transduction. Biol Reprod 1996;55:400–409.

44. Terranova PF, Hunter VJ, Roby KF, et al. Tumor necrosis factor-α in the female reproductive tract. Proc. Soc. Exp. Biol. Med. 1995;209:325–342.

45. Hunt JS, Chen HL, Bluethmann H. Placental abnormalities in tumor necrosis factor-α/lymphotoxin-α-deficient mice. Biol Reprod 1996;45(Suppl. 1):149.

46. Vince G, Shorter S, Starkey P, et al. Localization of tumour necrosis factor production in cells at the materno/fetal interface in human pregnancy. Clin Exp Immunol 1992;88:174–180.

47. Laham N, Van Dunne F, Abraham LJ, et al. Tumor necrosis factor-ß in human pregnancy and labor. J Reprod Immunol 1997;33:53–69.

48. Suzuki A, Enari M, Eguchi Y, et al. Involvement of Fas in regression of vaginal epithelia after ovariectomy and during an estrous cycle. Embo J 1996;15:211–215.

49. Bulmer JN, Morrison L, Johnson PM, et al. Immunohistochemical localization of interferons in human placental tissues in normal, ectopic, and molar pregnancy. Am J Reprod Immunol 1990;22:109–116.

50. Olah KS, Vince GS, Neilson JP, et al. Interleukin-6, interferon-γ, interleukin-8, and granulocyte-macrophage colony stimulating factor levels in human amniotic fluid at term. J Reprod Immunol 1996;32:89–98.

51. Peyman JA, Hammond GL. Localization of IFN-γ receptor in first trimester placenta to trophoblasts but lack of stimulation of HLA-DRA, -DRB, or invariant chain mRNA expression by IFN-γ. J Immunol 1992;149:2675–2680.

52. Lin H, Mosmann TR, Guilbert L, et al. Synthesis of T helper 2-type cytokines at the maternal-fetal interface. J Immunol 1993;151:4562–4573.

53. Platt JS, Hunt, JS. Immunoreactive interferon-γ in cycling and pregnant mouse uterus. Biol Reprod 1996;54(Suppl. 1):84.

54. Delassus S, Coutinho GC, Saucier C, et al. Differential cytokine expression in maternal blood and placenta during murine gestation. J Immunol 1994;152:2411–2420.

55. Chen HL, Kamath R, Pace JL, et al. Gestation-related expression of the interferon-γ receptor gene in mouse uterine and embryonic hematopoietic cells. J Leukocyte Biol 1994;55:617–625.

56. Chen H-L, Kamath R, Pace JL, et al. Expression of the interferon-γ receptor gene in mouse placentas is related to stage of gestation and is restricted to specific subpopulations of trophoblast cells. Placenta 15:109–121.

57. Yui J, Garcia-Lloret M, Wegmann TG, et al. Cytotoxicity of tumour necrosis factor-alpha and gamma-interferon against primary human placental trophoblasts. Placenta 1994;15:819–835.

58. Sheehan KCF, Schreiber RD. The synergy and antagonism of interferon-γ and TNF-α. In: Beutler B, ed. Tumor Necrosis Factors. New York: Raven Press, 1992:145–178.

59. Boehm KD, Kelley MF, Ilan J, et al. The interleukin 2 gene is expressed in the syncytiotrophoblast of the human placenta. Proc Natl Acad Sci USA 1989;86:656–660.

60. Chernicky CL, Tan H, Burfiend P, et al. Sequence of interleukin-2 isolated from human placental poly A+ RNA: possible role in maintenance of fetal allograft. Mol Reprod Dev 1996;43:180–186.

61. Wegmann TG, Lin H, Guilbert L, et al. Bidirectional cytokine interactions in the maternal-fetal relationship: is successful pregnancy a TH2 phenomenon? Immunol Today 1993;14:363–356.

62. Hunt JS. Prostaglandins, immunoregulation, and macrophage function. In: Immunological Obstetrics Coulam C, Faulk WP, McIntyre JA, eds. New York: Norton, 1992; 73–84.

63. Flynn A, Frike JH, Hilfiker ML. Placental mononuclear phagocytes as a source of interleukin-1. Science 1982;218:475–477.

64. Hu XL, Yang Y, Hunt JS. Differential distribution of interleukin-1α and interleukin-1ß proteins in human placenta. J Reprod Immunol 1992;22:257–268.

65. Librach CL, Feigenbaum SL, Bass KE, et al. Interleukin-1 beta regulates human cytotrophoblast metalloproteinase activity and invasion in vitro. J Biol Chem 1994;269:17125–17131.

66. Menon R, Swan KF, Lyden TW, et al. Expression of inflammatory cytokines (interleukin-1 beta and interleukin-6) in amniochorionic membranes. Am J Obstet Gynecol 1995;172:493–500.

67. Kauma SW, Walsh SW, Nestler JE et al. Interleukin-1 is induced in the human placenta by endotoxin and isolation procedures for trophoblasts. J Clin Endocrinol Metab 1992;75:951–955.

68. Miao D, Skibinski G, James K. The effects of human seminal plasma and PGE2 on mitogen induced proliferation and cytokine production of human splenic lymphocytes and peripheral blood mononuclear cells. J Reprod Immunol 1996;30:97–114.

69. Laird SM, Tuckerman E, Li TC, Bolton AE. Stimulation of human endodermal epithelial cell interleukin 6 production by interleukin 1 and placental protein 14. Human Reprod 1994;9:1339–1343.

70. Jauniaux E, Gulbis B, Schandene L, Collette J, Hustin J. Distribution of interleukin-6 in maternal and embryonic tissues during the first trimester. Mol. Human Reprod 1996;2:239–243.

71. Robertson SA, Seamark RF, Guilbert LJ, et al. The role of cytokines in gestation. Crit Rev Immunol 1994;14:239–292.

72. Krasnow JS, Tollerud DJ, Naus G, et al. Endometrial Th2 cytokine expression throughout the menstrual cycle and early pregnancy. Human Reprod 1996;11:1747–1754.

73. Stewart-Akers A, Krasnow JS, DeLoia JA. Decreased endometrial expression of interleukin (IL)-4 and IL-10 in women with implantation defects. Abstract, AAAAI/AAI/CIS Joint Meeting 1996.

74. De Moraes-Pinto MI, Vince GS, Flanagan BF, et al. Localization of IL-4 and IL-4 receptors in the human term placenta, decidua and amniochorionic membrane. Immunol 1997;90:87–94.

75. Kruse A, Rink L, Rutenfranz I, et al. Interferon and lymphokine production by human placental and cord blood cells. J Interferon Res 1992;12:113–117.

76. Spaziani EP, Lantz ME, Benoit RR, et al. The induction of cyclooxygenase-2 (COX-2) in intact human amnion tissue by interleukin-4. Prostaglandins 1996;51:215–223.

77. Greig PC, Herbert WN, Robinette BL, et al. Amniotic fluid interleukin-10 concentrations increase through pregnancy and are elevated in patients with preterm labor associated with intrauterine infection. Am J Obstet Gynecol 1995;173:1223–1227.

78. Mitchell MD, Trautman MS, Dudley DJ. Immunoendocrinology of preterm labour and delivery. Baillieres Clin Obstet Gynaecol 1993;7:553–575.

79. Roth I, Corry DB, Locksley RM, et al. Human placental cytotrophoblasts produce the immunosuppressive cytokine interleukin 10. J Exp Med 1996;184:539–548.

80. Krakauer T. IL-10 inhibits the adhesion of leukocytic cells to IL-1-activated human endothelial cells. Immunol Letters 1995;45:61–65.

81. Lysiak JJ, Hunt JS, Pringle GA, et al. Localization of transforming growth factor ß and its natural inhibitor decorin in the human placenta and decidua throughout gestation. Placenta 1995;16:221–231.

82. Tamada H, McMaster MT, Flanders KC, et al. Cell type-specific expression of transforming growth factor-β1 in the mouse uterus during the periimplantation period. Mol Endocrinol 1990;4:965–972.

83. Chen HL, Yelavarthi KK, Hu XL, et al. Identification of transforming growth factor-β1 mRNA in virgin and pregnant rats by in situ hybridization. J Reprod Immunol 1993;25:221–233.

84. Maeda H, Kuwahara H, Ichimura Y, et al. TGF-ß enhances macrophage ability to produce IL-10 in normal and tumor-bearing mice. J Immunol 1995;155:4926–4932.

85. Morrish DW, Bhardwaj D, Paras MT. Transforming growth factor ß1 inhibits placental differentiation and human chorionic gonadotropin and human placental lactogen secretion. Endocrinol 1991;129:22–26.

86. Graham CH, Lysiak JJ, McCrae KR, et al. Localization of transforming growth factor-β at the human fetal-maternal interface: role in trophoblast growth and differentiation. Biol Reprod 1992;46:561–572.

87. Chakraborty I, Das SK, Wang J, et al. Developmental expression of the cyclo-oxygenase-1 and cyclo-oxygenase-2 genes in the peri-implantation mouse uterus and their differential regulation by the blastocyst and ovarian steroids. J Mol Endocrinol 1996;16:107–122.

88. Yang ZM, Das SK, Wang J, et al. Potential sites of prostaglandin actions in the periimplantation mouse uterus: differential expression and regulation of prostaglandin receptor genes. Biol Reprod 1997;56:368–379.

89. Mitchell MC, Romero RJ, Edwin SS, et al. Prostaglandins and parturition. Reprod Fertil Dev 1995;7:623–632.

90. Adamson S, Edwin SS, LaMarche S, et al. Actions of interleukin-4 on prostaglandin biosynthesis at the chorion-decidual interface. Am J Obstet Gynecol 1993;169:1442–1447.

91. Cullingford TE, Pollard JW. Growth factors as mediators of sex steroid hormone action in the uterus during its preparation for implantation. In: Kahn SA, Stancel GM, eds. Protooncogenes and Growth Factors in Steroid Hormone Induced Growth and Differentiation. Boca Raton: CRC Press, 1994:13.

92. Robertson SA, Mayrhofer G, Seamark RF. Uterine epithelial cells synthesize granulocyte-macrophage colony-stimulating factor and interleukin-6 in pregnant and nonpregnant mice. Biol Reprod 1992;46:1069–1079.

93. Roby KF, Hunt JS. Mouse endometrial tumor necrosis factor-α mRNA and protein: localization and regulation by estradiol and progesterone. Endocrinology 1994;135:2780–2789.

94. Gilmore W, Weiner LP, Correale J. Effect of estradiol on cytokine secretion by proteolipid protein-specific T cell clones isolated from multiple sclerosis patients and normal control subjects. J Immunol 1997;158:446–451.

95. Ruiz C, Montes MJ, Abadia-Molina AC, et al. Phagocytosis by fresh and cultured human decidual stromal cells: opposite effects of interleukin-1α and progesterone. J Reprod Immunol 1997;33:15–26.

96. Piccinni MP, Giudizi MG, Biagiotti R, et al. Progesterone favors the development of human T helper cells producing Th2-type cytokines and promotes both IL–4 production and membrane CD30 expression in established Th1 cell clones. J Immunol 1995;155:128–133.

97. Schafer A, Pauli G, Friedmann W, et al. Human choriogonadotropin (hCG) and placental lactogen (hPL) inhibit interleukin-2 (IL-2) and increase interleukin-1 beta (IL-1 beta), -6 (IL-6) and tumor necrosis factor (TNF-α) expression in monocyte cell cultures. J Perinat Med 1992;20:233–240.

98. Feinberg BB, Anderson DJ, Steller MA, et al. Cytokine regulation of trophoblast steroidogenesis, J Clin Endocrinol Metab 1994;78:586–591.

99. Adamson E. Expression of proto-oncogenes in the placenta. Placenta 1987;8:449–466.

100. Hill JA. T-helper 1-type immunity to trophoblast: evidence for a new immunological mechanism for recurrent abortion in women. Human Reprod 1995;10(Suppl. 2):114–120.

10

CYTOKINES/GROWTH FACTORS IN THE HUMAN FALLOPIAN TUBE

Celeste M. Brabec and Joseph A. Hill

Brigham and Women's Hospital, Harvard Medical School, Boston, Massachusetts

The human fallopian tube (HFT) is the site of oocyte capture and migration, sperm migration, fertilization, and early embryonic development. The anatomy, histology, and physiology of the HFT all contribute important key background information to understanding cytokines in the human fallopian tube.

ANATOMY

The human adult fallopian tube is 9–11 cm long. The oviducts are formed embryologically from the paramesonephric ducts. The fimbriae, the most distal portion, have approximately 25 fingerlike extensions. The infundibulum, just proximal to the fimbriae, is approximately 1 cm long and narrows from 1 cm in diameter to 4 mm. The ampulla, proximal to the infundibulum and averaging 6 cm long, is believed to be the site of fertilization. Medial to the ampulla is the isthmus, which is approximately 2 cm long and is characterized by a relative thickening of the muscular wall. The in-

Cytokines in Human Reproduction, Edited by Joseph A. Hill
ISBN 0-471-35242-X Copyright © 2000 Wiley-Liss, Inc.

terstitial portion of the fallopian tube is 1 cm long and connects the tube to the uterine corpus. The HFT receives a dual blood supply from the ovarian uterine arteries, and is innervated in a complex network.

HISTOLOGY

Histologically, the fallopian tube is composed of three layers, the mucosa, serosa, and smooth muscle layer. The mucosa increases in structural complexity from its uterine to its tubal end. In its interstitial (most medial) portion, the mucosa exhibits five to six plicae (folds), whereas more distally the isthmus has 12 or more plicae with secondary folds. The ampulla and infundibulum have frondlike plicae with both secondary and tertiary branches. The mucosa, or epithelial layer, is a single layer of columnar cells and has at least three cell types. Secretory cells compose 55–65% of the mucosal layer. Secretory cells are columnar cells with ovoid nuclei perpendicular to the long axis of the cell. Ciliated cells account for 20% to 30% of the mucosal layer and are also columnar cells but are wider than secretory cells, with oval to round nuclei. Interciliary cells are columnar with thin, dark staining nuclei, and are thought to be a variant of the secretory cell.

Ciliated cells appear early during fetal development and are present until menopause. However, exogenous estrogen restores cilia and their ability to transport particulate matter. Early in the menstrual cycle, cells are low-lying and secretory cells are inactive. Periovulatory, secretory cells become columnar and project beyond ciliated cells. PAS-positive material most likely representing glycogen is discharged into the lumen at the time of ovulation. Simultaneous with ovulation, muscles of the fimbriae ovaricum contract, pulling the tube of the ipsilateral ovulating ovary toward the follicle. The fimbriae are thought to pick up the oocyte within minutes of its release from the ovary. Fimbriae are able to pick up oocytes from either ovary and from the pelvic cul-de-sac in the pouch of Douglas.

IMMUNOBIOLOGY OF THE HUMAN FALLOPIAN TUBE

Leukocyte Populations in the Human Fallopian Tube

It was not until the 1970s that lymphocytes were recognized in HFT mucosa. These basally located cells with round nuclei and dark chromatin were thought to be precursor or reserve cells for other cell types, but have since been identified as lymphocytes, originally by electron microscopy (1). The discovery of immune cells in the mucosal layer of HFT led to investigation into their further characterization and function.

Following the discovery of lymphocytes in the HFT, investigation into their location and numbers throughout the menstrual cycle was pursued. Lymphocytes in the epithelium appear to be more numerous in the secretory phase than in the proliferative phase. They are also in greater number in reproductive age women than in postmenopausal women or in cases of tubal pregnancies (2). The number of lymphocytes between phases of the menstrual cycle has been disputed (3). There appears to be no difference in lymphocyte numbers between specimens from normal women in proliferative phase and in women with purulent salpingitis. Lymphocytes appear to exist within the epithelium and are situated basally almost without exception. They appear to lie exclusively in an intercellular position. During the secretory phase, when lymphocytes have been noted to be most numerous, they appear in such great numbers that in places one can find lymphocytes along the base of the epithelial cells, whereas during the proliferative phase they are seldom seen. In pregnancy, numbers of pan T cells appear to be higher than in both phases of the menstrual cycle, and have been described as histologically forming a "string of pearls" (3). Complex interdigitations between lymphocytes and the adjacent epithelial cells have been observed with electron microscopy, suggesting an interaction between these cell types. These data were the first to demonstrate that lympho-epithelial relationships in the HFT are dynamic, and probably influenced by hormones.

In the 1980s, characterization of lymphocyte subtypes in the human fallopian tube was first performed. Using primary monoclonal antibodies, intraepithelial lymphocytes were identified as predominantly T-cytotoxic/suppressor (CD8) cells. Macrophages have also been identified but are rare within the epithelial layer. T helper cells (CD4), B cells, and natural killer cells are generally absent or rarely found within the epithelium. Within the subepithelium, however, macrophages, mast cells, T cells, B cells, infrequent plasma cells, and natural killer cells have been observed (4, 5). These data support the concept that the normal human fallopian tube is a form of mucosal associated lymphoid tissue (MALT).

Humoral Immune System in the Human Fallopian Tube

Most of the research done in the 1980s focused on investigation of the humoral immune system in the HFT. Immunoglobulins of most groups have been identified within the submucosa of the fallopian tube. Immunoglobulin A, secretory component (SC), and J chain-producing plasma cells have been identified in the subepithelium. Submucosal plasma cells of IgM and IgG classes appear less frequent than IgA. No menstrual cycle changes have been noted but infection appears to increase the numbers of plasma cells of all immunoglobulin classes by 16-fold, suggesting a local functional immune system (6–9).

Major Histocompatibility Complex Antigens in the Human Fallopian Tube

Major histocompatibility complex (MHC) class II antigens (human leukocyte antigens, HLA-DR, -DP, and -DQ) are expressed on columnar epithelium in the fallopian tube during the menstrual cycle. Initial reports indicated that a variety of tubal epithelial cells stained positive for DR-a and DR-b, but showed essentially no reactivity for DP or DQ. In contrast, in normal first trimester pregnancy and in ectopic pregnancy, tubal epithelium revealed uniformly intense staining reactivity for DR, DP, and DQ. At term, most cells again were pan-positive, with only a few cells DP- and

DQ-negative (10). These data suggest MHC class II expression may be mediated by hormones or some other trophoblast product.

Subsequent studies in nonpregnant women have revealed that preovulatory epithelial cells of the HFT stain positive for HLA-DR, -DP, and -DQ, but postovulatory HLA-DR is undetectable and -DP and -DQ are significantly lower than in preovulatory samples (11). This again suggests hormonal control, and perhaps a need for immunoreactivity against infection in the preovulatory phase, but optimal survival conditions for sperm and the foreign preimplantation embryo in the postovulatory phase.

Fallopian Tube Leukocyte Populations in Women with the Intrauterine Contraceptive Device

Characterization of leukocytes in the fallopian tubes of women with the intrauterine contraceptive device (IUCD) has been performed. Women with an IUCD appear to have higher numbers of leukocytes, T lymphocytes, B lymphocytes, granulocytes, monocytes, null cells, and IgA-, IgG-, and IgM-positive cells compared to controls (12). This suggests that the IUCD may disturb the immunologic function of the fallopian tube and any beneficial role it may play in fertilization.

Leukocyte Populations in Normal and Ectopic Tubal Pregnancy

As described above, in fallopian tubes from nonpregnant women, there is essentially no reactivity for the MHC Class II antigens DP or DQ, while a variable number of epithelial cells stain positive for DR molecules. In contrast, in normal first trimester pregnancy and in ectopic tubal pregnancy, the tubal epithelium shows intense reactivity for DR, DP, and DQ. At term, there is slight loss of DP, and DQ reactivity, but most cells continue to show DR, DP, and DQ reactivity (10).

In formalin-fixed tissues from ectopic pregnancy, chronic inflammatory cells of lymphocyte and histiocyte morphology are present at the implantation site, and show some tendency to aggregate around congested blood vessels. Plasma cells are rarely seen. Acute inflammatory cells appear in areas of tubal hemorrhage and necrosis.

In frozen tissues from ectopic pregnancy, abundant leukocytes have been identified in the basal layer of the epithelium that express the mature CD8 lymphocyte marker. In the interstitium, macrophages expressing Class II MHC antigens appear to be most populous, accounting for three-quarters of the total interstitial leukocytes. Other cells that can be identified in the interstitium include pan-T cells, CD8 cells, B cells, and granulocytes. Occasional cells react to antibody against the C3b complement receptor, expressed by monocytes, granulocytes, and a proportion of B cells (13).

CYTOKINES IN THE HUMAN FALLOPIAN TUBE

The identification of cytokines within human fallopian tubes has been documented only within the past 5 years. Prior to this time, little was known. This can be explained by several factors. First, the advent of molecular biology, enabling the type of studies required to document their presence, has been fairly recent (monoclonal and poly-clonal antibodies for immunohistochemistry, components for western and northern blotting, reverse transcription–polymerase chain reaction, and in situ hybridization). Secondly, from a practical standpoint, human fallopian tubes from reproductive-aged women are difficult to obtain, and because of the complex anatomy and histology of the tube, require the entire length of tube in order to perform comprehensive studies. The earliest studies involved identification of cytokines in the reproductive tract of other species, and eventually progressed to humans. Studies involving the female re-productive tract appear to have evolved in order of their accessibility, with the first studies involving the human uterus, placenta, cervix, and vagina, then ovary, and fi-nally, the fallopian tubes.

Only six cytokines/growth factors have been identified consistently within human fallopian tube mucosa to date. Many more cytokines have been shown to exist within human oviductal fluid. However, because of the difficulty in obtaining human tubal fluid, only one comprehensive cytokine study in human tubal fluid is currently in print.

HUMAN FALLOPIAN TUBE MUCOSA

Epidermal Growth Factor and Transforming Growth Factor α

Epidermal growth factor (EGF) was discovered in 1959 during experiments charac-terizing the effects of tumor extracts on nerve growth development. The human form was initially identified in urine of pregnant women. Cloning data suggest it is a 53 amino acid peptide cleaved from a 1217 amino acid precursor. EGF shares homology with TGF-α and *Vaccinia* virus P19. EGF works through a specific cell surface re-ceptor glycoprotein of approximately 170 kDa.

EGF is found in virtually all body fluids including milk, urine, saliva, and sweat. Binding has been demonstrated in virtually all cell types tested except those of hematopoetic lineage. EGF is reported to support growth and differentiation during fetal development and enhance epidermal growth and keratinization, in addition to multiple other functions. The human uterus was shown to contain EGF and its recep-tors, so it was natural that EGF and its structural and functional homologue TGF-α were among the first to be identified in the human fallopian tube.

EGF protein, TGF-α protein, and EGF/TGF-α receptor mRNA and protein have been identified in the human fallopian tube by immunohistochemistry, northern blot analysis, western blot analysis, and in situ hybridization. Intitial studies revealed that ampullary regions contain more than in the isthmus, proliferative phase more than se-cretory phase, and postmenopausal specimens contained the lowest amounts (14).

In later studies using immunohistochemistry, intense staining was noted in am-pullary epithelium, but only during the late follicular and luteal phases, with weak staining observed in the early follicular phase of the menstrual cycle. This was contra-dictory to earlier findings, but may be explained by more specific menstrual dating, whereas earlier studies had divided the cycle into only two phases. Quantitative reverse transcription and polymerase chain reaction studies also revealed higher levels during the late follicular and luteal phases compared to early follicular phase specimens. The expression of these growth factors was in proportion to increases in serum estradiol but not to progesterone levels. To demonstrate the potential biologic effects of these growth factors, experiments in two-cell murine embryos were performed in which they were co-cultured with human oviduct epithelial cells with and without the addition of blocking antibodies to various growth factors to determine the growth factor specificity of their findings. Co-culture promoted blastocyst formation, but this effect was abrogated by the addition of monoclonal antibodies to EGF and TGF-α. These data suggest a potential role for EGF and TGF-α in early embryonic development (15).

Another study demonstrating the presence of EGF, TGF-α, and their receptor by immunohistochemistry and RT-PCR again found higher levels of EGF and TGF-α during late proliferative and early to midsecretory phases compared to early proliferative or late secretory phases of the menstrual cycle. Reduced staining was found in postmenopausal specimens. These changes confirmed earlier suggestions of their regulation by ovarian steroids (16).

Estrogen appears to induce EGF, TGF-α, and their common receptor in vivo, and EGF and its receptor, but not TGF-α in vitro. This was demonstrated by treating postmenopausal women with estrogen preoperatively, and comparing fallopian tube RNA samples with specimens from untreated postmenopausal women using competitive PCR analysis. In vitro experiments using human tubal cells in culture indicated EGF involvement in estrogen induced cell growth using thymidine uptake. This effect could be abolished by adding monoclonal antibodies to EGF. These data suggest estrogen regulation of EGF and its receptor, and imply that EGF, but not TGF-α, may be involved in human tubal cell growth (17).

In summary, EGF, TGF-α, and their common receptor appear to be present in higher levels in fallopian tube mucosa during the late proliferative and early secretory phases of the menstrual cycle than during the late secretory or early proliferative phases. There are also higher levels of EGF and TGF in women of reproductive age than in postmenopausal women. The ampulla of the fallopian tube appears to contain higher levels of these factors than other areas of the fallopian tube. The concentration of these factors appears to be proportional to serum estradiol levels. Estrogen appears to induce EGF, TGF-α, and their common receptor in vivo.

Insulin-like Growth Factor 1–4 and Binding Proteins

Insulin-like growth factors (IGFs) are polypeptides with insulin-like growth promoting activities that are expressed in a variety of tissues. In the human uterus, expression of IGF-1 mRNA is greatest in the late proliferative phase of the menstrual cycle, and expression of mRNA for IGF-1 can be rapidly induced following administration of 17 B-estradiol in rats, mice, and pigs.

The expression of IGF binding proteins (IGFBPs) in the HFT was reported prior to expression of the proteins themselves. IGFBPs have been identified by northern and western blot analysis for RNA and protein, respectively. IGFBPs 2, -3, and -4 have been shown to be expressed in the HFT. IGFBP-1 mRNA has been detectable rarely (18).

The IGF proteins are also present in the HFT primarily in the epithelial lining of the tubes. Both ciliated and nonciliated tubal epithelial cells express IGF. Although there appears to be no difference in expression between regions of the tube, immunostaining intensity is cycle dependent, with considerably higher expression observed in the late proliferative and early secretory phase compared to the late secretory phase of the menstrual cycle. Very little staining has been detected in early proliferative and in postmenopausal specimens (19). The IGFs possibly mediate estrogen induced cellular mitosis in oviductal epithelium.

In summary, IGF 1-4 and IGFBPs 2-4 are present in the human fallopian tube and appear to be more abundant in the late proliferative and early secretory phases of the menstrual cycle, where they may mediate cellular mitosis of oviductal epithelium.

Transforming Growth Factor ß

Transforming growth factor (TGF-ß) has five subtypes (B1–5) and at least three receptor subtypes. TGF-ß has a wide range of biologic activities. With very few exceptions, all cells have surface receptors for, and respond to, TGF-ß. The nature of the response depends on cell type, growth conditions, state of cellular differentiation, and the presence of other growth factors. TGF-ß is an important modulator of cell growth, differentiation, and activities of a number of types of cells involved in both cellular and humoral immunity.

RT-PCR of total RNA from the HFT has revealed the presence of TGF-ß1, -2, and -3 and TGF-ß receptor Type I-III mRNA expression. Using in situ hybridization and immunohistochemistry, all tubal cell types express TGF-ß isoforms and Type II receptor mRNA and protein. Tubal epithelial cells appear to express more TGF-ß1 mRNA and TGF-ß1-3 proteins than other cell types. Both ciliated and nonciliated cells in the ampullary and isthmic regions of the fallopian tubes express mRNA and protein at a similar level. The intensity of immunostaining in fallopian tube epithelial cells appears to be higher in the mid to late proliferative and early to midsecretory phases compared to early proliferative and late secretory phases of the menstrual cycle (20). These data suggest a role for TGF-ß in a variety of tubal functions.

In summary, TGF-ß1-3 and TGF-ß receptor type II are present in the human fallopian tube. They are present in higher concentrations in mid to late proliferative phases and early to midsecretory phases compared to early proliferative or late secretory phases of the menstrual cycle.

Granulocyte Macrophage Colony Stimulating Factor and Its Receptors

Granulocyte macrophage colony stimulating factor (GM-CSF) is a 22 kDa glycoprotein that stimulates proliferation of multipotential progenitor cells and induces the proliferation, differentiation, and functional activation of granulocytes and macrophages. Its biologic activity is mediated through a specific cell surface receptor that consists of two interacting subunits, alpha and beta, encoded by two independent genes.

Human fallopian tubes express GM-CSF mRNA and protein, as well as MRNA for GM-CSF receptors (21). Tubal epithelial cells in the ampullary and isthmic regions of the fallopian tube appear to be the primary site of GM-CSF mRNA and protein expression. To a lesser extent, tubal stromal, smooth muscle, arterial endothelial, and arterial smooth muscle cells also express GM-CSF mRNA and protein. Observations using in situ hybridization and immunostaining indicate that the presence of both the mRNA and protein for GM-CSF appears to be cycle dependent, for levels of these factors are considerably higher during the mid to late proliferative and early to mid secretory phases of the menstrual cycle, and are reduced in the early proliferative and late secretory phases of the cycle (21). The physiological role of GM-CSF in oviductal tissue has not yet been determined.

Leukemia Inhibitory Factor

Leukemia inhibitory factor (LIF) may have an important role in early embryonic development and implantation. LIF mRNA has been reported to be expressed in the human fallopian tube with only a slight variation in staining observed across the menstrual cycle, but appears to be markedly elevated in association with an ectopic pregnancy (22). Levels of LIF appear to be higher in tubal mucosa than in other sites within the fallopian tube. LIF expression is more abundant in the more distal portions of the fallopian tube. Estradiol and progesterone levels have not been shown to modulate LIF expression in either fallopian tube epithelial or stromal cell cultures. IL-1α, TNF-β, and TGF-ß, however, have been shown to enhance LIF expression, with TGF-α enhancing expression by fourfold in stromal cells. The presence of LIF in the ampullary portion of the fallopian tube suggests a role for LIF in early embryonic development. Elevated expression in ectopic implantation and the marked induction of secretion by cytokines suggest a link between inflammation, LIF, and tubal ectopic pregnancies.

In summary, six cytokines/growth factors (EGF, TGF-α, IGF, TGF-ß, GM-CSF and LIF) have been identified in the human fallopian tube. Considering that tubal epithelial cells undergo cyclic morphological and biologic variations, one or a variety of cytokines, including those mentioned above, may play an important role in these activities. All these data suggest that fallopian tube-derived growth factors and cytokines may play a critical role at various stages of reproduction including fertilization and early embryonic development through the preimplantation period, in addition to having other biologic functions within the HFT.

HUMAN OVIDUCTAL FLUID

Investigation into tubal fluid components was initiated in the 1970s. Methods for collecting human tubal fluid in vivo for study have been devised and published. The amount of oviductal fluid collected has varied from 0.1 to 20 mL in a single day, with the majority of patients producing 1–2 mL per day. Human oviductal fluid volumes in the periovulatory period appear to be greatest, and lowest (less than 1 mL) prior to day

13 and after day 19 (23). Electrophoresis of tubal fluid proteins compared to autologous peripheral serum has been performed in selective cases. The biochemical analysis indicates that sodium and magnesium levels in tubal fluid are similar to serum, whereas potassium and chloride levels are higher than in serum, and calcium and magnesium are at the lower end of the normal range for serum. Sodium and chloride levels appear to be the same before and after ovulation, but potassium levels drop and calcium levels rise. Glucose is lower in the secretory phase compared to the proliferative phase. Protein concentrations appear to be lower in the periovulatory phase, when volumes appear to be greatest, and higher in the other phases of the menstrual cycle.

Similar rises in tubal fluid volumes in the late proliferative and early secretory phase have been described in other studies (24). Biochemical analysis of human tubal fluid has been used as the basis for the formulation of the culture media used in embryo culture systems for in vitro fertilization (25, 26).

In the only comprehensive study on cytokines in human tubal fluid, oviductal fluid was collected from multiparous women and cytokine levels were determined using commercially available ELISA kits. Significant levels of the immunosuppressive cytokines IL-10, TGF-ß1 (latent), and TGF-ß2 (latent) were detected. The active forms of TGF-B1 and TGF-B2 were not demonstrable. The cytokines IL-1RA, soluble IL-2Ra, IL-6, IL-8, IL-11, TNF-α, IFN-γ , MIP-1α, and stem cell factor (SCF) were present in detectable quantities. IL-2, IL-4, IL-12, LIF, TNF-ß, and GM-CSF have not been detected consistently or were detected only in negligible concentrations (27). The absence of IL-12 is notable because IL-12 is produced by antigen presenting cells with immune regulatory function important in generating TH-1 cells and cytotoxic lymphocytes.

The presence of pro-inflammatory cytokines IL-1ß, IL-2, IL-6, IL-8, TNF-α, MIP-1α and IFN-γ may play a role in defending the oviduct against infection. High levels of IL-10, IL-1RA, TGF-ß1, and TGF-ß2 may counterbalance the presence of pro-inflammatory cytokines. SCF is present in concentrations as high or higher than found in the sera of healthy controls, suggesting a potential role for this factor in the proliferation of cells of the preimplantation embryo. Any of these cytokines may also play a role in normal tubal motility, oocyte or sperm survival, fertilization, or early embryo development.

There are no published data to date regarding the potential changes in cytokine levels in human tubal fluid through the menstrual cycle.

THE POTENTIAL ROLE OF HUMAN OVIDUCTAL CYTOKINES IN REPRODUCTION

Tubal Motility

Tubal cilia at ovulation beat in the direction of the uterus in synchronized waves. During the course of ovum pickup, there appears to be a realignment of fimbriae in their relationship to the ovary. It is thought that, at the time of ovulation, the fimbria ovaricum contracts, pulling the tube in the direction of the rupturing follicle. At the same time, muscles in the paraovarian tissue also contract, pulling the ovary toward the tubal ostium. This anatomic realignment of the tube to the ovary has been documented in several laboratory species, but has not been fully substantiated in women.

Following ovulation, the ovum is surrounded by sticky cumulus cells and transported by the action of cilia along the surface of the fimbriated end of the tube. Muscular contraction of the fallopian tube is probably also quite important, because patients with Kartagener's syndrome, where cilia are structurally defective and immobile, have preserved, although impaired, fertility. The role of adrenergic innervation, prostaglandins, or cytokines has not been well defined but a few factors have been studied.

Macrophage stimulating protein (MSP) and its receptor RON tyrosine kinase have been implicated in tubal motility. RON has been localized at the apical surface of ciliated epithelia in the human airway and in the oviduct. MSP activation of RON increases ciliary beat frequency and might play a role in gamete motility through the fallopian tube facilitating fertilization (28).

The effects of γ-aminobutyric acid (GABA) have been examined on the spontaneous contractile activity of the ampullary region of the human fallopian tube in vitro. GABA increased the frequency and decreased the amplitude of contractions in both circular and longitudinal smooth muscle layers. In longitudinal muscle, this occurred independent of hormone status, whereas in circular muscle, amplitude was affected only in the follicular phase and in postmenopausal samples, but was unaffected in the luteal phase (29). These findings suggest that GABA receptors may be involved in the regulation of tubal motility, modulation of ovum transport and fertility.

Prostaglandin F-2α (PGF2α) has been shown to elicit an excitatory response in both muscle layers, whereas norepinephrine and isoproteronol decreased their activity. Oxytocin and indomethacin had relatively limited effects on the spontaneous motility of ampullary segments of the human fallopian tube (30).

These findings suggest the possibility that a number of autocrine, paracrine, endocrine, and other factors play a role in tubal motility. How these factors may be influenced by cytokines remains to be studied.

The Potential Effects of Tubal Cytokines on Sperm Function and Fertilization

Human oviductal fluid has been found to prolong sperm survival (31). Human oviductal cells and their conditioned medium maintain motility and hyperactivation of human sperm in vitro (32). Taurine and hypotaurine are necessary compounds for sperm capacitation, fertilization, and embryo development, and hypotaurine has a protective role against peroxidative damage. Both taurine and hypotaurine are synthesized and secreted in vitro by oviductal epithelial cells (33), and their role in both in vivo and in vitro fertilization needs more careful study. Human oviductal fluid appears to induce the acrosome reaction (34). Coincubation of human sperm with human oviductal epithelial cells induces sperm capacitation (35). There is evidence that human oviductal proteins bind to the surface of the entire sperm (36). In vitro studies comparing the sequential effects of human cervical mucus, oviductal fluid, and follicular fluid on sperm motility, hyperactivation, and the acrosome reaction have been reported (37). The complement system, including C3b, C1q, and CD46, has also been implicated in sperm–oocyte interaction (38–40).

Details regarding egg–sperm interaction are sparse, but as early as 1985, improved pregnancy rates were reported for human in vitro fertilization using medium based on the composition of human tubal fluid (41). Zona-free hamster ova penetration ability of human sperm with poor motility can be improved using human tubal fluid medium to process sperm compared with Ham's F-10 medium (42). In pigs, a factor(s) from oviductal secretion has been found to be required for the complete cortical granule reaction and in modification of the zona pellucida (43). Bovine studies indicate that oviductal fluid differentially affects sperm function, depending on the oviductal region and the stage of the estrous cycle at which the fluid was obtained (44). In one study, IFN-γ and TNF were shown to inhibit the ability of human sperm to penetrate hamster eggs (45). However, TNF has also been reported to have no interference with hamster penetration by human sperm (46). Different concentrations and individual susceptibilities to certain cytokines may explain these discrepancies. IL-6 has been detected in seminal plasma in significantly higher levels in infertile men compared to fertile men (47), suggesting that IL-6 may be associated with male infertility.

There is evidence of precontact sperm–egg communication (48). A number of factors have been studied for their potential role in egg–sperm attraction, binding, and penetration. Among these are serine/threonine-linked oligosaccharides (49), atrial natriuretic peptide (50), myelin basic protein (MAP) kinase (51), activators of protein kinase C (52), sperm protein PH-30 egg integrins (53–55), the zona pellucida binding proteins known as ZP1, ZP2, and ZP3 (56), and an unidentified follicular fluid factor (57). The role of cytokines in these and other potential sites of sperm–egg communication, fusion, and fertilization need further refinement.

The Potential Effects of Tubal Cytokines on the Pre-implantation Embryo

Once fertilized, the pre-implantation embryo spends 3–4 days in the human fallopian tube. A number of growth factors and cytokines have been examined for their effects on pre-implantation embryo development. Receptors for cytokines in human pre-implantation embryos appear to show stage-specific differential expression (58). Receptors for CSF-1, SCF, IL-6, LIF, and TNF-α have been documented in the human embryo. Effects of growth factors on pre-implantation mouse embryos have been studied, indicating that EGF, TGF-α, insulin, IGF-1, IGF-2, PDGF-A, PDGF-AB, and TGF-ß have tropic effects. The effects of CSF-1 are less clear (59). Many of these growth factors can be produced by embryos themselves. IL-6, IL-1ß, and IFN-γ are transcribed in the pre-implantation mouse embryo (60). Any of the cytokines produced by tubal epithelium or secreted into tubal fluid described earlier may affect human pre-implantation embryos. There may be sequential effects of cervical mucus, oviductal products, and follicular fluid on early embryos, and the exact nature of this response may vary with cytokine concentration, timing, receptor cell type, and the presence of other cytokines, but all evidence suggests a potential role for oviductal cytokines on early embryonic development.

FUTURE APPLICATIONS AND ANTICIPATED DEVELOPMENTS

The characterization of cytokines in the tissue and fluid of the human oviduct is just beginning to be explored. Much work is needed to investigate further the physiological implications of the cytokines documented to exist in HFT, and to look for the array of others not yet examined.

Research done to date in the human uterus and endometrium, and in the oviducts of other species, can provide valuable insight into which cytokines may be relevant in HFT studies. Investigations on preimplantation embryos and their receptors may also direct HFT research. Sperm research, including investigation into factors aiding capacitation and hyperactivation of sperm, can also direct the search for cytokines likely to be present in the female reproductive tract. Human fallopian tube cell culture and the use of co-culture systems in assisted reproduction may also direct the search for cytokines in the HFT.

Embryonic diapause, a phenomenon in some animal species but not in the human, is an enigma that might be explained by cytokine physiology in the female reproductive tract in affected animals.

Infection control in the oviduct and further understanding of ectopic pregnancy and endometriosis might be explained by cytokine physiology. Several animal studies already exist documenting abnormal tubal motility in the presence of peritoneal fluid from animals with endometriosis, suggesting the potential for cytokines to be detrimental in reproductive processes.

Ultimately, numerous cytokines will inevitably be discovered in the HFT and their functions more clearly understood. Adding to the complexity of this task is the difficulty in obtaining HFT specimens from reproductive-aged women, the dependence of their role with respect to concentration and timing of the presence of various cytokines, the possible need for egg, sperm, or embryo to elicit production of cytokines from the HFT, or the sequential effects of the journey through the female reproductive tract on egg, sperm, and embryo physiology. Understanding the potential factors that enable fertilization and successful reproduction may provide insight into devising preventitives and therapeutics for reproductive dysfunction and for the development of new contraceptive strategies.

REFERENCES

1. Pauerstein CJ, Woodruff JD. The role of the "indifferent" cell of the tubal epithelium. Am J Obstet Gynecol 1967;98:121–125.
2. Geppert M, Geppert J, Bohle A. On the lympho-epithelial relationships of the human oviduct. Virchows Arch 1977;373:133–142.
3. Boehme M, Donat H. Identification of lymphocyte subsets in the human fallopian tube. Am J Reprod Immunol 1992;28:81–84.
4. Morris H, Emms M, Visser T, et al. Lymphoid tissue of the normal fallopian tube—a form of mucosal-associated lymphoid tissue (MALT)? Int J Gynecol Pathol 1986;5:11–22.

5. Otsuki Y, Maeda Y, Magari S, et al. Lymphatics and lymphoid tissue of the fallopian tube: immunoelectronmicroscopic study. Anat Record 1989;225:288–296.

6. Kutteh WH, Hatch KD, Blackwell RE, Mestecky J. Secretory immune system of the female reproductive tract: I. Immunoglobulin and secretory component containing cells. Obstet Gynecol 1988;71:56.

7. Kutteh WH, Blackwell RE, Gore H, et al. Secretory immune system of the female reproductive tract II. Local immune system in normal and infected fallopian tube. Fertil Steril 1990;54:51.

8. Lee YS, Raju GC. Expression of IgA and secretory component in the normal and in adenocarcinomas of fallopian tube, endometrium and endocervix. Histopathology 1988;13:67–78.

9. Cooper MD, Dever C, Tempel K, et al. Characterization of lymphoid cells from the human fallopian tube mucosa. Adv Exp Med Biol 1987;216A:387–394.

10. Bulmer JN, Earl U. The expression of class II MHC gene products by fallopian tube epithelium in pregnancy and throughout the menstrual cycle. Immunology 1987,61(2):207–213.

11. Edelstam GA, Lundkvist OE, Klareskog L, et al. Cyclic variation of major histocompatibility complex call II antigen expression in the human fallopian tube epithelium. Fertil Steril 1992;57:1225.

12. Wollen AL, Sandvei R, Mork S, et al. In situ characterization of leukocytes in the fallopian tube in women with or without an intrauterine contraceptive device. Acta Obstet Gynaecol Scand 1994;73:103–112.

13. Earl U, Lunny DP, Bulmer JN. Leukocyte populations in ectopic tubal pregnancy. J Clin Pathol 1987,40:901–905.

14. Lei ZM, Rao CV. Expression of Epidermal growth factor (EGF) receptor and its ligands, EGF and Transforming Growth Factor-α, in human fallopian tubes. Endocrinology 1992;131:947.

15. Morishige K, Kurachi H, Amemiya K, et al. Menstrual stage-specific expression of epidermal growth factor and transforming growth factor-alpha in human oviduct epithelium and their role in early embryogenesis. Endocrinology 1993;133:199–207.

16. Chegini N, Zhao Y, McClean F. Expression of messenger ribonucleic acid and presence of immunoreactive proteins for epidermal growth factor (EGF), transforming growth factor alpha (TGFα) and EGF/TGFα receptors and 125I-EGF binding sites in human fallopian tube. Biol Reprod 1994;50:1049–1058.

17. Adachi K, Kurachi H, Homma H, et al. Estrogen induces epidermal growth factor (EGF) receptor and its ligands in human fallopian tube: involvement of EGF but no transforming growth factor alpha in estrogen-induced tubal call growth in vitro. Endocrinology 1995;136:2110–2119.

18. Giudice LC, Dsupin BA, Irwin J, et al. Identification of insulin like growth factor binding proteins in human oviduct. Fertil Steril 1992;57:294–301.

19. Pfeifer T, Chegini N. Immunohistochemical localization of insulin-like growth factor (IGF-1), IGF-1 receptor, and IGF binding proteins 1–4 in human fallopian tube at various reproductive stages. Biol Repro 1994;50:281–289.

20. Zhao Y, Chegini N, Flanders KC. Human fallopian tube expresses transforming growth factor (TGFß) isoforms, TGFß type I-III receptor messenger ribonucleic acid and protein, and contains 125I-TGFß-binding sites. J Clin Endo Met 1994;79:1177–1184

21. Zhao Y, Chegini N. Human fallopian tube espresses granulocyte-macrophage colongy

stimulating factor (GM-CSF) and GM-CSF alpha and beta receptors anad contain immunoreactive GM-CSF protein. J Clin Endo Met 1994, 79(2):662–665.

22. Keltz MD, Attar E, Buradagunta S, et al. Modulation of leukemia inhibitory factor gene expression and protein biosynthesis in the humana fallopian tube. Am J Obstet Gynecol 1996;175(6):1611–1619.

23. Lippes J, Enders RG, Pragay DA, et al. The collection of human fallopian tubal fluid. Contraception 1972;5:85–103.

24. Shams A, Rizk DG, Toppozada HK, et al. Human tubal fluid collection via vagina and its quantitative variations during the menstrual cycle. J Reprod Med 1977;18:61.

25. Borland RM, Biggers JD, Lechene CP, et al. Elemental composition of fluid in the human fallopian tube. J Reprod Fert 1980;58:479–482.

26. Quinn P, Kerm JF, Warnes GM. Improved pregnancy rate in human in vitro fertilization with the use of a medium based on the composition of human tubal fluid. Fertil Steril 1985;44:493.

27. Srivastava MD, Lippes J, Srivastava BI. Cytokines of the human reproductive tract. Am J Reprod Immunol 1996;36:157–166.

28. Sakomoto O, Iwama A, Amitani R, et al. Role of macrophage-stimulating protein and its receptor, RON tyrosine kinase, in ciliary motility. J Clin Invest 1997;99(4):701–709.

29. Laszlo A, Nadasy GL, Erdo SL, et al. Effects of GABA on the spontaneous muscular activity of the human fallopian tube ampullar segments in vitro. Acta Physiol Hung 1990;76(2):123–130.

30. Laszlo A, Nadasy GL, Monos E, Zsolnai B. Effect of pharmacological agents on the activity of the circular and longitudinal muscle layers of human fallopian tubal ampullar segments. Acta Physiol Hung 1988;72(1):123–133.

31. Zhu J, Barrat C, Lippes J, et al. Human oviductal fluid prolongs sperm survival. Fertil Steril 1994;61:360–366.

32. Yeung WSB, Ng VKH, Lau EYL, Ho PC. Human oviductal cells and their conditioned medium maintain the motility and hyperactivation of human spermatazoa in vitro. Human Reprod 1994;9:656–660.

33. Guerin P, Guillaud J, Menezo Y. Hypotaurine in spermatozoa and gential secretions and its production by oviduct epithelial cells in vitro. Human Reprod 1995;10:866–872.

34. De Jonge CJ, Barrat C, Radwanska E, Cooke I. The Acrosome Reaction-Inducing Effect of Human Follicular and Oviductal Fluid. J Androl 1993;14:359–365.

35. Vervancioglu, ME, Djahanabakhch O, Aitken RJ. Epithelial cell coculture and the induction of sperm capacitation. Fertil Steril 1994:61:1103–1108.

36. Lippes J, Wagh PV. Human oviductal fluid (hOF) proteins. Evidence for hOF proteins binding to human sperm. Fertil Steril 1989;51:89–94.

37. Zhu J, Barratt C, Lippes J, et al. The sequential effects of human cervical mucus, oviductal fluid and follicular fluid on sperm function. Fertil Steril 1994;61:1129–1135.

38. Anderson DJ, Abbott AF, Jack RM. The role of complement component C3b and its receptors in sperm-oocyte interaction. Proc Natl Acad Sci USA 1993;90:10051–10055.

39. Okabe M, Matzno S, Nagira T, et al. A human sperm antigen possibly involved in binding and/or fusion with zona-free hamster eggs. Fertil Steril 1990;54:1211–1126.

40. Fusi F, Bronson RA, Hong Y, et al. Complement component C1q and its receptor are involved in the interaction of human sperm with zona free hamster eggs. Mol Reprod Dev 1991;29:180–188.

41. Quinn P, Kerin JF, Warnes GM. Improved pregnancy rate in human in vitro fertilization with the use of a medium based on the composition of human tubal fluid. Fertil Steril 1985;44(4):493–498.

42. Cai XQ, Marik JJ. Comparison of the effects on penetration capacity of human spermatozoa between using Ham's F-10 medium and a medium based on the composition of human tubal fluid. Andrologia 1990;22(6):539–542.

43. Kim NH, Funahashi H, Abeydeera LR, et al. Effects of oviductal fluid on sperm penetration and cortical granule exocytosis during fertilization of pig oocytes in vitro. J Reprod Fertil 1996;107(1):79–86.

44. Grippo AA, Way AL, Killian GJ. Effect of bovine ampullary and isthmic oviductal fluid on motility, acrosome reaction and fertility of bull spermatozoa. J Reprod Fertil 1995;105(1):57–64.

45. Hill JA, Cohen J, Anderson DJ. The effects of lymphokines and monokines on human sperm fertilizing ability in the zona free hamster egg penetration test. Am J Obstet Gynecol 1989;160:1154–1159.

46. Wincek TJ, Meyer TK, Meyer MR, Kuehl TJ. Absence of a direct effect of recombinant tumor necrosis factor-alpha on human sperm function and murine preimplantation development. Fertil Steril 1991;56(2):332–339.

47. Naz RK, Kaplan P. Increased levels of interleukin-6 in seminal plasma of infertile men. J Androl 1994; 15(3):220–227.

48. Eisenbach M, Ralt D. Precontact mammalian sperm-egg communication and role in fertilization. Am J Physiol 1992;262:C1095–1101.

49. Litscher ES, Wassarman PM. Characterization of mouse ZP3-derived glycopeptide, gp55, that exhibits sperm receptor and acrosome reaction-inducing activity in vitro. Biochemistry 1996;35:3980–3985.

50. Zamir N, Riven-Kreitman R, Manor M, et al. Atrial natriuertic peptide attracts human spermatozoa in vitro. Biochem Biophys Res Commun 1993;197:116–122.

51. Moos J, Visconti PE, Moore GD, et al. Potential role of mitogen-activated protein kinase in pronuclear envelope assembly and disassembly following fertilization of mouse eggs. Biol Reprod 1995; 53:692–699.

52. Moore GD, Kopf GS, Schultz RM. Differential effect of activators of protein kinase C on cytoskeletal changes in mouse and hamster eggs. Dev Biol 1995;170:519–530.

53. Myles DG. Molecular mechanisms of sperm-egg membrane binding and fusion in mammals. Dev Biol 1993;158:35–45.

54. Moos J, Faundes D, Kopf GS, Schultz RM. Composition of the human zona pellucida and modifications following fertilization. Human Reprod 1995;10:2467–2471.

55. Evans JP, Schultz RM, Kopf GS. Mouse sperm-egg plasma membrane ineractions: analysis of roles of egg integrins and the mouse sperm homologue of PH-30 (fertilin) beta. J Cell Sci 1995;108:3267–3278.

56. Evans JP, Schultz RM, Kopf GS. Identification and localization of integrin subunits in oocytes and eggs of the mouse. Mol Reprod Dev 1995;40:211–220.

57. Ralt D, Goldenberg M, Fetterfhol P, et al. Sperm attraction to a follicular factor(s) correlates with human egg fertilizability. Proc Natl Acad Sci USA 1991; 88:2840–2844.

58. Sharkey AM, Dellow K, Blayney M, et al. Stage-Specific Expression of Cytokine and Receptor Messenger Ribonucleic Acids in Human Preimplantation Embryos. Bio Reprod 1995;53:955–962.

59. Adamson ED. Activities of growth factors in preimplantation embryos. J Cell Biochem 1993;53:280–297.

60. Rothstein JL, Johnson D, DeLoia JA, et al. Gene expression during preimplantation mouse development. Genes Devel 1992;6:1190–1201.

61. Harvey MB, Leco KJ, Panlilio MY, et al. Roles of growth factors during peri-implantation development. Mol Human Reprod 1995;10:712–718.

62. Smotrich DB, Stillman RJ, Widra EA, et al. Immunocytochemical localization of growth factors and their receptors in human pre-embryos and fallopiain tubes. Eur Soc Hum Reprod Embryol 1995;184–190.

63. Kaye PL, Harvey MB. The role of growth factors in preimplantation development. Prog Growth Factor Res 1995;6:1–24.

64. Slager HG, Inzen W, Eijnden AJ, et al. Transforming Growth Factor-ß in the early mouse embryo:implications for the regulation of muscle formation anad implantation.Dev Gen 1993;14:212–224.

65. Larson RC, Ignotz GG, Currie WB. Transforming Growth Factor B and Basaic Fibroblsat Growth Factor Synergistically Promote Early Bovine Embryo Development During the Fourth Cell Cycle. Mol Reprod Dev 1992;33:432–435.

66. Lim J, Bongso A, Ratnam S. Mitogenic and Cytogenetic Evaluation of Transforming Growth Factor-B on Murine Preimplantation Embryonic Development in vitro. Mol Reprod Dev 1993;36:482–487.

67. Rappolee DA, Brenner CA, Schultz R, et al. Developmental expression of PDGF, TGF-α, and TGF-ß genes in preimplantation mouse embryos. Science 1988;1823–1825.

68. Analysis of the expression of growth factor, interleukin-1, and lactoferrin genes and the distribution of inflammatory leukocytes in the preimplantation mouse oviduct. Biol Reprod 1994;51:597–606.

69. Watson AJ, Watson PH, Panilio MA, et al. A growth factor phenotype map for ovine preimplantation development. Biol Reprod 1994;50:725–733.

70. Paria BC, Jones KL, Flanders KC, Dey SK, Localization and binding of transforming growth factor-B isoforms in mouse preimplantation embryos and in delayed and activated blastocysts. Devel Biol 1992;151:91–104.

71. Paria BC, Dey SK. Preimplantation embryo development in vitro: cooperative interactions among embryos and the role of growth factors. Proc Natl Acad Sci USA 1990;87:756–760.

72. Leukemia inhibitory factor significantly enhances the blastocyst formation rates of human embryos cultured in serum-free medium. Am Soc Human Reprod Embryol 1995;191–196.

73. Kauma SW, Matt DW. Coculture Cells that express leukemia inhibitory facotr (LIF) enhance mouse blastocyst development in vitro. J Assist Reprod Gen 1995;12:153–156.

74. Larson RC, Ignotz GG Currie WB. Platelet derived growth factor (PDGF) stimulates development of bovine embryos during the fourth cell cycle. Development 1992;115:821–826.

75. Morishige KI, Kurachi H, Amemiya K, et al. Menstrual stage specific expression of epidermal growth factor and transforming growth factor-α in human oviduct epithelium and their role in early embryogenesis. Endocrinology 1993;133:199–207.

76. Takeuchi K, Nagata Y, Sandow B, et al. Primary culture of human fallopian tube epithelial cells and co-culture of early mouse pre-embryos. Mol Reprod Dev 1992;32:236–242.

77. Hoshi K, Kanno Y, Katayose H, et al. Coculture of Mouse embryos with cryopreserved human oviduct epithelial cells. J Assist Reprod Gen 1994;11:367–372.

78. Robertson SA, Seamark RF, Guilbert LG, Wegmann TG. The role of cytokines in gestation. Crit Rev Immunol 1994;14:239–292.

79. Schultz RM, Kopf GS. Molecular basis of mammalian egg interaction. Curr Top Dev Biol 1995;30:21–62.

80. Wassarman PM, Litscher ES. Sperm-egg recognition mechanisms in mammals. Curr Top Dev Biol 1995;30:1–19.

81. Hillier SG, ed. Scientific Essentials of Reproductive Medicine. WB Saunders Company, 1996

82. Kurman RJ, ed. Blaustein's Pathology of the Female Genital Tract. Springer-Verlag, 1994.

11

CYTOKINES IN THE PERITONEAL ENVIRONMENT

Emre Seli and Aydin Arici

Yale University School of Medicine,
New Haven, Connecticut

The peritoneal environment is an immunologically dynamic milieu that links the reproductive and immune systems. Fallopian tubes and ovaries are bathed in peritoneal fluid (PF). Oocytes are exposed to the peritoneal environment even after they are captured by the fimbria because the fallopian tube is a conduit freely communicating with the peritoneal cavity. Spermatozoa are exposed to PF factors before and during fertilization. The embryo undergoes early development in the fallopian tube where it may also be exposed to the cellular and soluble components of PF.

In this chapter, the peritoneal environment and its cellular constituents are defined, as well as the cytokines and growth factors found in the peritoneal environment (Table 11.1). The source and fluctuation of these secreted factors throughout the menstrual cycle is defined, as is their potential involvement in peritoneum-related conditions affecting reproduction.

Cytokines in Human Reproduction, Edited by Joseph A. Hill
ISBN 0-471-35242-X   Copyright © 2000 Wiley-Liss, Inc.

Table 11.1. Cytokine and growth factor levels in the peritoneal fluid. Effects of endometriosis and menstrual cycle phase

Cytokine Growth Factor	Level in Endometriosis[a]	Effect of Menstrual Phase[a]	Reference
IL-1	↑	NA (all samples from the proliferative phase)	Fakih et al. (14)
	↑	Not mentioned	Hill and Anderson (47)
	↑	NA (all samples from the late proliferative phase)	Taketani et al. (44)
	↔	NA (all samples from the peri-ovulatory phase)	Mori et al. (51)
	↔	↔	Awadalla et al. (48)
	↔	Not mentioned	Koyama et al. (50)
	↔	NA (all samples from the proliferative phase)	Keenan et al. (49)
IL-2	↔	NA (all samples from the proliferative phase)	Keenan et al. (49)
IL-5	↑	Not mentioned	Koyama et al. (50)
IL-6	↑	Not mentioned	Rier et al. (64)
	↑	Not mentioned	Koyama et al. (50)
	↔ (In nonendometriosis pelvic adhesions: ↑)	↔	Buyalos et al.(62)
	↔	Not mentioned	Boutten et al. (61)
	↔	Not mentioned	Keenan et al. (63)
IL-8	↑	Not mentioned	Arici et al. (74)
	↑	↔	Ryan et al. (73)
IL-10	↔	Not mentioned	Rana et al. (76)
MCP-1	↑	Proliferative > secretory	Arici et al. (81a in press)
RANTES	↑	↔	Khorram et al. (87)
GRO-α	↑	↔	Oral et al. (79)
TNF-α	↑	↔	Eisermann et al. (92)
	↑	Not mentioned	Halme et al. (15)
	↑	NA (all samples from the late proliferative phase)	Taketani et al. (44)
	↑	Not mentioned	Mori et al. (52)
	↑	NA (all samples from the secretory phase)	Rana et al. (76)
	↔	↔	Vercellini et al. (93)
	↔	NA (all samples from the proliferative phase)	Keenan et al. (49)
IFN-γ	↔	↔	Khorram et al. (87)
	↔	Not mentioned	Keenan et al. (63)
M-CSF	↑	NA	Fukaya et al. (104)
TGF-ß	↑	↔	Oosterlynck et al. (108)
EGF	↔	Secretory > proliferative	De Leon et al. (34)
	↔	Secretory > proliferative	Huang et al. (116)
bFGF	↔	↔	Huang et al. (116)
	↔	↔	Seli et al. (126a)
IGFs	Not evaluated for levels in endometriosis	↔	Giudice et al. (118)

[a] ↔, no difference; ↑, increased; NA, not applicable.

PERITONEAL ENVIRONMENT

Peritoneum is the most extensive serous membrane in the body with a surface area equivalent to that of the skin (1). Peritoneum consists of two layers: a loose connective tissue layer that contains collagen, elastic fibers, fat cells, and macrophages, and a mesothelial layer consisting of squamous cells. The human peritoneal cavity normally contains 5–20 mL of straw-colored fluid that varies widely depending on the physiological conditions. Peritoneal fluid arises primarily from two different sources, plasma transudate and ovarian exudate. Other contributing sources include tubal fluid, retrograde menstruation, and immune and inflammatory cell secretions. In women PF volume is maximum following ovulation and depends on follicular activity, corpus luteum vascularity, and hormone production.

Peritoneal fluid also reflects the intraperitoneal pathological conditions that may affect reproductive events. Changes in PF volume and concentration of a variety of cells, hormones, and other compounds have been characterized in women with endometriosis and during the normal menstrual cycle (2). Cellular and biochemical constituents of PF have been suggested to play an important role in the pathogenesis of endometriosis (3, 4). Components of the PF may adversely interact with ovulatory function, gamete transport or survival, sperm–ovum interaction, early embryonic development, and implantation (5). Thus PF abnormalities associated with endometriosis may also be linked to endometriosis associated infertility.

Peritoneal fluid volume may be altered in various pathological conditions. A review of 17 studies on the PF volume in endometriosis has revealed conflicting results (6). Five of the 17 studies found increased PF volume in endometriosis, and 11 found no difference. The largest study suggested an increase in the PF volume in endometriosis throughout the menstrual cycle (2). However, two other well designed studies performed between cycle days 8–12 and 13–18, failed to demonstrate increased PF volume among women with endometriosis (7, 8). Cycle day variations, improperly selected control groups, and different collection techniques may explain the discrepancies found in these studies. Overall, there are suggestive findings that the volume of PF may be modestly increased in women with endometriosis compared to the volume in women without this disease. However, PF volume appears to be of little clinical importance because it correlates poorly with infertility.

Cells in the Peritoneal Fluid

Peritoneal fluid contains a variety of free floating cells subject to change with pathological conditions. Hill et al. (9) used monoclonal antibodies rather than histological morphology to identify cell types in PF, and reported that women with early stages of endometriosis had the most significant elevations of total leukocytes, macrophages, helper T cells, and natural killer (NK) cells compared to fertile controls. These cells may be chemotactically attracted to the peritoneal cavity in response to the disease or their increased presence may represent the primary abnormality.

Macrophages. Macrophages are attracted to the peritoneal environment more abundantly than any other cell type. Macrophage directed host defense mechanisms resulting in recognition, phagocytosis, and destruction of microorganisms are well known. Macrophages also promote cellular growth and viability through secretion of growth factors and cytokines. Macrophages digest and process peritoneal debris such as sperm and endometrial tissue and present antigens to lymphocytes. Macrophages also are capable of secreting various substances such as growth factors, cytokines, prostanoids, complement components, and hydrolytic enzymes. Furthermore, macrophages release low levels of reactive oxygen metabolites, such as superoxide anion, hydrogen peroxide, and singlet oxygen.

Normally, PF contains leukocytes in concentration of 0.5 to 2.0 × 10^6/mL of which 85% are macrophages (10). Their concentration appears to fluctuate throughout the menstrual cycle, being highest during menstruation. The association between macrophages and endometriosis has been investigated extensively. Haney et al. (11) first reported an increase in peritoneal macrophages in infertile women with endometriosis. Subsequent studies of the PF of women with this disorder have confirmed an increased number, concentration, and activation of macrophages (12, 13). The extent of endometriosis generally does not appear to correlate with macrophage count, although a tendency toward higher numbers has been observed in women with minimal to mild stages of disease (12).

Macrophages can induce chemotaxis and proliferation of cells involved in inflammation, tissue repair, and neovascularization, such as neutrophils, monocytes, fibroblasts, and endothelial cells, by secreting factors such as interleukin (IL)-1, IL-6, IL-8, tumor necrosis factor-α (TNF-α), macrophage-derived growth factor, monocyte chemoattractant protein-1 (MCP-1), RANTES, transforming growth factor ß (TGF-ß), and platelet derived growth factor (PDGF) and thus play a critical role in inflammation and adhesion formation in the peritoneal cavity. Peritoneal fluid levels of these factors are also elevated in endometriosis (3, 14, 15). Macrophage products may be responsible for growth or maintenance of ectopic endometrium. Surrey and Halme (16) demonstrated that PF from women with endometriosis stimulated cell proliferation in endometrial stromal cell culture. Further support for this concept was demonstrated by studies indicating that peritoneal macrophages from women with endometriosis produce substantially more fibronectin, a growth factor for fibroblasts, than macrophages from healthy women (17). Macrophage products also may contribute to inflammation, adhesion formation, and infertility resulting from other inflammatory conditions such as trauma and infection.

Granulocytes and Lymphocytes. Neutrophils, normally present in small numbers, are greatly increased in PF in association with pelvic inflammatory conditions. Peritoneal fluid from patients with endometriosis has been shown to be chemotactic for neutrophils. Recently neutrophil chemoattractant cytokines such as IL-8 and GROα were found to be increased in the PF of women with endometriosis. Like neutrophils, lymphocytes constitute only a minority of cells found in the peritoneal cavity under normal conditions. Significantly higher numbers of T cells and NK cells, but few B lymphocytes and no plasma cells, have been observed in the PF of women with endometriosis compared to numbers of these cells in PF from those without disease (18).

Natural killer cells represent a cell population whose functional activities arise from the basic responsibility of safeguarding the biologic system from foreign antigen invasion. Peritoneal NK cell activity appears to be decreased in endometriosis with less activity in more severe forms of the disease (19). However, despite decreased NK cell activity in the PF of women with endometriosis, the percentage of peripheral NK cells in these women may be unchanged (20) or even increased (9). Why NK activity is decreased in the PF of women with endometriosis must be clarified. One possibility is that this effect is a result of soluble factors contained in the sera and PFs of the affected women. Natural killer cell activity of women without endometriosis has been reported to be decreased following addition of sera or PF of women with endometriosis (21).

Mesothelial Cells. The mesothelium is a simple layer of squamous epithelium lining the peritoneal cavity. Mesothelial cells are capable of producing cytokine-growth factors, either constitutively (IL-1, IL-6, IL-8, MCP-1, granulocyte colony stimulating factor, macrophage colony stimulating factor [M-CSF]) or in response to a variety of stimuli, including TNF-α, IL-1, and epidermal growth factor (EGF) (22). In addition, these cells secrete CA-125 from their apical surfaces (23). These findings suggest that mesothelial cells play an important role in the regulation of peritoneal inflammation and tissue regeneration.

Endometrial Cells. Retrograde menstruation is quite common. Polishuk and Sharf, performing culdoscopy during menstruation, found blood-stained PF in 50% of women (24). Others have reported that approximately 90% of normal women experience retrograde menstruation, with 70% exhibiting grossly bloody PF during menstruation (25). However, the existence of red blood cells in PF during menstruation does not necessarily correlate with retrograde transport of viable endometrial cells. Studies analyzing the incidence of endometrial cells in PF are conflicting, varying from 0% to 59% (26). Several investigators have found endometrial tissue in the PF of women with or without endometriosis with equal frequency (27, 28). Only one study has identified endometrial tissue more frequently in the PF of women with endometriosis (29). The classic theory of Sampson explains the histogenesis of endometriosis as endometrial implantation resulting from retrograde seeding of endometrial cells during menstruation. Data showing that retrograde transport of viable endometrial cells during menstruation occurs in most women with patent tubes suggest that other factors besides the mere presence of endometrial cell reflux is critical for the pathogenesis of endometriosis.

SOLUBLE SUBSTANCES IN THE PERITONEAL FLUID

Prostaglandins

Prostaglandins (PGs) are the most extensively studied molecules in PF to date (30, 31). There are several sources of PGs in the PF, including macrophages, the peritoneal surface, ovarian follicles, and endometriotic implants (31). Owing to their short half-life, physiologically active PGs are infrequently measured; instead, PG metabolites have been studied. PGEM, PGFM, 6-keto-PGF$_{1\alpha}$, and thromboxane (TX)B$_2$ have been measured as representatives of their active precursors including PGE, PGF_2, PGI, and TXA_2, respectively. Under physiological conditions, no significant cyclic variation of PG levels has been found (2).

Studies reporting levels of $PGF_{2\alpha}$ and PGE_2 in the PF of women with and without endometriosis are contradictory. Some of these studies have reported no difference (32), whereas others have found elevated levels throughout the menstrual cycle (33), or only in the secretory phase (34). Drake et al. measured stable metabolites of TXA_2 and PGI in PF, and observed an increase in the PF of women with endometriosis over controls (35). They suggested that these mediators of smooth muscle contraction might cause infertility by altering tubal function. On the other hand, Badawy et al. (36) and Dawood et al. (37) were unable to substantiate cycle-dependent changes in the PF concentrations of PGs, nor were there differences between patients with unexplained infertility and those with endometriosis. Moon et al. documented the presence of $PGF_{2\alpha}$ in ectopic endometrium (38). In primate animal studies, increased PF levels of $PGF_{2\alpha}$ but not PGE_2 were associated with moderate and severe endometriosis (39).

In summary, data on the levels of TXB_2, 6-keto-PGF_{1a}, and PGF_{2a} in the PF of women with endometriosis are conflicting, but suggestive that they may be elevated. The question of whether these compounds can act as markers or even causal factors in reduced fertility remains unknown.

Cytokines

Cytokines are a heterogeneous group of soluble regulatory polypeptides that are released from cells that regulate cell growth, differentiation, and/or function by binding to specific cellular receptors. They exert autocrine and paracrine effects, but unlike hormones they are produced by a variety of cell types that are not localized in a distinct gland and act on many different types of target cells. Cytokine activities are various and include proliferation and differentiation of immune cells, growth of connective tissue and endothelial cells, induction of release of hormones, enzymes, and acute phase proteins, enhancement of various cytotoxic activities, regulation of immunoglobulin secretion and isotype, chemotaxis, and direct antiviral and tumoricidal effects (40). Expression of biologic activity is achieved at very low concentrations by binding of cytokines to specific, saturable, high-affinity receptors on the plasma membrane of the cell. Additionally, cytokines may either induce or downregulate the production of other cytokines. A subgroup of cytokines, chemokines, are potent leukocyte chemotactic factors, each with a distinct but partially overlapping spectrum of action. Chemokines are further subdivided, according to the position of the first two cysteines, as C-X-C or C-C (41). The C-X-C chemokines are neutrophil chemoattractants (e.g., IL-8) whereas C-C chemokines are predominantly monocyte chemoattractants (e.g., MCP-1, RANTES).

Much evidence points toward an interaction between the immune system and reproduction. Macrophages and other cellular constituents of the peritoneal environment secrete cytokines in response to a variety of inflammatory stimuli. Cytokines may affect reproduction at various levels including gonadal function, gamete function, fertilization and embryo development, implantation, and postimplantation survival of the conceptus. Many cytokines such as IL-1 and TNF-α can have detrimental effects on reproductive cells, especially sperm and embryos, when present at an appropriate place, time, and concentration (42, 43). Taketani et al. reported that medical treatment of endometriosis not only decreased inflammatory cytokine levels, but also concurrently eliminated embryotoxicity of the peritoneal fluid of women with endometriosis (44).

Interleukin-1. Interleukin-1 is a 17 kDa, pleiotropic, pro-inflammatory cytokine, secreted by mononuclear phagocytes, endothelial cells, epithelial cells, and fibroblasts. IL-1 has stimulatory and regulatory effects on the growth and differentiation of numerous cell types. The IL-1 system is composed of IL-1α, IL-1β, and an inhibitor, IL-1 receptor antagonist (IL-1RA). Although IL-1α and IL-1β are encoded by different genes and have different amino acid sequences, both are recognized by the same receptor on target cells and produce the same biologic effects (45).

There are conflicting observations as to the in vitro effect of IL-1 on early reproductive events (14, 42, 43). Interleukin-1 inhibits mouse embryo development in vitro, but only at very high concentrations ($>10^6$ U/mL). Interleukin-1 also impairs the oocyte penetrating capacity of sperm, in both the hamster and the human (46). However, IL-1 does not appear to affect sperm motion parameters significantly (42).

Seven well designed studies have compared IL-1 activity in the PF and women with or without endometriosis with conflicting results. Four of these studies have reported that IL-1 activity was increased in the PF of women with endometriosis (14, 44, 47, 51), whereas the other three reported no difference (48–50). Fakih et al., using a bioassay system, found elevated IL-1 activity in the PF of women with minimal and mild endometriosis compared to normal women undergoing tubal ligation (14). Hill and Anderson, using radioimmunoassay, observed elevated (>1 U/mL) levels of IL-1β in PF from 5 of 26 women with endometriosis compared to none of eight fertile controls, and none of eight women with unexplained infertility (47). Taketani et al. found that IL-1 levels in the PF of women with untreated endometriosis were higher compared to women with medically treated endometriosis and to women without endometriosis (44). Mori et al. detected increased IL-1β levels in early endometriosis compared to fertile controls. On the other hand IL-1β levels in PF of women with moderate to severe endometriosis were not different from controls. On the contrary, Awadalla et al. reported that PF IL-1 activity did not differ between infertile patients with or without endometriosis, but they did not evaluate the levels in fertile controls (48). Koyama et al. compared IL-1 levels in the PF of women with endometriosis to those with other pathologies and found no difference (50). Recently, Keenan et al. found that IL-1 levels in PF of women with and without endometriosis were not different (49). Between those six studies, only one (48) evaluated PF IL-1 levels according to menstrual phases and found no difference between samples collected during the proliferative and secretory phases. Other studies have reported that progression of endometriosis was associated with higher levels of IL-1RA mRNA rather than IL-1ß in peritoneal macrophages (51). In endometriosis, IL-1 may induce adhesion formation by its stimulatory effect on fibroblast proliferation and collagen deposition while causing infertility by its embryotoxic effects.

IL-1 levels in PF are elevated in acute pelvic inflammatory disease (52). Experimentally, IL-1 administration caused increased adhesion formation in rats after cecal abrasion (53). In vitro, IL-1 induced ultrastructural changes in fibroblasts that resulted in alterations of focal adhesions in monolayers (54). This may be one of the mechanisms by which IL-1 can rapidly modulate cell–matrix interactions during inflammation and wound healing. Interleukin-1 also stimulates ICAM-1 mRNA expression in human peritoneal mesothelial cells (55). Finally, preoperative intravenous administration of anti-IL-1 antibody has been observed to diminish adhesion formation in rats (56). The majority of the adhesion stimulatory effect of IL-1 is likely due to its stimulation of macrophages to secrete fibrogenic factors such as PDGF and TGF-ß.

Interleukin-2. IL-2 is a 15 kDa cytokine that stimulates lymphocyte proliferation and activation of NK cells. The production of IL-2 by T cells is stimulated by IL-1. IL-2 was detected (>2 U/mL) in the PF from 3 of 23 women with endometriosis, compared to 0 of 8 fertile controls and 6 of 8 women with unexplained infertility (47). Recently, Keenan et al. were not able to detect IL-2 in either PF or macrophage conditioned media of women with endometriosis (49). Neither of these studies evaluated menstrual cycle differences.

Kovacs et al. reported that conditioned media from IL-2-treated human peripheral blood leukocytes induced higher fibroblast proliferation and collagen synthesis than non-IL-2-treated leukocyte media. In leukocytes mRNA expression of the fibrogenic growth factors TGF-ß and PDGF increased following treatment with IL-2 (57). Later, this same group investigated the effects of IL-2 on rat peritoneal macrophages and found that PDGF-A and -B chain mRNA expressions was upregulated but had no effect on TGF-ß1 mRNA expression (58).

Interleukin-6. Interleukin-6 is a 26 kDa cytokine produced by macrophages, T and B cells, fibroblasts, endothelial cells, endometrial stromal cells, and several other cell types (59). The biologic activities of IL-6 are numerous and include regulation of immunocompetent cell growth and differentiation, induction of acute phase proteins, and stimulation or inhibition of cell growth depending on the target cell type (61). Recent evidence suggests that this cytokine plays an active role in reproductive physiology, including regulation of ovarian steroid production and early implantation events (60).

Five studies investigated the levels of IL-6 in PF with conflicting results. Boutten et al. detected IL-6 in the PF, but IL-6 levels in patients with minimal or mild endometriosis and fertile and infertile controls was not different (61). Buyalos et al. reported no difference between IL-6 levels in the PF from women with and without endometriosis, although they found increased levels in women with pelvic adhesions (62). In a more recent study, Keenan et al. (63) reported that, although there was no difference in the PF levels of IL-6 between women with and without endometriosis, levels of IL-6 were significantly higher in macrophage conditioned media of women with endometriosis compared to those without endometriosis. However, in two other studies, IL-6 levels in PF correlated with the severity of endometriosis, while the levels of IL-6 soluble receptor decreased (50, 64).

Interleukin-6 is produced by peritoneal leukocytes. Leukocytes obtained from patients with mild endometriosis produced more IL-6 compared to leukocytes from women with severe endometriosis. Similarly, leukocytes obtained from patients with nonendometriotic pelvic adhesions produced more IL-6 compared to controls (65).

Many investigators suggest an association between pelvic adhesions and IL-6. Interleukin-6 levels were found to be higher in the PF of women with pelvic adhesions compared to controls (62). This study failed to substantiate increased levels of IL-6 in the PF of women with endometriosis. Interleukin-6 levels are also increased in the PF of women with bacterial peritonitis (66). In rats, IL-6 increased and anti-IL-6 decreased with experimentally induced peritoneal adhesions, although anti-IL-6 antibodies had no significant effect on wound healing (67).

Interleukin-8. Interleukin-8 is a 8 kDa chemoattractant, activating factor for neutrophils (68) and a potent angiogenic factor (69). IL-8 is produced by a number of cells, including monocytes (70), endothelial cells, fibroblasts, mesothelial, and endometrial cells (71).

Peritoneal fluid of women with endometriosis has been reported to have increased neutrophil chemotactic activity compard to PF of women without this disease (72). One of the candidates for this activity is IL-8. IL-8 concentrations have been reported to be higher in the PF of women with endometriosis than in controls. IL-8 levels have also been shown to correlate with the stage of the disease (73, 74). We have recently shown that IL-8 induces the proliferation of endometrial stromal cells in vitro (74a). This factor has thus been speculated to play a role in the pathogenesis of endometriosis. Interleukin-8 levels have not been shown to vary in the PF collected during different menstrual cycle phases (73).

The angiogenic properties of IL-8 suggest that this chemokine may be important in adhesion formation. Interleukin-8 has been reported to affect intercellular adhesion in primary fibroblast cultures suggesting an additional role for IL-8 in adhesion formation (75).

Interleukin-10. Interleukin-10, also known as cytokine synthesis inhibitory factor, is secreted by the Th2 subset of T cells and blocks activation of cytokine synthesis by Th1 T cells, activated monocytes, and NK cells. The levels of IL-10 in the PF from women with and without endometriosis are not different (76). IL-10 has been reported to reduce postoperative adhesion formation in mice (72).

Growth-Regulated α. This chemokine, GROα, was orginially named "melanocyte growth stimulating activity" owing to its mitogenic activity on melanocytes. Later, this factor was found to be a more potent chemoattractant for neutrophils than IL-8. It is expressed by activated monocytes, neutrophils, fibroblasts, and endothelial cells (78). We have recently reported that GROα is present in the PF and its concentration increases in moderate and severe endometriosis, but levels of GROα do not vary between the phases of the menstrual cycle (79).

Monocyte Chemotactic Protein-1. Monocyte chemotactic protein-1 is a 8 kDa chemotactic and activating factor specific for monocytes/macrophages. It is secreted by a number of cells including monocytes, lymphocytes, fibroblasts, endothelial cells (80), and endometrial cells (81). Its secretion is regulated by IL-1, TNF-α, and interferon-γ (IFN-γ).

Peritoneal fluid from patients with endometriosis has increased chemotactic activity for macrophages (72). The presence of this chemotactic stimulus increases macrophage number and activation, resulting in the secretion of a variety of cytokines. MCP-1 levels are elevated in PF of women with endometriosis. In addition, the levels of MCP-1 were significantly higher in the PF from women who had untreated endometriosis than in women who had medical treatment with gonadotropin releasing hormone analogues. Proliferative phase levels of MCP-1 are significantly higher than levels in PF collected during the secretory phase (81a).

MCP-1 may also play a role in adhesion formation. We have recently found that MCP-1 levels are increased in the PF of women with intra-peritoneal adhesions. On the other hand the presence of adhesions had no incremental effect of PF MCP-1 levels in women with endometriosis (81b). Using a mice adhesion model we also showed that MCP-1 mRNA expression is increased during adhesion formation. Moreover, animals treated with anti-MCP-1 antibody developed significantly less adhesions (81c). The effect of MCP-1 on adhesion formation may be hormonally regulated. Peritoneal adhesion formation is inhibited by estradiol (81d). In stimulated murine fibroblast cultures expression of MCP-1 is down-regulated by low and high physiological concentrations of estradiol offering a potential mechanism by which estradiol may be inhibiting peritoneal adhesions (83).

RANTES. RANTES is a newly discovered 8 kDa T cell specific cytokine of the chemokine superfamily (85). RANTES is a selective chemoattractant for monocytes and T-lymphocytes (86). Peritoneal fluid concentrations of RANTES have been reported to be elevated in women with endometriosis with PF levels correlating with the severity of the disease not differing between proliferative and secretory phases (87).

Tumor Necrosis Factor. Tumor necrosis factor α (TNF-α) is another cytokine with a wide range of biologic effects. It is secreted as a 26 kDa membrane-bound precursor that is cleaved proteolytically to a mature 17 kDa form (88). It is secreted primarily by macrophages and monocytes and mediates macrophage cytotoxicity against susceptible cell (89). It is a pleiotropic factor that exerts a variety of effects including proinflammation, growth promotion, growth inhibition, immunomodulation, angiogenesis, and cellular toxicity (88). It stimulates the proliferation of human fibroblasts in vitro (90), activates neutrophils (91), and stimulates fibrin deposition in tumor vasculature. Tumor necrosis factor α also affects sperm motility in vitro, but only at very high concentrations (42) and may also be embryotoxic (43).

Tumor necrosis factor α levels in PF of women have been evaluated in seven studies. Eisermann et al. first documented the presence of TNF-α in PF (92). In that study, the mean concentration of TNF-α in women with extensive endometriosis was elevated, but the highest values were seen in women with acute pelvic inflammatory disease. Halme studied TNF-α activity in PF obtained from tubal ligation, unexplained infertility, pelvic adhesion, and endometriosis cases. The mean level of TNF-α was higher in women with endometriosis than in fertile women, although there was no difference between the levels in fertile versus infertile women or in the presence versus absence of endometriosis (15). In this same study, TNF-α secretion was reported to be higher in peritoneal macrophage cultures obtained from these women with endometriosis compared to the levels from in vitro cultures of women without disease (15). Mori et al. also reported elevated levels of PF TNF-α in acute pelvic inflammatory disease and in stage I, II, III, and IV endometriosis (52). Taketani et al. reported that PF levels of TNF-α were increased in women with untreated endometriosis compared to infertile women without endometriosis or to women with medically treated endometriosis (44). On the other hand, Vercellini et al. did not demonstrated any difference in TNF-α levels in either plasma or PF from infertile women with and without endometriosis (93). Keenan et al. also reported no difference in PF levels of TNF-α between women with and without endometriosis, although they observed increased levels in conditioned media of peritoneal macrophages from women with endometriosis (49). More recently, Rana et al. reported elevated levels of TNF-α in PF of women with endometriosis (76). Only two of these studies evaluated PF TNF-α levels according to the menstrual cycle phase and found no significant change (92, 93).

Tumor necrosis factor α also enhances the adhesion of endometrial stromal cells to mesothelial cells in vitro (94) and stimulates ICAM-1 expression in murine and human peritoneal mesothelial cells (55, 95). These data suggest that TNF-α may play a role in the pathogenesis of endometriosis and adhesion formation.

The severity of postoperative adhesion formation correlates with PF and serum TNF-α concentrations in rats with experimentally induced bowel injury (96). Anti-TNF-α antibodies together with anti-IL-1 antibodies administered preoperatively increases protection against adhesion formation (56). An additional mechanism by which TNF-α may contribute to fibrosis and adhesion formation is its inhibitory effect on collagen phagocytosis (97).

Interferon-γ. Interferon-γ is a 23 kDa homodimer that is produced primarily by activated T lymphocytes (98). It is toxic to a variety of virally infected and neoplastic cells and can interfere with cell growth by disrupting the structural organization of the plasma membrane cytoskeletal complex (98).

Interferon-γ may adversely affect many aspects of reproductive processes including sperm motility (42), fertilization (99), and embryo development (43). It also inhibits in vitro blastocyst implantation at concentrations as low as 1000 U/mL (100) and proliferation of endometrial epithelial cells (101). Two studies have reported that IFN-γ is present in human PF but IFN-γ levels neither differ between women with and without endometriosis nor vary in regards to the phase of the menstrual cycle (63, 87).

Macrophage Colony Stimulating Factor. Macrophage colony stimulating factor (M-CSF or CSF-1) is involved in the differentiation of monocytes to become phenotypically activated macrophages and can serve as a chemotactic factor for blood monocytes. This growth factor has been identified in the PF of women at a consistently higher concentration than found in plasma (102). The concentration of M-CSF has also been reported to be significantly higher in the PF of women patients with endometriosis compared to levels in women without endometriosis (103).

Other Growth Factors

Growth factors comprise a wide group of proteins produced by a variety of cells and act in both paracrine and autocrine fashion. These factors are able to affect the growth and differentiation of cells and act alone or in synergy with other factors. Although many growth factors are named after their originally observed biologic action, they are generally involved in a wide range of actions including stimulation of cell growth, inhibition of cellular proliferation, and alterations of cellular functions. Division between cytokines and growth factors is arbitrary because their functions commonly overlap and they are generally grouped together.

Transforming Growth Factor ß. Transforming growth factor ß (TGF-ß) is a 25 kDa peptide mainly produced by macrophages, platelets, osteoblasts, and activated lymphocytes (104). Beside its growth regulating properties, TGF-ß is one of the most potent chemoattractants for human monocytes, as well as macrophages and fibroblasts, and an inducer of fibrosis and angiogenesis, indicating that it is an important mediator of tissue repair (105). Furthermore TGF-ß has immunomodulatory activity profoundly inhibiting T cell, B cell, and NK cell functions (106, 107).

Ooesterlynck et al. demonstrated that TGF-ß activity is increased in the PF of women with endometriosis compared to both fertile and infertile women without endometriosis (108). They suggested that decreased NK cell activity frequently observed in the PF of women with endometriosis may be secondary to increased PF TGF-ß. Hammond et al. (109) demonstrated that TGF-ß induced proliferation of human endometrial cells. One of the sources of TGF-ß in the PF may be endometrial implants because both the mRNA and the protein are expressed by human endometrial stromal and epithelial cells (109) and TGF-ß has been demonstrated by immunohistochemistry in surgically induced endometriotic implants in the rat model (110). PF TGF-ß levels have been reported to be independent of the phase of the menstrual cycle.

As an important mediator of tissue repair, TGF-ß is expected to play a role in adhesion formation. Experimentally, TGF-ß increased peritoneal adhesion formation in rats subjected to surgical injury to the uterine horns (111). Fibrous adhesive tissues from the peritoneum of rats with surgically induced injury showed stronger immunostaining for TGF-ß1, 2, and 3 compared to intact peritoneum (112).

Platelet-Derived Growth Factor. Platelet-derived growth factor (PDG-F) is a well characterized secretory product of activated macrophages that plays a major role in the inflammatory response, serving in part as a potent mitogen for fibroblasts and angiogenic precursor cells, and as a chemotactic agent for monocytes, neutrophils, and fibroblasts (113). PDGF is a 30 kDa protein that consists of two subunits, A and B, connected by interchain disulfide bonds (113). The subunits may be combined as homodimers or heterodimers, giving rise to three dimeric forms (PDGF-AA, PDGF-AB, and PDGF-BB). These isoforms bind to two different classes of receptors, a and b (114).

Halme et al. (3) demonstrated that peritoneal macrophages isolated from patients with endometriosis released growth factor activity in vitro to a greater extent than those derived from women without disease. Recent evidence suggests that this macrophage derived growth factor may be similar to PDGF (115).

Epidermal Growth Factor. Epidermal growth factor (EGF) is a single peptide with a molecular weight of 5 kDa. It acts as a mitogen for most epithelial cells including keratinocytes, epithelial cells, and fibroblasts. Two studies, 10 years apart, have investigated EGF in the PF (34, 116). Both studies identified EGF in PF and reported that PF levels of EGF from women with and without endometriosis were not different. Both studies indicated that EGF levels were higher in the secretory compared to the proliferative phase of the menstrual cycle.

Epidermal growth factor has been shown by immunohistochemistry to be present in all cell types found in intraperitoneal fibrous adhesions. It is also present in experimentally injured tissues of the rat, suggesting a role in peritoneal repair after injury and in the formation of fibrous adhesions (117). Epidermal growth factor also enhances adhesion of peritoneal macrophages to mesothelial cells, although it does not cause an increase in ICAM-1 expression (95).

Insulin-Like Growth Factors. Insulin-like growth factor-I (IGF-I) and IGF-II are mitogens that can promote differentiation. Insulin-like growth factors circulate bound to IGF binding proteins (IGFBPs), which regulate their actions on target tissues. Giudice et al. (118) have reported that human PF contains IGF-I, IGF-II, IGFBP-1, -2, -3, -4, and IGFBP-3 protease. Peritoneal fluid IGF levels were approximately 60% of paired serum levels, and PF levels of IGFBP-2 and IGFBP-3 were approximately half of their serum concentrations. The IGF system may be one of several growth factor systems in PF that has the capacity to stimulate endometrial cellular proliferation.

Fibroblast Growth Factor. Basic fibroblast growth factor (bFGF) is an 18 kDa heparin-binding protein with autocrine and paracrine angiogenic and mitogenic effects (119). Basic FGF is mitogenic for eutopic (120) and ectopic (121) endometrial stromal cells. It is also expressed by eutopic and ectopic endometrial stromal and epithelial cells (122, 123). Secretion of bFGF by endometrial adenocarcinoma cells increases in response to estradiol, and this increase is inhibited by progesterone (124). Basic FGF expression increases in the atrophic endometrium after menopause (125) and returns to normal levels following hormone replacement therapy (126). Huang et al. have found that bFGF levels in PF from women with or without endometriosis do not differ significantly. There is also no difference in PF bFGF levels collected during the cycle (116). We recently confirmed these findings and also showed that bFGF inhibits the development of pre-implantation murine embryos but only at concentrations 10 to 100 times higher than the levels detected in PF (126a).

REFERENCES

1. diZerega GS, Rodgers KE. Peritoneum. In: diZerega GS, Rodgers KE, ed. The Peritoneum. New York: Springer-Verlag, 1992:1–25.

2. Syrop CH, Halme J. Cyclic changes of peritoneal fluid parameters in normal and infertile patients. Obstet Gynecol 1987;69:416–418.

3. Halme J, White C, Kauma S, et al. Peritoneal macrophages from patients with endometriosis release growth factor activity in vitro. J Clin Endocrinol Metab 1986;66:1044–1049.

4. Koutsilieris M, Allaire-Michaud L, Fortier M, et al. Mitogen(s) for endometrial-like cells can be detected in human peritoneal fluid. Fertil Steril 1991;56(5):888–893.

5. Ramey JW, Archer DF. Peritoneal fluid: its relevance to the development of endometriosis. Fertil Steril 1993;60:1–14.

6. Hurst BS, Rock JA. The peritoneal environment in endometriosis. In: Thomas EJ, Rock JA, ed. Modern Approaches to Endometriosis. Norwell, MA: Kluver Academic, 1991:79–96.

7. Rock JA, Dubin NH, Ghodgaonkar PB, et al. Cul-de-sac fluid volume and prostanoid concentration during the proliferative phase of the cycle days 8 to 12. Fertil Steril 1982;37:747–750.

8. Rezai N, Ghodaonkar RB, Zacur HA, et al. Cul-de-sac fluid in women with endometriosis: fluid volume and prostanoid concentration during the proliferative phase of the cycle days 13–18. Fertil Steril 1987;48:29–32.

9. Hill JA, Faris HMP, Schiff I, et al. Characterization of leukocyte subpopulations in the peritoneal fluid of women with endometriosis. Fertil Steril 1988;50:216–222.

10. vanFurth R, Raebum JA, vanZwet TI. Characteristics of human mononuclear phagocytes. Blood 1979;54:485–500.

11. Haney AF, Muscato JJ, Weinberg JB. Peritoneal fluid cell populations in infertility patients. Fertil Steril 1981;35:696–698.

12. Olive DL, Weinberg JB, Haney AF. Peritoneal macrophages, and infertility: the association between cell number and pelvic pathology. Fertil Steril 1985;44:772–777.

13. Dunselman GA, Hendrix MG, Bouckaert PX, et al. Functional aspects of peritoneal macrophages in endometriosis of women. J Reprod Fertil 1988;1988:707–710.

14. Fakih H, Bagget B, Holtz G, et al. Interleukin-1: possible role in the infertility associated with endometriosis. Fertil Steril 1987;47:213–217.

15. Halme J. Release of tumor necrosis factor-alpha by human peritoneal macrophages in vivo and in vitro. Am J Obstet Gynecol 1989;161:1718–1725.

16. Surrey ES, Halme J. Effect of peritoneal fluid from endometriosis patients on endometrial stromal cell proliferation in vitro. Obstet Gynecol 1990;76:792–797.

17. Kauma S, Clark MR, White C, et al. Production of fibronectin by peritoneal macrophages and concentration of fibronectin in peritoneal fluid from patients with or without endometriosis. Obstet Gynecol 1988;72:13–18.

18. Dmowski WP, Gebel HM, Braun DP. The role of cell-mediated immunity in pathogenesis of endometriosis. Acta Obstet Gynecol Scand 1994;159:7–14.

19. Oosterlynck DJ, Meulman C, Waer M, et al. The natural killer activity of peritoneal fluid lymphocytes is decreased in women with endometriosis. Fertil Steril 1992;58:290–295.

20. Oosterlynck DJ, Cornillie FJ, Waer M, et al. Women with endometriosis show a defect in natural killer activity resulting in a decreased cytotoxicity to autologous endometrium. Fertil Steril 1991;56:45–51.

21. Kanzaki H, Wang H-S, Kariya M, et al. Suppression of natural killer cell activity by sera from patients with endometriosis. Am J Obstet Gynecol 1992;167:257–261.

22. Lanfrancone L, Borasctu D, Gtuara P, et al. Human peritoneal mesothelial cells produce many cytokines and are activated and stimulated to grow by IL-1. Blood 1992;80:2835–2842.

23. Zeillemaker AM, Verbrugh HA, Honyckvan-Papendrecht AAGM, et al. CA-125 secretion by peritoneal mesothelial cells. J Clin Pathol 1994;47:263–265.

24. Polishuk WZ, Sharf M. Culposcopic findings in primary dysmenorrhea. Obstet Gynecol 1965;26:746–748.

25. Halme J, Hammond MG, Hulka JF, et al. Retrograde menstruation in healthy women and in patients with endometriosis. Obstet Gynecol 1984;64:151–154.

26. Kruitwagen RFPM, Poels LG, Willemsen WNP, et al. Endometrial epithelial cells in peritoneal fluid during early follicular phase. Fertil Steril 1991;55:297–303.

27. Koninckx PR, Ide P, Vanderbroucke W, et al. New aspects of the pathopysiology of endometriosis and associated infertility. J Reprod Med 1980;24:257–263.

28. Bartosik D, Jacobs SL, Kelly LJ. Endometrial tissue in peritoneal fluid. Fertil Steril 1986;46:796–800.

29. Badawy SZ, Cuenca V, Marshall L, et al. Cellular components in peritoneal fluid in infertile patients with and without endometriosis. Fertil Steril 1984;42:704–708.

30. Rock JA, Hurst BS. Clinical significance of prostanoid concentration in women with endometriosis. In: Chadha DR, Buttram VC, ed. Current Concepts in Endometriosis. New York: Alan R. Liss, 1990:61–80.

31. Ylikorkala O, Viinikka C. Prostaglandins in endometriosis. Acta Obstet Gynecol Scand 1983;113:105–107.

32. Chacho KJ, Chacho MS, Andresen PJ, et al. Peritoneal fluid in patients with and without endometriosis: prostanoids and macrophages and their effect on the spermatozoa penetration assay. Am J Obstet Gynecol 1986;154:1290–1296.

33. Badawy SZA, Marshall L, Cuenca V. Peritoneal fluid prostaglandins in various stages of the menstrual cycle: role in infertile patients with endometriosis. Int J Fertil 1985;30:48–53.

34. DeLeon FD, Vijayakumar R, Brown M, et al. Peritoneal fluid volume, estrogen, progesterone, prostaglandin, and epidermal growth factor concentrations in patients with and without endometriosis. Obstet Gynecol 1986;68:189–194.

35. Drake TS, O'Brien WF, Ramwell PW, et al. Peritoneal fluid thromboxane B2 and 6-keto-prostaglandin F1 in endometriosis. Am J Obstet Gynecol 1981;140:401–404.

36. Badawy SZA, Marshall L, Gabal AA, et al. The concentration of 13, 14-dihydro-15-keto prostaglandin F2 and prostaglandin E2 in peritoneal fluid of infertile patients with and without endometriosis. Fertil Steril 1982;38:166–170.

37. Dawood MY, Khan-Dawood FS, Wilson L. Perioneal fluid prostaglandins and prostanoids in women with endometriosis, chronic pelvic inflammatory disease, and pelvic pain. Am J Obstet Gynecol 1984;148:391–395.

38. Moon YS, Leung PCS, Yuen BH, et al. Prostaglandin F1 in human endometriotic tissue. Am J Obstet Gynecol 1981;141:344–345.

39. Schenken RS, Asch RH, Williams RF, et al. Etiology of infertility in monkeys with endometriosis: luteinized unruptured follicles, luteal phase defects, pelvic adhesions, and spontaneous abortions. Fertil Steril 1984;41:122–130.

40. Arai KI, Lee F, Miyajiima A, et al. Cytokines: coordination of immune and inflammatory responses. Ann Rev Biochem 1990;59:783–836.

41. Oppenheim JJ, Zachariae OC, Mukaida N, et al. Properties of the novel proinflammatory supergene "intercrine" cytokine family. Ann Rev Immunol 1991;617–648.

42. Hill JA, Haimovici F, Politch J, et al. Effect of soluble products of activated lymphocytes and macrophages (lymphokines and monokines) on human sperm motion parameters. Fertil Steril 1987;47:460–465.

43. Hill JA, Haimovici F, Anderson DJ. Products of activated lymphocytes and macrophages inhibit mouse embryo development in vitro. J Immunol 1987;139:2250–2254.

44. Taketani Y, Kuo TM, Mizuno M. Comparison of cytokine levels and embryo toxicity in peritoneal fluid in infertile women with untreated or treated endometriosis. Am J Obstet Gynecol 1992;167:265–270.

45. Dower SK, Kronheim SR, Hopp TP, et al. The cell surface receptors of interleukin 1a and interleukin 1b are identical. Nature 1986;324:266–268.

46. Sueldo CE, Kelly E, Montoro L, et al. Effect of interleukin-1 on gamete interaction and mouse embryo development. J Reprod Med 1990;35:868–872.

47. Hill JA, Anderson DJ. Lymphocyte activity in the presence of peritoneal fluid from fertile women and infertile women with and without endometriosis. Am J Obstet Gynecol 1989;161:861–864.

48. Awadalla SG, Friedman CH, Haq AU, et al. Local peritoneal factors: their role in infertility associated with endometriosis. Am J Obstet Gynecol 1987;157:1207–1214.

49. Keenan JA, Chen TT, Chadwell NL, et al. IL-1ß, TNF-α, and IL-2 in peritoneal fluid and macrophage conditioned media of women with endometriosis. Am J Reprod Immunol 1995;34:381–385.

50. Koyama N, Matsuura K, Okamura H. Cytokines in the peritoneal fluid of patients with endometriosis. Int J of Gynecol Obstet 1993;43:45–50.

51. Mori H, Sawairi M, Nakagawa M, et al. Expression of interleukin-1 (IL-1) beta messenger ribonucleic acid (mRNA) and IL-1 receptor antagonist mRNA in peritoneal macrophages from patients with endometriosis. Fertil Steril 1992;57:535–542.

52. Mori H, Sawairi M, Nakagawa M, et al. Peritoneal fluid interleukin-1 beta and tumor necrosis factor in patients with benign gyecologic disease. Am J Reprod Immunol 1991;26:62–67.

53. Herslag A, Ottemess IG, Bliven ML, et al. The effect of interleukin-1 on adhesion formation in the rat. Am J Obstet Gynecol 1991;165:771–774.

54. Qwarnstrom EE, MacFarlane SA, Page RC, et al. Interleukin 1 beta induces rapid phosphorylation and redistribution of talin: a possible mechanism for modulation of fibroblast focal adhesion. Proc Natl Acad Sci USA 1991;88:1232–1236.

55. Liberek T, Topley N, Luttman W, et al. Adherence of neutrophils to human peritoneal mesothelial cells: role of intercellular adhesion molecule-1. J Am Soc Nephrol 1996;7:208–217.

56. Kaidi AA, Nazzal M, Gurchumelidze T, et al. Preoperative administration of antibodies against tumor necrosis factor-alpha (TNF-alpha) and interleukin-1 (IL-1) and their impact on peritoneal adhesion formation. American Surgeon. 1995;61:569–572.

57. Kovacs EJ, Brock B, Silber IE, et al. Production of fibrogenic cytokines by interleukin-2–treated peripheral blood leukocytes: expression of transforming growth factor-beta and platelet-derived growth factor B chain genes. Obstet Gynecol 1993;82:29–36.

58. Kovacs EJ, VanStedum S, Neuman JE. Selective induction of PDGF gene expression in peritoneal macrophages by interleukin-2. Immunobiology 1994;190:263–274.

59. Le J, Vileck J. Interleukin 6: multifunctional cytokine regulating immune response. Lab Invest 1989;61:588–602.

60. Gorospe WC, Hughes FM, Spangelo BL. Interleukin-6: effects on and production by rat granulosa cells in vitro. Endocrinology 1992;130:1750–1752.

61. Boutten A, Dehoux M, Edelman P. IL-6 and acute phase plasma proteins in peritoneal fluid of women with endometriosis. Clin Chim Acta 1992;210:187–195.

62. Buyalos RP, Funari VA, Azziz R, et al. Elevated interleukin-6 levels in peritoneal fluid of patients with pelvic pathology. Fertil Steril 1992;58:302–306.

63. Keenan JA, Chen TT, Chadwell NL, et al. Interferon-gamma (IFN-γ) and interleukin-6 (IL-6) in peritoneal fluid and macrophage-conditioned media of women with endometriosis. Am J Reprod Immunol 1994;32:180–183.

64. Rier SE, Zarmakoupis PN, Hu X, et al. Dysregulation of interleukin-6 responses in ectopic endometrial stromal cells: correlation with decreased soluble receptor levels in peritoneal fluid of women with endometriosis. J Clin Endocrinol Metab 1995;80:1431–1437.

65. Rier SE, Parsons AK, Becker JL. Altered interleukin-6 production by peritoneal leukocytes from patients with endometriosis. Fertil Steril 1994;61:294–299.

66. Pruimboom WM, Bac DJ, vartDijk AP, et al. Levels of soluble intercellular adhesion molecule 1, eicosanoids and cytokines in ascites of patients with liver cirrhosis, peritoneal cancer and spontaneous bacterial peritonitis. International Journal of Immunopharmacology 1995;17:375–384.

67. Saba AA, Kaidi AA, Godziachvili V, et al. Effects of interleukin-6 and its neutralizing antibodies on pertioneal adhesion formation and wound healing. American Surgeon 1996;62:569–572.

68. Baggiolini M, Walz A, Kunkel SL. Neutrophil-activating peptide-1/interleukin-8, a novel cytokine that activates neutroptuls. J Clin Invest 1989;84:1045–1049.

69. Koch AE, Polverini PJ, Kunkel SL, et al. Interleukin-8 as a macrophage-derived mediator of angiogenesis. Science 1992;258:1798–1801.

70. Yoshimura TK, Matsushima K, Oppenheim JJ, et al. Neutroptul chemotactic factor produced by lipopolysaccharide (LPS)-stimulated human blood mononuclear leukocytes: partial characterization and separation from interleukin-1 (IL-1). J Immunol 1987;139:788–793.

71. Arici A, Head JR, MacDonald PC, et al. Regulation of interleukin-8 gene expression in human endometrial cells in culture. Mol Cell Endocrinol 1993;94:195–204.

72. Leiva MC, Hasty LA, Pfeifer S, et al. Increased chemotactic activity of peritoneal fluid in patients with endometriosis. Am J Obstet Gynecol 1993;168:592–598.

73. Ryan IP, Tseng JF, Schriock ED, et al. Interleukin-8 concentrations are elevated in peritoneal fluid of women with endometriosis. Fertil Steril 1995;63:929–932.

74. Arici A, Tazuke SI, Attar E, et al. Interleukin-8 concentration in peritoneal fluid of patients with endometriosis and modulation of interleukin-8 expression in human mesothelial cells. Mol Human Reprod 1996;2(1):40–45.

74a. Arici A, Seli E, Zeyneloglu HB, Senturk LM, Oral E, Olive DL. Interleukin-8 induces proliferation of endometrial stromal cells: a potential autocrine growth factor. J Clin Endocrinol Metab 1998;83:1201–1205.

75. Dunlevy JR, Couchman JR. Interleukin-8 induces motile behavior and loss of focal adhesions in primary fibroblasts. J Cell Sci 1995;108:311–321.

76. Rana N, Braun DP, House R, et al. Basal and stimulated secretion of cytokines by peritoneal macrophages in women with endometriosis. Fertil Steril 1996;65:925–930.

77. Montz FJ, Holschneider CH, Bozuk M, et al. Interleukin-10: ability to minimize postoperative intraperitoneal adhesion formation in a murine model. Fertil Steril 1994;61:1136–1140.

78. Wen D, Rowland A, Derynck R. Expression and secretion of gro/MGSA by stimulated human endothelial cells. EMBO J 1989;8:1761–1766.

79. Oral E, Seli E, Bahtiyar MO, et al. Growth-regulated a expression in the peritoneal environment with endometriosis. Obstet Gynecol 1996;88:1050–1056.

80. Sica A, Wang JM, Colotta F, et al. Monocyte chemotactic and activating factor gene expression induced in endothelial cells by IL-1 and tumor necrosis factor. J Immunol 1990;144:3034–3038.

81. Arici A, MacDonald PC, Casey ML. Regulation of monocyte chemotactic, protein-1 gene expression in human endometrial cells in culture. Mol Cell Endocrinol 1995;107:189–197.

81a. Arici A, Oral E, Attar E, Tazuke S, Olive DL. Monocyte chemotactic protein-1 concentration in peritoneal fluid of women with endometriosis and its modulation of expression in mesothelial cells. Fertil Steril 1997;67:1065–1072.

81b. Zeyneloglu HB, Senturk LM, Seli E, Oral E, Plive DL, Arici A. The role of moncyte chemotactic protein-1 in intraperitoneal adhesion formation. Hum Reprod 1998;13:1194–1199.

81c. Zeyneloglu HB, Seli E, Senturk LM, Gutierrez LS, Olive DL, AriciA. The effect of monocyte chemotactic protein 1 in intraperitoneal adhesion formation in a mouse model. Am J Obstet Gynecol 1998;179:438–443.

81d. Frazier-Jessen MR, Mott FJ, Witte PL, Kovacs EJ. Estrogen suppression of abdominal connective tissue deposition in a murine model of peritoneal adhesion formation. J Immunol 1998;156(8):3036–3042.

82. Kovacs EJ, DiPietro LA. Fibrogenic cytokines and connective tissue production. FASEB J 1994;8:854–861.

83. Kovacs EJ, Faunce DE, Ramer-Quinn DS, et al. Estrogen regulation of JE/MCP-1 mFNA expression in fibroblasts. J Leukocyte Biol 1996;59:562–568.

84. Frazier-Jessen MR, Kovacs EJ. Estrogen modulation of JE/monocyte chenioattractant protein-1 mRNA expression in murine macrophages. J Immunol 1995;154:1838–1845.

85. Schall TJ. Biology of the RANTES/SIS cytokine family. Cytokine 1991;3:165–183.

86. Schall TJ, Bacon K, Toy KJ, et al. Selective attraction of monocytes and T lymphocytes of the memory phenotype by cytokine RANTES. Nature 1990;347:669–671.

87. Khorram O, Taylor RN, Ryan IP, et al. Peritoneal fluid concentrations of the cytokine RANTES, correlate with the severity of endometriosis. Am J Obstet Gynecol 1993; 169:1545–1549.

88. Jue DM, Sherry B, Leudke C, et al. Processing of newly synthesized cachectin/tumor necrosis factor in endotoxtin stimulated macrophages. Biochemistry 1990; 29:8371–8379.

89. Urban JL, Shepard HM, Rothstein JL, et al. Tumor necrosis factor: a potent effector molecule for tumor cell killing by activated macrophages. Proc Natl Acad Sci USA 1986;83:5233–5237.

90. Sugarman BJ, Aggarwal BB, Hass PE, et al. Recombinant human tumor necrosis factor-alpha: effects on proliferation of normal and transformed cells in vitro. Science 1985;230:943–945.

91. Shalaby MR, Aggarwal BB, Rinderknecht E, et al. Activation of human polymorphonuclear neutrophil function by interferon gamma and tumor necrosis factor. J Immunol 1985;35:2069–2073.

92. Eisermann J, Gast MJ, Pineda J, et al. Tumor necrosis factor in peritoneal fluid of women undergoing laparoscopic surgery. Fertil Steril 1988;50:573–579.

93. Vercellini P, Benedetti FD, Rossi E, et al. Tumor necrosis factor in plasma and peritoneal fluid of women with and without endometriosis. Gynecol Obstet Invest 1993;36:39–41.

94. Zhang R, Wild R, Ojago J. Effect of tumor necrosis factor-a on adhesion of human endometrial stromal cells to peritoneal mesothelial cells: an in vitro system. Fertil Steril 1993;59:1196–1201.

95. Muller J, Yostuda T. Interaction of murine peritoneal leukocytes and mesothelial cells: in vitro model system to survey cellular events on serosal membranes during inflammation. Clin Immunol Immunopathol 1995;75:231–238.

96. Kaidi AA, Gurchumelidze T, Nazzal M, et al. Tumor necrosis factor-alpha: a marker for peritoneal adhesion formation. J Sur Res 1995;58:516–518.

97. Chou DH, Lee W, McCulloch CA. TNF-alpha inactivation of collagen receptors: implications for fibroblast function and fibrosis. J Immunol 1996;156:435–4362.

98. Ijzermans JNM, Marquet RL. Interferon gamma: a review. Immunobiology 1989;179: 456–464.

99. Wang E, Pfeffer LM, Tamm I. Interferon increases the abundance of submembranous microfilaments in the HeLa-S3 cells in suspension culture. Proc Natl Acad Sci USA 1981;78:6281–6285.

100. Hill JA, Cohen J, Anderson DJ. The efects of lymphokines and monokines on human sperm fertilizing ability in the zona-free hamster egg penetration test. Am J Obstet Gynecol 1989;160:1154–1159.

101. Haimovici F, Hill JA, Anderson DJ. The effects of soluble products of activated lymphocytes and macrophages on blastocyst implantation events in vitro. Biol Reprod 1991;44:69–75

102. Tabibzadeh SS, Satyawaroop PG, Rao PN. Antiproliferative effect of interferon-g in human endometrial cells in vitro: potential local growth modulatory role in endometrium. J Clin Endocrinol Metab 1988;67:131–138.

103. Weinberg JB, Haney AF, Xu FJ, et al. Peritoneal fluid and plasma levels of human macrophage colony-stimulating factor in relation to peritoneal macrophage content. Blood 1991;78:513–516.

104. Fukaya T, Sugawara J, Yostuda H, et al. The role of macrophage colony stimulating factor in the peritoneal fluid in infertile patients with endometriosis. Tohuku J Exp M 1994;172:221–226.

105. Sporn MB, Robeerts AB, Wakefield LM, et al. Transforming growth factor b: biological function and chemical structure. Science 1986;233:532–534.

106. Yang EY, Moses HL. Transforming growth factor b1 induced changes in cell migration, proliferation, and angiogenesis in the ctucken chorioallantoic membrane. J Cell Biol 1990;111:731–741.

107. Rook AH, Kehrl JH, Wakefield LM, et al. Effects of transforming growth factor b on the functions of natural killer cells: depressed cytolytic activity and blunting of interferon responsiveness. J Immunol 1986;136:3916–3920.

108. Oosterlynck DJ, Meuleman C, Waer M, et al. Transforming growth factor-beta activity is increased in peritoneal fluid from women with endometriosis. Obstet Gynecol 1994;83:287–292.

109. Hammond MG, Oh ST, Anners J, et al. The effect of growth factors on the proliferation of human endometrial stromal cells in culture. Am J Obstet Gynecol 1993;168:1131–1136.

110. Marshbum PB, Arici AM, Casey ML. Expression of transforming growth factor-bl 1TGF-ß1) mRNA and the modulation of DNA synthesis by TGF-ß1 in human endometrial cells. Am J Obstet Gynecol 1994;170:1152–1158.

111. Chegini N, Gold LI, Williams RS. Localization of transforming growth factor beta isoforms TGF-beta 1, TGF-beta 2, and TGF-beta 3 in surgically induced endometriosis in the rat. Obstet Gynecol 1994;83:455–461.

112. Williams RS, Rossi AM, Chegini N, et al. Effect of transforming growth factor beta on postoperative adhesion formation and intact peritoneum. J Surg Res 1992;52:65–70.

113. Chegini N, Gold LI, Williams RS, et al. Localization of transforming growth factor beta isoforms TGF-beta 1, TGF-beta 2, and TGF-beta 3 in surgically induced pelvic adhesions in the rat. Obstet Gynecol 1994;83:449–454.

114. Ross R, Raines EW, Bowen-Pope DF. The biology of platelet derived growth factor. Cell 1986;46:155–169.

115. Heldin CH, Backstrom G, Ostman A, et al. Binding of differrent dimeric forms of PDGF to human fibroblasts: evidence for two separate receptor types. EMBO J 1988;7:1387–1393.

116. Huang JC, Papasakelariou C, Dawood MY. Epidermal growth factor and basic fibroblast growth factor in peritoneal fluid of women with endometriosis. Fertil Steril 1996;65:931–934.

117. Chegini N, Simms J, Williams RS, et al. Identification of epidermal growth factor, transforming growth factor-alpha, and epidermal growth factor receptor in surgically induced pelvic adhesions in the rat and intraperitoneal adhesions in the human. Am J Obstet Gynecol 1994;171(2):321–327.

118. Giudice LC, Dsupin BA, Gargosky SE, et al. The insulin-like growth factor system in human peritoneal fluid: its effect on endometrial stromal cells and its potential relevance to endometriosis. J Clin Endocrinol Metab 1994;79:1284–1293.

119. Folkman J, Klagsbrun M. Angiogenic factors. Science 1987;235:442–444.

120: Irwin JC, Utian WH, Eckert RL. Sex steroids and growth factors differentially regulate the growth and differentiation of cultured human endometrial stromal cells. Endocrinology 1991;129:2385–2392..

121. Taketani Y, Mizuno M. Hormonal regulation of 1the cell growth in an endometriotic cell culture system. Arch Gynecol Obstet 1992;251:29–34.

122. Zhang L, Rees MC, Bicknell R. The isolation and long-term culture pf normal human endometrial epithelium and stroma. J Cell Sci 1995;108:323–331.

123. Ferriani RA, Charnock-Jones DS, Prentice A, et al. Immunohistochemical localization of acidic and basic fibroblast growth factors in normal endometrium or endometriosis and the detection of their mRNA by polymerase chain reaction. Human Reprod 1993;8:11–16.

124. Presta M. Sex hormones modulate the synthesis of basic fibroblast growth factor in human endometrial adenocarcinoma cells: implications for the neovascularisation of normal and neoplastic endometrium. J Cell Physiol 1988;137:593–597.

125. Rusnati M, Casarotti G, Pecorelli S, et al. Basic fibroblast growth factor in ovulatory cycle and postmenopausal human endometrium. Growth Fact 1990;3:299–307.

126. Rusnati M, Casarotti G, Pecorelli S, et al. Estro-progestinic replacement therapy modulates the levels of basic fibroblast growth factor (bFGF) in postmenopausal endometrium. Gynecol Oncol 1993;48:88–93.

126a. Seli E, Zeynelglu HB, Senturk LM, Bahtiyar OM, Olive DL, Arici A. Basic fibroblast growth factor: peritoneal and follicular fluid levels and its effect on early embryonic development. Fertil Steril 1998;69:1145–1148.

12

CYTOKINES IN ENDOMETRIOSIS

Isabelle P. Ryan, Ellen S. Moore, and Robert N. Taylor

University of California, San Francisco, California

Endometriosis is a common gynecologic disorder, affecting at least 10% of reproductive-aged women, and is characterized by the growth of endometrial tissue outside the uterine cavity. The association of endometriosis with pelvic pain and impaired fecundity has been recognized since the 1920s (1). However, the hypothesis that this condition directly causes these symptoms has not been proved, and the mechanisms by which endometriosis might mediate pain and infertility have not been fully characterized. Although the prevalence of pelvic endometriosis is greater in infertile than fertile women (2), and the fecundity of women with endometriosis appears to be less than that of normal women (3, 4), prospective studies establishing that the development of endometriosis antecedes infertility have never been performed. The effect of endometriosis on the success of assisted reproductive techniques also is controversial. However, some studies suggest that the presence of this clinical condition has a negative impact on implantation and pregnancy rates even when fertilization occurs extracorporally (5–7).

Cytokines in Human Reproduction, Edited by Joseph A. Hill
ISBN 0-471-35242-X   Copyright © 2000 Wiley-Liss, Inc.

Implantation of Endometrial Fragments

Although multiple theories exist regarding the etiology of the disease, the implantation hypothesis of Sampson (1) is the most widely accepted, although with some disagreement (8). Recent studies have supported the Sampson theory by documenting that retrograde menstruation (9) and peritoneal spillage of viable endometrial epithelial cells (10) occur frequently in cycling women. The attachment and adhesion of shed endometrial cells to peritoneal and subperitoneal surfaces are likely to involve the expression of extracellular membrane adhesion molecules and their co-receptors (11).

Ovarian Hormone Responsiveness of Endometriosis

That the progression of endometriosis depends on ovarian endocrine function has been recognized for decades. Symptoms do not occur until menarche and typically regress spontaneously following menopause. Surgical or pharmacological castration has been effective as treatment for symptomatic endometriosis in women not desiring fertility. Like the normal, eutopic endometrium from which these implants appear to arise, endometriosis lesions respond to ovarian steroid hormones. DiZerega and colleagues used a primate model to demonstrate that estrogen and/or progestin treatment promoted the maintenance of experimentally induced endometriosis (12). Radioligand binding assays to quantify estrogen and progesterone receptors in endometriosis lesions by Jänne et al. (13) suggested that both steroid receptor types had characteristic affinities, but were present in lower concentrations in endometriosis implants than in normal endometrium. A concern about the latter conclusion is that peritoneal and fibroblast cells associated with endometriosis lesions have low to undetectable steroid receptor concentrations and would be expected to dilute these receptors in implant homogenates. Immunohistochemical studies of steroid receptors have been performed in endometriosis using steroid fluorochrome derivatives (14) and monoclonal anti-receptor antibodies (15). These studies demonstrated that endometriosis implants express specific estrogen and progesterone receptors in both glandular epithelium and stroma. In contrast to normal endometrium, receptor content in implants was noted to be heterogeneous, and did not undergo predictable changes in response to the ovarian cycle. Studies from our laboratory comparing isolated endometriosis and normal endometrial cells in culture indicate that their estrogen receptor concentrations and affinity do not differ (16). Functional evidence for the ovarian steroid hormone dependence of endometriosis was afforded by prospective, randomized clinical trials, comparing objective and subjective responses of the lesions before and after administration of pituitary downregulating doses of a GnRH analogue that suppressed ovarian estrogen and progesterone production (17).

Neovascularization and Growth of Endometriosis Implants

As discussed above, the retrograde menstruation hypothesis of Sampson (1) is the most widely accepted hypothesis of endometriosis histogenesis. Shed endometrial fragments are believed to accumulate in the dependent portions of the pelvis and adhere to the peritoneal surface. Microscopic defects allow the cells to contact the submesothelial matrix (18) where they proliferate, spread, and grow, sometimes invading deeply into the subperitoneal space.

Folkman has demonstrated that tumor implants are not capable of growing beyond a volume of 2–3 mm^3 unless they develop a new blood supply (19). The sprouting and formation of a new vascular supply is termed angiogenesis. This is a complex process that includes the proteolytic degradation of extracellular matrix, proliferation of endothelial cells, and their migration and formation into capillary tubules supplying the angiogenic stimulus. Such an "angiogenic switch" also may be critical for the growth and progression of an endometriosis implant (20).

Oosterlynck et al. (21) used the chick chorioallantoic membrane bioassay to show that pelvic fluid from women with endometriosis had more angiogenic activity than pelvic fluid from normal controls. We confirmed this observation using an in vitro model of endothelial cell proliferation. [^{3}H]Thymidine incorporation into nascent cellular DNA (22) demonstrated that peritoneal fluid from women with endometriosis contains significantly more angiogenic activity than pelvic fluid from normal controls. Using this in vitro bioassay, we did not observe differences among the clinical stages of endometriosis (23).

Cytokines and Growth Factors Associated with Endometriosis

In recent years it has become apparent that steroid hormone actions on uterine tissues are not direct but are effected by paracrine mediators such as cytokines and growth factors (24, 25). Cytokines and growth factors are proteins or glycoproteins typically secreted by leukocytes or other cells into the extracellular environment where they exert their effects on the same cells (autocrine activity) or nearby cells (paracrine activity). Some of these proteins can circulate or traverse body cavities and thus may exert endocrine activities as well. In specific cases, cytokines exist in cell membrane associated forms where they act on adjacent cells (juxtacrine activity). Cytokines are key mediators of intercellular communication within the immune system. They have pleiotropic activities on a variety of target cells, exerting proliferative, cytostatic, chemoattractant, or differentiative effects. Most cytokines have high molar biological activities and are coupled to intracellular signaling and second messenger pathways via specific high-affinity receptors on target cell membranes. The cytokine and growth factor nomenclature reflects the historical description of biologic activity rather than a systematic relationship based on molecular structure. In Table 12.1 are grouped several cytokines and growth factors of interest to scholars of endometriosis according to superfamily homologies based on genomic organization and structural motifs.

Owing to their potency in low concentrations, the elaboration of cytokines within tissue microenvironments is very tightly regulated. Because of its clinical accessibility and proximity to the site of endometriosis growth, peritoneal fluid has been evaluated as an indicator of the in vivo milieu of endometriosis lesions. Although pelvic fluid is a complex medium containing and influenced by multiple cell types, we and other investigators (26) have found this to be a useful biologic fluid to define local, intercellular mediators of the inflammatory reaction associated with endometriosis. Evaluation of soluble cytokines and growth factors in pelvic fluid has been extended by the identification of these proteins within endometriosis implants

Table 12.1. Cytokine and growth factor families, based on genomic and protein structure (172)

Family	Cytokine/Growth Factor	Approx. Mol. Weight (kDa)	Receptor characteristics
Chemokine superfamily	RANTES	8	7-Transmembrane,
	IL-8	8	G-protein linked
	MCP-1	8–18	receptors
Epidermal growth factor superfamily	EGF	6	Tyrosine kinase
	TGF-α	6	
Hematopoietin superfamily	IL-1α and ß	17	jak-stat protein
	IL-6	23–26	associated receptors
	IFN-γ	20, 25	
	M-CSF	40–90	
	GM-CSF	18–22	
Platelet derived growth factor superfamily	PDGF	32	"Split" tyrosine kinase
	VEGF	35–45	
Transforming growth factor-ß superfamily	TGF-ß	25	Serine/threonine kinase
Others	FGFs	18–24	"Split" tyrosine kinase
	IGFs	7	Heterotetrameric tyrosine kinase
	TNF-α	17	Phospholipase and sphingomyelinase activation

per se. Studies using immunohistochemistry, mRNA hybridization, and cell culture techniques have documented that ectopic endometrial tissues can produce potent inflammatory and growth promoting proteins in situ. In this chapter we review the evidence that selected cytokines and growth factors, known to be produced by eutopic endometrial tissues, also are synthesized by endometriosis implants and may contribute to pro-inflammatory, mitogenic, and ultimately pathogenic activities within the peritoneal environment.

CYTOKINES

Interleukin-1

The cytokine interleukin-1 (IL-1) plays a central role in the regulation of inflammation and immune responses, and has been implicated in several disease processes including diabetes and rheumatoid arthritis. Although originally recognized as a product of activated monocytes and macrophages, it now is known to affect the activation of T lymphocytes and differentiation of B lymphocytes and other progenitor cells. Other paracrine and endocrine effects of IL-1 also have been characterized in non-hematopoietic cells, including osteoclasts, hepatocytes, and cells of the central nervous system (27).

Two receptor agonists, IL-1α and IL-1ß, are encoded by different genes and are synthesized as 31 kDa precursors, which are then cleaved to generate 17 kDa mature forms of IL-1. These two proteins, although sharing only 18–26% amino acid homology, bind to the same receptors and have comparable biologic activities. A related protein is the IL-1 receptor antagonist (IL-1ra). IL-1ra blocks the binding of both IL-1α and ß to IL-1 receptor type I. IL-1ra has been identified in two forms, a secreted form (sIL-1ra) and an intracellular form (icIL-1ra). The latter form is preferentially expressed in epithelial cells (28).

The IL-1 receptor (IL-1R) family also consists of numerous proteins with low amino acid homology. This includes IL-1R type I (80 kDa), IL-1R type II (68 kDa), and the recently described IL-1R accessory protein (IL-1R AcP) (27). Many cells coexpress both receptors. All three IL-1 isoforms can bind to both IL-1Rs, but IL-1ß preferentially binds IL-1RII. Only the IL-1RI appears to transduce a signal in response to IL-1 (27).

In the endometrium, the IL-1 system has been implicated as an important mediator of embryo implantation. The human embryo secretes both IL-1 isoforms (29, 30), and increased concentrations of IL-1 in embryo cultures correlate with improved implantation rates in in vitro fertilization (30). IL-1RI mRNA is expressed in endometrial epithelial cells and immunoreactive IL-1RI is present predominantly in luminal epithelium, with greatest staining in the secretory phase (31, 32). Functional IL-1R binding by its ligands has been demonstrated in epithelial cell cultures, where it is associated with increased PGE_2 synthesis (33). However, IL-1ß is specifically detected only in endothelial cells of spiral arteries and isolated stromal cells, and gene expression occurs only in the mid to late secretory phase (32). The receptor antagonist, IL-1ra, is localized to the glandular epithelium and expressed throughout the menstrual cycle both at the mRNA and protein levels, with greatest protein expression in the follicular phase. The IL-1 system represents a highly compartmentalized and regulated system of communication between the embryo, which secretes ligands, and the endometrial epithelium, which expresses both receptors and receptor antagonist peptide. The importance of these interactions has been demonstrated by the blocking of successful implantation in mice with the administration of exogenous IL-1ra (34).

IL-1 has been isolated from the peritoneal fluid of patients with endometriosis. Results have been inconsistent, with some investigators demonstrating elevated concentrations in patients with endometriosis (35–38) and others finding no elevation (39–41). Mori et al. (42) showed increased levels of IL-1ß mRNA expression in peritoneal macrophages from patients with mild endometriosis and increased levels of IL-1ra mRNA expression in macrophages from patients with moderate to severe endometriosis. These data suggest that there is a switch in gene expression with progression of disease. A different pattern of IL-1ra expression was observed in endometrium. In paired samples of eutopic endometrium and peritoneal implants analyzed for IL-1ra protein, eutopic samples showed glandular epithelial immuno-staining whereas peritoneal implants were negative for IL-1ra (43). Several investi-gators have shown a direct correlation between propagation of inflammation, abnormal cellular differentiation, and the absence of IL-1ra (43). Thus dysregulation of the IL-1 system may contribute to the inflammation of endometriosis and subse-quent sequelae.

Interleukin-6

The pleiotropic cytokine interleukin-6 (IL-6) is an important regulator of inflamma-tion and immunity that serves as a physiological link between the endocrine and the immune systems. Like IL-1, IL-6 modulates secretion of other cytokines, promotes T cell activation and B cell differentiation, and inhibits growth of various human cell lines. It is a 23–26 kDa phosphoglycoprotein that exists in several isoforms and is produced by a number of cell types including monocytes, macrophages, fibroblasts, endothelial cells, keratinocytes, vascular smooth muscle cells, and endometrial ep-ithelial and stromal cells (44–47). In addition, IL-6 is produced by several endocrine glands, including the pituitary and pancreas.

IL-6 initiates its biologic effects through binding to a high-affinity receptor com-plex consisting of two membrane glycoproteins: a low affinity 80 kDa membrane-bound receptor (IL-6R) and a receptor associated protein of 130 kDa (gp130) that is required for high-affinity binding and signal transduction. Additionally, a soluble form of the IL-6R has been identified (IL-6sR). This form of the receptor apparently arises from proteolytic cleavage of the membrane-bound IL-6R and has been shown to augment ligand activity (48–50).

Endometrial stromal and epithelial cells produce IL-6 in response to steroid hor-mones and other immunologic agents. Endometrial stromal cell IL-6 protein is in-duced by IL-1α or ß, tumor necrosis factor, platelet derived growth factor and interferon-γ (46, 47). Additionally, estradiol-17ß appears to strongly inhibit IL-1-induced endometrial stromal cell expression of IL-6 (45). Because estrogen typically enhances proliferation in endometrial epithelium, it is proposed that estrogen causes epithelial cell proliferation by limiting the synthesis of epithelial cell inhibitors such as IL-6 (45). Similarly, Zarmakoupis et al. have found that IL-6 inhibits proliferation of human endometrial stromal cells, and that this growth inhibition depends on cell density, suggesting that IL-6 may play a role in epithelial–stromal interactions gov-erning the regulation of normal uterine function (51). Indeed, Tabibzadeh et al. (45) have suggested that IL-6 fluctuations during the menstrual cycle reflect an inverse re-lationship to estrogen action; estrogen concentrations are high in the proliferative phase of the cycle, but IL-6 levels are low. Conversely, estrogenic activity is low dur-ing the secretory phase of the cycle, whereas IL-6 levels are high.

Endometriosis is characterized by the ectopic implantation and proliferation of en-dometrial cells. A long-standing debate is whether these cells are intrinsically differ-ent from eutopic endometrial cells or whether they become modified by an ensuing immune response following ectopic implantation. Because IL-6 is a potent immune cell mediator with growth regulatory activities, alterations in the local production of this cytokine within the peritoneal environment may contribute to the pathogenesis of endometriosis.

In vitro studies suggest that there is a dysregulation of IL-6 response in peritoneal macrophages (52, 53), endometrial stromal cells (54), and peripheral blood macrophages (44, 55) of patients with endometriosis. As proposed by Rier et al., endometriosis implants may be resistant to growth inhibition by IL-6 due to a decreased expression of cell surface IL-6R. This may be the cause of lower concentrations of IL-6 soluble receptor (IL-6sR) in the peritoneal fluid of these patients (56). However, it should be noted that other investigators have reported an increased concentration of IL-6sR in the peritoneal fluid of patients with endometriosis (57). Furthermore, conflicting results have been reported on the level of immunoreactive IL-6 detected in the peritoneal fluid of patients with endometriosis, with some investigators demonstrating elevated concentrations (39, 40, 56), and others finding no elevation (44, 53, 58). Our studies in peritoneal fluid (Table 12.2) failed to demonstrate statistically significant differences among control and endometriosis patients (23). It is likely that these inconsistent findings are related to antibody specificity.

Interleukin-8

Interleukin 8 (IL-8) is a member of the α or "C-X-C" chemokine family, a group of small peptide inflammatory mediators characterized by four conserved cysteine residues. In all members of this subfamily the first cysteine residues are separated by a variable amino acid. IL-8 recruits and activates polymorphonuclear leukocytes and T lymphocytes, and induces expression of several adhesion molecules (59). It also has been shown to have angiogenic activity (59). IL-8 is an 8 kDa peptide that is produced by a variety of cell types, including monocytes, lymphocytes, fibroblasts, epithelial

Table 12.2. Cytokine and growth factor concentrations in pelvic peritoneal fluid (PF)

		Endometriosis Stage [a]				
	Control	I–II	III–IV	(P)	ρ value [b] (P)	n^c
PF vol. (ml)	10.0±3.1	10.1±1.1	10.0±2.6	0.23	-0.22 (0.29)	15
IL-6 (pg/ml)	44±28	41±26	98±39	0.44	0.17 (0.32)	12
IL-8 (pg/ml)	15±7	152±105	380±131	0.03	0.51 (<0.01)	9
RANTES (ng/ml)	0.6±0.3	7.8±7.2	29.1±16.9	<0.01	0.54 (<0.01)	12
TNF-α^d (U/ml)	10±2	85±12	250±70	0.02	0.55 (<0.01)	
IFN-γ^e (pg/ml)	155±9	143±6	142±5	0.54	-0.20 (0.30)	12
VEGF (pg/ml)	71±9	68±8	111±11	0.04	0.47 (0.03)	7

[a] Revised AFS endometriosis stage.

[b] Spearman (ρ) correlation coefficient and level of significance (P).

[c] Matched independent observations in each clinical group.

[d] Adapted from Eisermann et al. (90). A matched analysis was not performed; however, 10 controls, 35 stage I–II and 11 stage II–IV endometriosis cases were studied by the authors.

[e] interferon-γ.

and endothelial cells in response to a variety of proinflammatory stimuli (e.g., IL-1, TNF-α, LPS) (60). Biologic activity is exerted by binding to two distinct but homologous receptors, type I and type II, that share 77% amino acid homology. Both of these are members of the G protein coupled receptors. Although the type I receptor specifically binds IL-8, the type II receptor also can bind other members of the chemokine family (61). A red blood cell receptor also has been described, although this chemokine receptor is not active on neutrophils and may represent a clearance factor for IL-8 and other chemokines (62).

In the human endometrium and decidua, hormonal (endocrine) and local (paracrine) control of leukocyte migration have been demonstrated (63, 64). Furthermore, there is a cyclical regulation of angiogenesis and neovascularization that occurs following menstruation. Thus two phenomena suggest a role of IL-8 in endometrial physiology. In vivo, IL-8 protein is selectively localized to the perivascular smooth muscle cells, independent of menstrual cycle phase (65). In vitro, IL-8 gene expression and protein secretion were documented in cultured endometrial stromal cells stimulated with IL-1α, TNF-α, or serum (66). Furthermore, co-incubation with progesterone caused an increase in mRNA synthesis and stability (67). Cultured epithelial cells also express IL-8 mRNA, although steady-state concentrations in stromal cells were higher (66). These data indicate that endometrial stromal and epithelial cells have the potential to secrete IL-8 upon stimulation by other cytokines, and may contribute to recruitment of leukocytes or neovascularization.

In endometriosis, we have shown that IL-8 protein is present in the peritoneal fluid of patients with endometriosis and documented a correlation between IL-8 concentration and endometriosis stage (68). We hypothesize that IL-8 derived from pelvic macrophages and endometriosis implants may contribute to the pathogenesis of endometriosis either by promoting the neovascularization, and hence proliferation of ectopic endometrial implants, or by the recruitment and activation of leukocytes to the peritoneal cavity. Our pelvic fluid findings are supported by the study of Rana et al., who have shown increased levels of IL-8 secreted by peritoneal macrophages from patients with endometriosis (69).

RANTES

Regulated on activation, normal T cell expressed and secreted (RANTES) is a cytokine of the ß or "C-C" chemokine family. Members of this family have the first two of four cysteine residues adjacent to each other. The RANTES gene encodes a 10 kDa intracellular and an 8 kDa secreted protein (70). RANTES is a chemoattractant for monocytes, memory T cells, and eosinophils. Although the original studies identified RANTES secretion by hematopoietic cells, it also has been shown to be secreted by some epithelial and mesenchymal cells. RANTES may be an important mediator in both acute and chronic inflammation. There are numerous potential binding sites for transcription factors that regulate this gene, and both early- and late-activating transcription factor complexes have been described (71). Four ligand receptors have been identified thus far, all G protein coupled receptors with seven transmembrane domains, and these share homology with the C-X-C chemokine receptors (72).

In normal endometrium, RANTES protein immunolocalization predominates in the stromal compartment (73). In vitro, stromal cell cultures synthesize RANTES mRNA and secrete protein when induced by TNF-α stimulation, although epithelial cells synthesize neither transcripts or protein (74). The discrepancy between basal RANTES expression in vivo and in vitro, and the requirement of cytokine stimulation in cultured cells for expression of RANTES, may indicate that cytokines from resident immune cells provide paracrine tissue effects in vivo. In cultures of purified cells, TNF-α must be added exogenously to effect significant RANTES gene expression.

In endometriosis, the pattern of RANTES protein distribution was similar to that found in normal endometrium (73). However, an important distinction between normal endometrial stromal cell cultures and those derived from endometriomas is that under similar conditions, endometrioma-derived stromal cell cultures secrete significantly greater concentrations of RANTES (74). In this way, peritoneal implants may contribute to the increased pelvic fluid concentrations of RANTES seen in patients with moderate and severe endometriosis (75). We have proposed that secretion of RANTES by ectopic implants provides a mechanism for peritoneal leukocyte recruitment.

Monocyte Chemotactic Protein-1

Monocyte chemotactic protein 1 (MCP-1), also known as monocyte chemotactic and activating factor (MCAF), is a ß or "C-C" chemokine. MCP-1 exists as multiple species that differ in size due to post-translational modification (76). Two related monocyte chemoattractants, MCP-2 and MCP-3, show 62% and 72% homology with MCP-1. Although originally described as a monocyte chemoattractant, MCP-1 also is chemoattractant for basophils (77). Numerous cell types express MCP-1 upon induction or activation by pro-inflammatory cytokines. Specific receptors for MCP-1 on monocytes have been reported, some of which also bind RANTES.

Investigators have documented the presence of MCP-1 mRNA in endometrial tissue from normal patients, as well as cultured cells from these biopsies. MCP-1 is expressed in normal endometrium and eutopic endometrium of women with endometriosis (78). IL-1ß stimulation of epithelial cell cultures resulted in a dramatic upregulation of MCP-1 in cells from eutopic endometrium of patients with endometriosis (78). No such expression was found in epithelial cells from normal patients, or in stromal cell cultures. These data suggest that MCP-1 expression may be regulated at the translational level in specific cell and tissue types. In endometrial cell cultures derived from endometriosis implants, IL-1ß induced MCP-1 expression in both stromal and epithelial cells (79), further suggesting that there may be site-specific differences in the expression of this monocyte chemoattractant.

Tumor Necrosis Factors

The tumor necrosis factors (TNFs) play a central role in the syndrome of septic shock, and it is from studies of this syndrome that we understand their biology. TNFs are pleiotropic cytokines with a range of beneficial and injurious effects, depending on the quantity produced, their tissue localization, the local activity of TNF-binding proteins, and their hormonal and cytokine milieu. Two receptor agonists have been identified. TNF-α or cachectin, and TNF-ß or lymphotoxin, are two related proteins, sharing about 30% amino acid homology, that bind to the same receptors. TNF-α, a 17 kDa peptide, is initially expressed as a membrane bound protein, from which the soluble form is derived by cleavage of the extracellular domain. By contrast, TNF-ß, a 25 kDa glycosylated peptide, is processed and secreted in a manner typical of other secreted proteins (80).

TNF-α is produced by neutrophils, activated lymphocytes, macrophages, NK cells, and other nonhematopoietic cells, whereas TNF-ß is produced by lymphocytes. Although these were initially identified for their ability to kill certain cell lines, their primary function is in their ability (along with IL-1) to initiate the cascade of cytokines and other factors associated with inflammatory responses. In contrast to their similar biologic activities, the regulation of the expression and processing of these two factors is quite different.

Two distinct TNF receptors have been identified. Virtually all cells except erythrocytes show the presence of one or both of these receptor types. TNF receptor II (TNF RII or type A) is a 75 kDa transmembrane protein. The other receptor, TNF receptor I (TNF RI or type B), is a 55 kDa transmembrane protein. Both receptor types have high affinities for TNF-α and TNF-ß. The extracellular domains of the two receptors show similarities, but the intracellular domains are apparently unrelated (81), suggesting possible different signal transduction pathways. Both receptors also exist in soluble forms, which are produced by the proteolytic cleavage of the extracellular domain. The biologic role of the soluble TNF receptors is not well defined, but these may modulate TNF activity either by binding and inhibiting the ligand or by stabilizing the ligand and augmenting its activities (82).

In the human endometrium, TNF-α has been implicated in the normal physiology of endometrial proliferation and shedding. Both TNF-α mRNA and protein are expressed in normal endometrium throughout the menstrual cycle. The greatest expression of protein and message is in the epithelial cells, with most staining during the secretory phase (83–85). Staining of stromal cells is also detected, predominantly in the proliferative phase of the cycle, suggesting differential local and hormonal regulation of this cytokine (83, 84). Short-term cultures of fresh explants secrete immunoreactive TNF-α protein, in increasing concentrations from the proliferative to menstrual phases of the cycle (86). In vitro, epithelial cell TNF-α secretion is modulated by IL-1, progesterone, and PP14 (87). TNF-α has been shown to increase prostaglandin production by cultured endometrial epithelial cells (88) and to promote the adherence of cultured stromal cells to mesothelial cells (89). This latter finding suggests that the presence of TNF-α in pelvic fluid may promote adherence of ectopic endometrium to the peritoneum, promoting implant formation.

Numerous investigators have shown that TNF-α concentrations are elevated in the peritoneal fluid of patients with endometriosis, and that these correlate with the stage of disease (36, 69, 90–92). The source of the elevated concentration of this cytokine in the pelvic fluid of endometriosis patients is not clear, but in vitro studies suggest that peritoneal macrophages (41, 69) and peripheral blood monocytes (55) from these patients also have upregulated TNF-α protein secretion. Because of its importance in other inflammatory processes, it is likely that this cytokine plays a role in the pathogenesis of endometriosis.

Interferon-γ

Interferon (IFN)-γ is a pleiotropic, pro-inflammatory cytokine with anti-viral, antiproliferative, and immunomodulatory effects. IFN-γ can be expressed as a 20 or 25 kDa glycoprotein with little sequence homology to IFN-α or ß. The two IFN-γ isoforms are glycosylated at different amino acid sites, but in neither case is glycosylation required for biologic activity (93). This cytokine is produced by a number of immune cells, including activated CD4+ and CD8+ T cells, and natural killer cells. The precise regulators of IFN-γ gene expression are still undefined; however its primary physiological stimuli are the antigens presented in the context of major histocompatibility class I or II proteins, and products of activated T cells and macrophages (e.g., IL-2, IL-12, and TNF-α) (94). Recently, IFN-γ secretion by T cells was shown to be inhibited by IL-10 (95). Most of the activities attributed to IFN-γ are believed to be mediated by IFN-γ induced proteins. The appearance of these latter proteins is a consequence of IFN-γ binding to a specific receptor that is distinct from the receptor for IFN-α or ß. The IFN-γ receptor is expressed on the surfaces of all cell types except erythrocytes and shows homology to the superfamily of cytokine receptors (93).

The general biology of IFN-γ is vast and includes promotion of both humoral and cell mediated immunity, regulation of TNF-α production, and participation in cellular recruitment. IFN-γ works synergistically with TNF-α to mediate septic shock and is implicated in the development of autoimmune diseases (94). Finally, IFN-γ is the principal inducer of class II MHC antigen expression on most cell types (excluding B cells).

In contrast, the precise physiological role of IFN-γ in normal human endometrium is relatively unknown. It is postulated that IFN-γ opposes the mitogenic effect of estrogen via a paracrine, antiproliferative action (96). Lymphoid cells may increase the local concentration of IFN-γ, exerting a cytostatic effect on normal epithelial cells and inducing HLA-DR expression (97). Consequently, IFN-γ might limit the cellular growth of the endometrium throughout the menstrual cycle, particularly in the basal layer where a greater density of lymphoid aggregates has been noted. This hypothesis is supported by the low proliferative activity and the presence of HLA-DR expression in the basal layer of the human endometrium.

IFN-γ is a potent activator of macrophages, and as several investigators have shown, the peritoneal fluid of patients with endometriosis has increased concentrations of activated macrophages (98). However, peritoneal fluid concentrations of IFN-γ are not significantly elevated in patients with endometriosis (53, 75). Although this may suggest that IFN-γ does not play a role in macrophage activation in these patients, it should be noted that soluble IFN-γ concentrations in peritoneal fluid samples may underestimate the actual concentrations in vivo, owing to the ubiquity of its receptor and high rate of cellular uptake. Within endometriosis implants themselves, more T lymphocytes and macrophages have been documented than the number found in eutopic endometrium (99). Additionally, in situ hybridization studies reveal that mRNA expression for IFN-γ is significantly greater in leukocytes of ectopic implants than of eutopic tissues (99). Protein localization studies reveal that the receptor for IFN-γ is present in glandular epithelium of ectopic endometrium, suggesting a possible paracrine role for resident leukocytes and IFN-γ in regulating cell proliferation in endometriosis. Other effects of IFN-γ that may contribute to infertility include embryotoxicity and adverse effects on sperm motility (100).

Colony Stimulating Factors

Colony stimulating factors (CSF) are cytokines that were initially identified by their ability to stimulate in vitro colony formation by hematopoietic progenitor cells. Three have retained their CSF designation and are distinguished by their effects on the generation, proliferation, migration, and activation of target cells: granulocytes (G-CSF), macrophages (M-CSF), and both granulocytes and macrophages (GM-CSF). Two of these, M-CSF and GM-CSF, have been studied in endometriosis. Natural M-CSFs are 40–90 kDa glycosylated, homodimeric proteins. A soluble M-CSF can be released by intracellular proteolytic cleavage and secretion of the longer prepropeptides. A juxtacrine interaction between membrane bound M-CSF and the M-CSF receptor also is possible. The receptor is a high affinity cell surface protein encoded by the c-*fms* proto-oncogene (101).

Little is known about the role of M-CSF in the endometrium. In vitro, stromal cells secrete immunoreactive M-CSF, and this effect can be enhanced by progesterone but not by estrogen. Epithelial cultures also secrete M-CSF, but this response does not appear to be hormonally regulated (102). In endometriosis, immunoreactive M-CSF is detected in the peritoneal fluid of affected patients, and concentrations correlate with disease stage (103).

GM-CSF is an 18–22 kDa glycoprotein, which mediates its effects via interactions with two cell surface receptors: a high-affinity complex composed of α and ß subunits, and a low-affinity complex (104). The role of GM-CSF in normal human endometrial physiology has not been explored. In endometriosis, GM-CSF was localized in matched implant and eutopic endometrial biopsy specimens. Endometrial biopsy specimens from control patients also were compared (105). GM-CSF protein was expressed in epithelial cells of all three biopsy sources, with increased expression in the ectopic implant biopsies during the secretory phase (105). It is postulated that M-CSF and GM-CSF in endometriosis lesions may activate peritoneal macrophages, and in this way contribute to the inflammatory cascade of the peritoneal environment.

GROWTH FACTORS

Growth Factor Expression in Endometrium and Endometriosis

Several human endometrial growth factors with known angiogenic and/or endometrial cell mitogenic activity have been identified and are discussed in the following section. Although their precise effects on endometriosis are generally unknown at the current time, these are potential regulators of endometriosis implant growth and modulators of secretion of inflammatory proteins and cytokines.

Vascular Endothelial Growth Factor

Vascular endothelial growth factor (VEGF), also known as vascular permeability factor and vasculotropin, is one of the most potent and specific angiogenic factors. The biochemistry and molecular biology of VEGF are well described (106). VEGF binds to a family of tyrosine kinase receptors inluding Flt-1 and KDR, leading to dimer formation, autophosporylation of the receptor, and, as for FGF, activation of mitogen activated protein kinases (107). With the exception of human trophoblast cells, which develop an endothelial phenotype during endovascular invasion, expression of VEGF receptors is restricted to vascular endothelial cells. Although the precise signaling pathway for VEGF remains unknown, VEGF receptor activation leads to a rapid increase in intracellular Ca^{2+} and inositol trisphosphate concentrations in endothelial cells.

The regulation of bioavailable VEGF is controlled at the transcriptional and posttranslational levels. Four distinct mRNA species arising via differential splicing of a primary VEGF transcript have been identified and characterized. The most common VEGF transcripts encode proteins comprising 165 and 121 amino acid residues that form glycosylated homodimers of about 45 and 35 kDa, respectively. Longer forms of VEGF (189 and 206), despite containing identical hydrophobic signal sequences, are not actively secreted into the extracellular milieu (106). Instead, the relatively basic carboxyl termini of these isoforms cause them to become reversibly associated with heparan sulfate proteoglycans of the extracellular matrix. These bound isoforms may have juxtracrine effects. Release of bioactive VEGF fragments from this extracellular reservoir can be effected by heparin, hypoxia, or plasmin cleavage (108).

In the endometrium the 165 and 121 variants appear to be the predominant isoforms (109, 110); however, only semiquantitative RT-PCR methods were used. A novel endometrial mRNA transcript predicting a 145 residue protein was reported by Charnock-Jones et al. (109), but this finding was not confirmed by Torry et al. (110) and no protein corresponding to this transcript has been demonstrated.

VEGF mRNA was detected in normal endometrium by RNase protection analyses and its expression was found to be highest during the secretory phase of the menstrual cycle (110, 111). VEGF protein was localized predominantly in endometrial glands whereas stromal staining was less abundant and more diffuse (110–112). Expression of the VEGF gene in normal human endometrial (111) and adenocarcinoma (109) cells is acutely upregulated by estradiol in vitro as it is in rodent uterus in vivo (113, 114). Other factors are known to upregulate VEGF expression including hypoxia (115), IL-1ß (116), PDGF and TGF-ß (117), EGF (118), and PGE_2 (119).

The physiological roles of VEGF in cycling endometrium include neovascularization and implantation. VEGF-induced angiogenesis allows repair of the endometrium following menstruation (114). It also appears to increase microvascular permeability, permitting the formation of a fibrin matrix for endothelial migration and proliferation (120). As a result, increased fluid and protein extravasation cause local edema, which helps to prepare the endometrium for embryo implantation (111).

The expression of VEGF by endometriosis implants provides a mechanism for the neovascularization that is commonly observed around these lesions (121). VEGF immunostaining was observed in the epithelium of endometriosis implants (111) and increased concentrations of soluble VEGF in pelvic fluid from patients with endometriosis has been reported (111, 122). A summary of our results is shown in Table 12.2, where peritoneal fluid levels of VEGF were found to correlate significantly with the stage of endometriosis ($\rho = 0.47$, $P = 0.03$). The cellular sources of VEGF in peritoneal fluid have not been precisely defined. Although evidence exists for production of this factor by endometriosis lesions (111), activated peritoneal macrophages also have the capacity to synthesize and secrete VEGF (123).

Fibroblast Growth Factors

Fibroblast growth factors (FGFs) are a family of nine heparin binding proteins ranging in size from 18 to 24 kDa that include the prototypic acidic and basic FGFs (FGF 1 and 2) as well as keratinocyte growth factor (FGF 7). The FGFs are mitogenic for a variety of cell types and play crucial roles in normal development and tumorigenesis. FGFs are particularly important as angiogenic peptides (19). Interestingly, FGF 1 and 2 do not contain obvious signal sequences, yet they become associated with heparan sulfate proteoglycan moieties on the extracellular matrix where they exert juxtacrine effects on adjacent target cells. Up to five different FGF receptors have been identified. These are transmembrane glycoprotein tyrosine kinase receptors that dimerize following ligand activation.

In human endometrium FGF 2 has been localized in the epithelial glands and perivascular adventitia (124), where it is likely to mediate angiogenic activity. An early report indicated that levels of FGF 2 did not change during the normal menstrual cycle (125); however, a more recent study did show an increase in FGF 1 and 2 during the secretory phase (126). Both FGF 7 and its receptor mRNA are expressed in the human endometrium throughout the menstrual cycle. FGF 7 mRNA levels are high in endometrial stromal cells whereas levels of its receptor predominate in the epithelial cell-enriched fractions (127). This observation suggests that FGF 7 may play a paracrine role in endometrial epithelial growth.

Huang et al. (128) measured FGF 2 by enzyme immunoassay and observed lower peritoneal fluid concentrations of FGF 2 in women with advanced stages of endometriosis, but these were not statistically different from normal controls.

Platelet Derived Growth Factor

Platelet derived growth factor (PDGF), the major growth promoting component in serum, is chemotactic and a potent mitogen for cells of mesenchymal origin, including endothelial cells, although the latter effect appears to be indirect (129). PDGF was initially identified and purified from human platelets (130, 131) but now is known to be produced by a variety of different cell types, particularly macrophages (132). PDGF is a cationic 32 kDa glycoprotein consisting of two polypeptide chains linked by disulfide bonds. The subunits of the dimer, termed A and B, share 60% sequence homology and are encoded by two distinct genes. PDGF is biologically active in any of three possible dimeric isoforms: AA, AB, and BB. PDGF purified from human platelets consists of about 70% AB and 30% BB isoforms (133). Like VEGF (see above), the A chain of PDGF undergoes differential splicing and may generate subunits with different functional properties (134).

Two distinct receptors for PDGF exist and are referred to as type α and type ß. The type α receptor binds all three PDGF isoforms with equal and high ($K_d = 0.1$ nM) affinity. The type ß receptor binds PDGF BB with high affinity and PDGF AB with lower affinity ($K_d = 1$ nM), but does not bind PDGF AA (135). The receptors are monomeric transmembrane glycoproteins of 180 kDa, each with an intrinsic intracellular tyrosine kinase domain. Ligand-induced activation of the receptor stimulates receptor phosphorylation, phosphoinositol turnover, Ca^{2+} mobilization, arachidonic acid release, enhanced expression of c-*myc* and c-*fos*, DNA synthesis, and cell mitosis (136).

Normal human endometrium expresses PDGF ligand subunits and receptors in vivo (137, 138), and both stromal (139) and epithelial (140) cells derived from this source proliferate in vitro in response to PDGF. Human peritoneal fluid (141) and media conditioned by activated peritoneal macrophages (142) contain mitogenic activity that has many of the biochemical characteristics of PDGF. Pelvic fluid and purified PDGF were noted to stimulate [^{3}H]thymidine incorporation into the nascent DNA of human endometrial stromal cell cultures (139). These findings suggest that PDGF, derived from macrophages or pelvic endometriosis implants might contribute to stimulate the growth and progression of endometriosis lesions.

Transforming Growth Factor ß

Transforming growth factor ß (TGF-ß) is a disulfide linked dimer of 25 kDa. Three isoforms exist, as well as the related activin and inhibin proteins and müllerian inhibiting substance. Virtually all cell types possess TGF-ß receptors containing at least three general classes of subunits (types I, II, and III) which are incompletely characterized (143). As a result, TGF-ß has a variety of biologic activities that include both growth stimulatory and inhibitory effects. It appears to play important roles in tissue morphogenesis and development, and thus is likely to be important in the cyclic regeneration of the human endometrium. It also is an important modulator of macrophage and NK cell function (144). Like PDGF, TGF-ß appears to have an indirect effect on angiogenesis and inconsistent actions on endothelial cell proliferation (19).

Early studies of human endometrial tissue indicated that variable levels of TGF-ß mRNA were expressed throughout the menstrual cycle (145). Epithelial and stromal cells isolated from normal human endometrium were found to express TGF-ß mRNA transcripts corresponding to all three isoforms (146) and secreted immunoreactive TGF-ß protein into their conditioned media. In keeping with an increased level of TGF-ß3 mRNA in proliferative endometrium, the addition of estradiol to endometrial stromal cell cultures increased the steady-state concentration of TGF-ß3 mRNA in these cells (147). Human endometrial cells also express TGF-ß receptor mRNAs

(148) and binding proteins (146). Co-culture experiments suggest that endometrial stromal cell production of TGF-ß is an active paracrine suppressor of epithelial stromelysin production (149). At low concentrations (<12.5 ng/mL) TGF-ß increased endometrial stromal cell proliferation, although this effect was lost at higher ligand concentrations (146, 150). Curiously, rat endometrial stromal cells exposed to 0.02–20 ng/mL TGF-ß1 demonstrated a dose-dependent increase in apoptotic cell death (151).

Oosterlynck et al. (152) used a cell growth inhibition bioassay to quantify concentrations of TGF-ß in the pelvic fluid of 26 women with endometriosis and 26 women without endometriosis. The variance of the data was high, but using a paired statistical analysis the authors demonstrated that TGF-ß concentrations were elevated in the endometriosis cases and speculated that at the mean concentration observed in endometriosis cases (11.4 ± 3.3 ng/mL), TGF-ß might act as a mitogen for endometriosis implants.

Insulin-like Growth Factors

The insulin-like growth factors (IGFs) and their receptors and binding proteins (IGF-BPs) represent a complex system of growth regulating factors in human endometrium. The IGFs are nonglycosylated peptides 7 kDa in size and evolutionary relatives of insulin. The IGF type I receptor (IGF-I-R) is structurally similar to the classical insulin receptor. It forms a heterotetrameric transmembrane complex that binds IGF-I and -II ligands with high affinity (1–5 nM) and signals cellular mitogenesis via tyrosine kinase domains in its ß-subunits (153). The IGF type II receptor is a single membrane spanning protein identical to the mannose-6-phosphate receptor that also binds IGFs with high affinity. Although it is believed that IGF-II-R does not transduce a mitogenic signal, mice carrying null mutations of the related IGF-II-XR gene manifest a specific reduction in placental growth (154). Six forms of human IGFBPs, ranging in size from 24 to 45 kDa, have been identified. These proteins serve as IGF transporters and modulate local bioactive IGF concentrations. The bioactivity of the IGFBPs in turn may be modulated by endogenous serine proteases (155).

In human endometrium IGF-I is expressed predominantly in the proliferative phase of the cycle whereas IGF-II is abundant during the secretory phase (156). Some controversy exists as to the localization of these products within the endometrial tissue. In situ hybridization analyses by Zhou et al. (157) suggest that IGF-I and II transcripts were found predominantly in the stroma, whereas the two receptors were more abundant in the epithelium. Immunoreactive IGF-I and IGF-I-R proteins were reported to be localized predominantly in the glandular epithelium of this tissue (158). IGFBPs 1-6 mRNA and protein have been identified in human endometrial tissue and cells (155, 157). Interestingly, the mitogenic effect of IGF-I on endometrial stromal cell cultures was significantly less than that induced by PDGF or EGF (158); however, as noted above, modulation by IGFBPs might alter these effects in vivo.

Direct studies of the IGF system in endometriosis are very limited. Tang et al. (158) describe more heterogeneous and localized glandular immunostaining of IGF-

I-R in endometriosis patients compared to normal subjects. IGF I and II and IGFBPs 2 and 3 (155, 159) have been identified in pelvic fluid from normal subjects but no studies of peritoneal fluid from endometriosis patients have been reported to date. Whether this growth factor system plays a specific role in the pathophysiology of endometriosis remains to be proven.

Epidermal Growth Factor

Epidermal growth factor (EGF) was the first peptide growth factor to be identified (160) and belongs to a family of proteins that includes TGF-α, heparin-binding EGF, and amphiregulin. These proteins are synthesized as 160 kDa precursors that are proteolytically cleaved to yield mature soluble peptides 6 kDa in size. The EGF family precursors contain transmembrane domains and may act as cell surface associated juxtacrine mitogens (161). EGF is a mitogen for epithelial and mesenchymal cells, and TGF-α has angiogenic activity (19). The mitogenic signals of these peptides are transduced via a 170 kDa transmembrane tyrosine kinase receptor (EGF-R). In the endometrium EGF and EGF-R appear to mediate estrogen induced proliferative effects through the coupling of signaling pathways (25, 162). An excellent review of the uterine physiology of this pathway was compiled by Giudice (163).

Immunostaining for EGF (164) and EGF-R (165) was observed in normal endometrial and endometriosis glands and stroma. Using isolated stromal cells from normal endometrium and endometriomas, Mellor and Thomas (166) reported that cells derived from endometriosis tissues had less mitogenic response to EGF than normal endometrial stromal cells. Unfortunately, their data were not normalized to cell number so direct comparisons between the cell cultures are difficult to interpret. Peritoneal fluid concentrations of EGF were estimated by De Leon et al. (167) using a radioreceptor assay, and no differences were found between normal and endometriosis patients. Similar findings were reported recently by Huang et al. (128) using a more sensitive enzyme immunoassay. Interestingly, only 52% of patients had immunodetectable concentrations of EGF even after a fivefold concentration of pelvic fluid.

SUMMARY

Clinical studies supporting a direct relationship between lesion volume and the pain (168, 169) or infertility (170, 171) symptoms of endometriosis remain controversial. Recent evidence suggesting that the symptoms associated with endometriosis are the result of local peritoneal inflammatory reactions may explain this conundrum. Increased concentrations of activated pelvic macrophages and lymphocytes and the elevated levels of specific cytokines and growth factors reviewed above support this hypothesis. The precise roles of these soluble factors are currently unknown, but we propose that a complex network of locally produced cytokines and growth factors modulate the growth and inflammatory behavior of ectopic endometrial implants. The secretion of pro-inflammatory and mitogenic proteins by endometriosis lesions and associated immune cells into the peritoneal microenvironment participates in a cascade of events resulting in implant proliferation and invasion, the recruitment of capillaries to the growing lesions, and further chemoattraction of leukocytes to these foci of peritoneal inflammation. Future therapeutic strategies to ameliorate the inflammatory reaction associated with endometriosis should target these potentially pathological proteins, but we must not ignore the likely physiological actions of many of the same bioactive molecules in normal eutopic endometrial function.

REFERENCES

1. Sampson J. Peritoneal endometriosis due to menstrual dissemination of endometrial tissue into the peritoneal cavity. Am J Obstet Gynecol 1927;14:422–429.

2. Drake T, Grunert G. The unsuspected pelvic factor in the infertility investigation. Fertil Steril 1980;34:27–31.

3. Olive D, Haney A. Endometriosis-associated infertility: a critical review of therapeutic approaches. Obstet Gynecol Surv 1986;41:538–555.

4. Jansen R. Minimal endometriosis and reduced fecundability: prospective evidence from an artificial insemination donor program. Fertil Steril 1986;46:141–143.

5. Simón C, Gutierrez A, Vidal A, et al. Outcome of patients with endometriosis in assisted reproduction: results from in-vitro fertilization and oocyte donation. Human Reprod 1994;9:725–729.

6. Tanbo T, Omland A, Dale P, et al. In vitro fertilization/embryo transfer in unexplained infertility and minimal peritoneal endometriosis. Acta Obstet Gynecol Scand 1995;74:539–543.

7. Brizek C, Schlaff S, Pellegrini V, et al. Increased incidence of aberrant morphological phenotypes in human embryogenesis: an association with endometriosis. J Assist Reprod Genet 1995;12:106–112.

8. Redwine D. Mülleriosis: the single best-fit model of the origin of endometriosis. J Reprod Med 1988;33:915–920.

9. Halme J, Hammond M, Hulka J, et al. Retrograde menstruation in healthy women and in patients with endometriosis. Obstet Gynecol 1984;64:151–154.

10. Kruitwagen R, Poels L, Willemsen W, et al. Endometrial epithelial cells in peritoneal fluid during the early follicular phase. Fertil Steril 1991;55:297–303.

11. Evers J. The defense against endometriosis. Fertil Steril 1996;66:351–353.

12. DiZerega G, Barber D, Hodgen G. Endometriosis: role of ovarian steroids in intiation, maintenance and suppression. Fertil Steril 1980;33:649–653.

13. Jänne O, Kauppila A, Kokko E, et al. Estrogen and progestin receptors in endometriosis lesions: comparison with endometrial tissue. Am J Obstet Gynecol 1981;41:562–566.

14. Bergqvist A, Jeppsson S, Ljungberb O. Histochemical demonstration of estrogen and progesterone binding in endometriotic tissue and in uterine endometrium: a comparative study. J Histochem Cytochem 1985;33:155–161.

15. Lessey B, Metzger D, Haney A, et al. Immunohistochemical analysis of estrogen and progesterone receptors in endometriosis: comparison with normal endometrium during the menstrual cycle and the effect of medical therapy. Fertil Steril 1989;51:409–415.

16. Ryan I, Schriock E, Taylor R. Isolation, characterization, and comparison of human endometrial and endometriosis cell *in vitro*. J Clin Endocrinol Metab 1994;78:642–649.

17. Schriock E, Monroe S, Henzl M, et al. Treatment of endometriosis with a potent agonist of gonadotropin-releasing hormone (nafarelin). Fertil Steril 1985;44:583–588.

18. Van der Linden P, de Goeif A, Dunselman G, et al. Endometrial cell adhesion in an in vitro model using intact amniotic membranes. Fertil Steril 1996;65:76–80.

19. Folkman J. Clinical applications of research on angiogenesis. N Engl J Med 1995;333: 1757–1764.

20. Gordon J, Shifren J, Foulk R, et al. Angiogenesis in the human female reproductive tract. Obstet Gynecol Surv 1995;50:688–697.

21. Oosterlynck D, Meuleman C, Sobis H, et al. Angiogenic activity of peritoneal fluid from women with endometriosis. Fertil Steril 1993;59:778–782.

22. Taylor R, Heilbron D, Roberts J. Growth factor activity in the blood of women in whom preeclampsia develops is elevated from early pregnancy. Am J Obstet Gynecol 1990;163:1839–1844.

23. Taylor R, Ryan I, Moore E, et al. Angiogenesis and macrophage activation in endometriosis. Ann NY Acad Sci 1997:1997;828:194–207.

24. Sirbasku D, Leland F, Benson R. Properties of a growth factor activity present in crude extracts of rat uterus. J Cell Biochem 1981;107:345–358.

25. Nelson K, Takahashi T, Bossert N, et al. Epidermal growth factor replaces estrogen in the stimulation of female genital-tract growth and differentiation. Proc Natl Acad Sci USA 1991;88:21–25.

26. Ramey J, Archer D. Peritoneal fluid: its relevance to the development of endometriosis. Fertil Steril 1993;60:1–14.

27. Bankers-Fulbright J, Kalli K, McKean D. Interleukin-1 signal transduction. Life Sci 1996;59:61–83.

28. Haskill S, Martin G, Van Le L, et al. cDNA cloning of an intracellular form of the human interleukin 1 receptor antagonist associated with epithelium. Proc Natl Acad Sci USA 1991;88:3681–3685.

29. Baranao R, Piazza A, Rumi L, et al. Predictive value of interleukin-1ß in supernatants of human embryo culture. American Fertility Society Meeting 1992:O-007[abstract].

30. Sheth K, Roca G, Al-Sedairy S, et al. Prediction of successful embryo implantation by measuring interleukin-1-alpha and immunosuppressive factor(s) in preimplantation embryo culture fluid. Fertil Steril 1991;55:952–957.

31. Simón C, Piquette G, Frances A, et al. Interleukin-1 type I receptor messenger ribonucleic acid expression in human endometrium throughout the menstrual cycle. Fertil Steril 1993;59:791–796.

32. Simón C, Piquette G, Frances A, et al. Localization of interleukin-1 type I receptor and interleukin-1 beta in human endometrium throughout the menstrual cycle. J Clin Endocrinol Metab 1993;77:549–555.

33. Tabibzadeh S, Kaffka K, Satyaswaroop P, et al. Interleukin-1 (IL-1) regulation of human endometrial function: presence of IL-1 receptor correlates with IL-1-stimulated prostaglandin E_2 production. J Clin Endocrinol Metab 1990;70:1000–1006.

34. Simón C, Frances A, Piquette G, et al. The immune mediator interleukin-1 receptor antagonist (IL-1ra) preevents embryo implantation. Endocrinology 1994;134:521–528.

35. Mori H, Sawairi M, Nakagawa M, et al. Peritoneal fluid interleukin-1ß and tumor necrosis factor in patients with benign gynecologic disease. Am J Reprod Immunol 1991;26:62–67.

36. Taketani Y, Kuo T, Mizuno M. Comparison of cytokine levels and embryo toxicity in peritoneal fluid in infertile women with untreated or treated endometriosis. Am J Obstet Gynecol 1992;167:265–270.

37. Hill J, Anderson D. Lymphocyte activity in the presence of peritoneal fluid from fertile women and infertile women with and without endometriosis. Am J Obstet Gynecol 1989;161:861–864.

38. Fakih H, Baggett B, Holtz G, et al. Interleukin-1: a possible role in the infertility associated with endometriosis. Fertil Steril 1987;47:213–217.

39. Koyama N, Matsuura K, Okamura H. Cytokines in the peritoneal fluid of patients with endometriosis. J Reprod Med 1993;43:45–50.

40. Ueki M, Tsurunaga T, Ushiroyama T, et al. Macrophage activation factors and cytokines in peritoneal fuid from patients with endometriosis. Asia-Oceania J Obstet Gynaecol 1994;20:427–431.

41. Keenan J, Chen T, Chadwell N, et al. IL-1ß, TNF-α, and IL-2 in peritoneal fluid and macrophage-conditioned media of women with endometriosis. Am J Reprod Immunol 1995;34:381–385.

42. Mori H, Sawairi M, Nakagawa M, et al. Expression of interleukin-1 (IL-1) beta messenger ribonucleic acid (mRNA) and IL-1 receptor antagonist mRNA in peritoneal macrophages from patients with endometriosis. Fertil Steril 1992;57:535–542.

43. Sahakian V, Anners J, Haskill S, et al. Selective localization of interleukin-1 receptor antagonist in eutopic endometrium and endometriotic implants. Fertil Steril 1993;60:276–279.

44. Boutten A, Dehoux M, Edelman P, et al. IL6 and acute phase plasma proteins in peritoneal fluid of women with endometriosis. Clin Chim Acta 1992;210:187–195.

45. Tabibzadeh S, Santhanam U, Sehgal P, et al. Cytokine-induced production of IFN-ß$_2$/IL-6 by freshly explanted human endometrial stromal cells. J Immunol 1989;142:3134–3139.

46. Laird S, Li T, Bolton A. The production of placental protein 14 and interleukin 6 by human endometrial cells in culture. Human Reprod 1993;8:793–798.

47. Laird S, Tuckerman E, Li T, et al. Stimulation of human endometrial epithelial cell interleukin 6 production by interleukin 1 and placental protein 14. Human Reprod 1994;9:1339–1343.

48. Fey G, Hattori M, Hocke G, et al. Gene regulation by interleukin 6. Biochimie 1991;73: 47–50.

49. Hibi M, Murakami M, Saito M, et al. Molecular cloning and expression of an IL-6 signal transducer, gp130. Cell 1990;63:1149–1157.

50. Yamasaki K, Taga T, Hirata Y, et al. Cloning and expression of the human interleukin-6 (BSF-2/IFN beta 2) receptor. Science 1988;241:825–828.

51. Zarmakoupis P, Rier S, Maroulis G, et al. Inhibition of human endometrial stromal cell proliferation by interleukin 6. Human Reprod 1995;9:2395–2399.

52. Rier S, Parsons A, Becker J. Altered interleukin-6 production by peritoneal leukocytes from patients with endometriosis. Fertil Steril 1994;61:294–299.

53. Keenan J, Chen T, Chadwell N, et al. Interferon-gamma (IFN-γ) and interleukin-6 (IL-6) in peritoneal fluid and macrophage-conditioned media of women with endometriosis. Am J Reprod Immunol 1994;32:180–183.

54. Tseng J, Ryan I, Murai J, et al. Interleukin-6 secretion *in vitro* is up-regulated in ectopic and eutopic endometrial stromal cells from women with endometriosis. J Clin Endocrinol Metab 1996;81:1118–1122.

55. Braun D, Gebel H, House R, et al. Spontaneous and induced synthesis of cytokines by peripheral blood monocytes in patients with endometriosis. Fertil Steril 1996;65:1125–1129.

56. Rier S, Zarmakoupis P, Hu X, et al. Dysregulation of interleukin-6 responses in ectopic endometrial stromal cells: correlation with decreased soluble receptor levels in peritoneal fluid of women with endometriosis. J Clin Endocrinol Metab 1995;80:1431–1437.

57. Schroder W, Gaetje R, Baumann R. Interleukin-6 and soluble interleukin-6 receptor in peritoneal fluid and serum of patients with endometriosis. Clin Exp Obstet Gynecol 1996;23:10–14.

58. Buyalos R, Funari V, Azziz R, et al. Elevated interleukin-6 levels in peritoneal fluid of patients with pelvic pathology. Fertil Steril 1992;58:302–306.

59. Koch A, Polverini P, Kunkel S, et al. Interleukin-8 as a macrophage-derived mediator of angiogenesis. Science 1992;258:1798–1801.

60. Clark D. Cytokines, decidua, and early pregnancy. Oxf Rev Reprod Biol 1993;15:83–111.

61. LaRosa G, Thomas K, Kaufmann M, et al. Amino terminus of the interleukin-8 receptor is a major determinant of receptor subtype specificity. J Biol Chem 1992;267:25402–25406.

62. Neote K, Darbonne W, Ogez J, et al. Identification of a promiscuous inflammatory peptide receptor on the surface of red blood cells. J Biol Chem 1993;268:12247–12249.

63. Lea R, Clark D. Macrophages and migratory cells in endometrium relevant to implantation. Baillieres Clin Obstet Gynecol 1991;5:25–29.

64. Bulmer J, Longfellow M, Ritson A. Leukocytes and resident blood cells in endometrium. Ann NY Acad Sci 1991;622:57–68.

65. Crichley H, Kelly R, Kooy J. Perivascular location of a chemokine interleukin-8 in human endometrium: a preliminary report. Human Reprod 1994;9:1406–1409.

66. Arici A, Head J, MacDonald P, et al. Regulation of interleukin-8 gene expression in human endometrial cells in culture. Mol Cell Endocrinol 1993;94:195–204.

67. Arici A, MacDonald P, Casey M. Progestin regulation of interleukin-8 mRNA levels and protein synthesis in human endometrial stromal cells. J Steroid Biochem Mol Biol 1996;58:71–76.

68. Ryan I, Tseng J, Schriock E, et al. Interleukin-8 concentrations are elevated in peritoneal fluid of women with endometriosis. Fertil Steril 1995;63:929–932.

69. Rana N, Braun D, House R, et al. Basal and stimulated secretion of cytokines by peritoneal macrophages in women with endometriosis. Fertil Steril 1996;65:925–930.

70. Schall T, Jongstra J, Dyer B, et al. A human T cell-specific molecule is a member of a new gene family. J Immunol 1988;141:1018–1025.

71. Ortiz D, Krensky A, Nelson P. Kinetics of transcription factors regulating the RANTES chemokine gene reveal a developmental switch in nuclear events during T-lymphocyte maturation. Mol Cell Biol 1996;16:202–210.

72. Horuk R. Molecular properties of the chemokine receptor family. Trends Pharmacol Sci 1994;15:159–165.

73. Hornung D, Ryan I, Chao V, et al. Immunolocalization and regulation of the chemokine RANTES in human endometrial and endometriosis tissues and cells. J Clin Endocrinol Metab 1997;82:1621–1628.

74. Ryan I, Tseng J, Schall T, et al. RANTES chemokine expression is upregulated in stromal cells cultured from humen endometriosis tissues. J Soc Gynecol Invest 1996:#S32[abstract].

75. Khorram O, Taylor R, Ryan I, et al. Peritoneal fluid concentrations of the cytokine RANTES correlate with the severity of endometriosis. Am J Obstet Gynecol 1993;169:1545–1549.

76. Graves D, Jiang Y. Chemokines, a family of chemotactic cytokines. Crit Rev Oral Biol Med 1995;6:109–118.

77. Kuna P, Reddigari S, Schall T, et al. Characterization of the human basophil response to cytokines, growth factors, and histamine releasing factors of the intercrine/chemokine family. J Immunol 1993;150:1932–1943.

78. Akoum A, Lemay A, Brunet C, et al. Secretion of monocyte chemotactic protein-1 by cytokine-stimulated endometrial cells of women with endometriosis. Fertil Steril 1995;63:322–328.

79. Akoum A, Lemay A, Brunet C, et al. Cytokine-induced secretion of monocyte chemotactic protein-1 by human endometriotic cells in culture. Am J Obstet Gynecol 1995;172:594–600.

80. Nedwin G, Naylor S, Sakaguchi A, et al. Human lymphotoxin and tumor necrosis factor genes: structure, homology and chromosomal localization. Nucleic Acids Res 1985;13:6361–6373.

81. Dembic Z, Loetscher H, Gubler U, et al. Two human TNF receptors have similar extracellular, but distinct intracellular, domain sequences. Cytokine 1990;2:231–237.

82. Aderka D, Angelmann H, Maor Y, et al. Stabilization of the bioactivity of tumor necrosis factor by its soluble receptors. J Exp Med 1992;175:323–329.

83. Tabibzadeh S. Ubiquitous expression of TNF-α/cachectin immunoreactivity in human endometrium. Am J Reprod Immunol 1991;26:1–4.

84. Hunt J, Chen H, Hu X, et al. Tumor necrosis factor-α messenger ribonucleic acid and protein in human endometrium. Biol Reprod 1992;47:141–147.

85. Philippeaux M, Piguet P. Expression of tumor necrosis factor-alpha and its mRNA in the endometrial mucosa during the menstrual cycle. Am J Pathol 1993;143:480–486.

86. Tabibzadeh S, Zupi E, Babaknia A, et al. Site and menstrual cycle-dependent expression of proteins of the tumour necrosis factor (TNF) receptor family, and BCL-2 oncoprotein and phase specific production of TNFα in human endometrium. Human Reprod 1995;10:277–286.

87. Laird S, Tuckerman E, Sarvelos H, et al. The production of tumor necrosis factor alpha (TNF-alpha) by human endometrial cells in culture. Human Reprod 1996;11:1318–1323.

88. Chen D, Yang Z, Hilsenrath R, et al. Stimulation of prostaglandin (PG) F2 alpha and PGE2 release by tumor necrosis factor-alpha and interleukin-1 alpha in cultured human luteal phase endometrial cells. Human Reprod 1995;10:2773–2780.

89. Zhang R, Wild R, Ojago J. Effect of tumor necrosis factor-alpha on adhesion of human endometrial stromal cells to peritoneal mesothelial cells: an in vitro system. Fertil Steril 1993;59:1196–1201.

90. Eisermann J, Gast M, Pineda J, et al. Tumor necrosis factor in peritoneal fluid of women undergoing laparoscopic surgery. Fertil Steril 1988;50:573–579.

91. Kupker W, Felberbaum R, Bauer O, et al. Significance of tumor necrosis factor alpha (TNF-alpha) in endometriosis. Geburtshilde Frauenheilkd 1996;56:239–242.

92. Liang X, Hu L, Wu P. Tumor necrosis factor in peritoneal fluid of infertile women with endometriosis and its relation to sperm motility. Chin J Obstet Gynecol 1994;29:524–526, 573.

93. Lundell D, Narula S. Structural elements required for receptor recognition of human interferon-gamma. Pharm Therap 1994;64:1–21.

94. Farrar M, Schreiber R. The molecular cell biology of interferon-γ and its receptor. Ann Rev Immunol 1993;11:571–611.

95. Fiorentino D, Bond M, Mosmann T. Two types of mouse T helper cells. IV: TH2 clones secrete a factor that inhibits cytokine production of TH1 clones. J Exp Med 1989;170:2081–2095.

96. Tabibzadeh S, Satyaswaroop P, Rao P. Antiproliferative effect of interferon-γ in human endometrial epithelial cell in vitro: potential local growth modulatory role in endometrium. J Clin Endocrinol Metab 1988;67:131–138.

97. Tabibzadeh S, Gerber M, Satyaswaroop P. Induction of HLA-DR antigen expression in human endometrial epithelial cells in vitro by recombinant γ-interferon. Am J Pathol 1986;125:90–96.

98. Halme J, Becker S, Wing R. Accentuated cyclic activation of peritoneal macrophages in patients with endometriosis. Am J Obstet Gynecol 1984;148:85–90.

99. Klein N, Pergola G, Tekmal R, et al. Cytokine regulation of cellular proliferation in endometriosis. Ann NY Acad Sci 1994;734:322–332.

100. Hill J. Immunological factors in endometriosis and endometriosis-associated reproductive failure. Med Clin North Am 1992;3:583–596.

101. Sherr C, Roussel M, Rettenmier C. Colony-stimulating factor-1 receptor (c-fms). J Cell Biochem 1988;38:179–187.

102. Kariya M, Kanzaki H, Hanamura T, et al. Progesterone-dependent secretion of macrophage colony-stimulating factor by human endometrial stromal cells of nonpregnant uterus in culture. J Clin Endocrinol Metab 1994;79:86–90.

103. Fukaya T, Sugawara J, Yoshida H, et al. The role of macrophage colony stimulating factor in the peritoneal fluid in infertile patients with endometriosis. Tohoku J Exp Med 1994;172:221–226.

104. Sakamoto K, Mignacca R, Gasson J. Signal transduction by granulocyte-macrophage colony-stimulating factor and interleukin-3 receptors. Receptors and Channels 1994;2:175–181.

105. Sharpe-Timms K, Bruno P, Penney L, et al. Immunohistochemical localization of granulocyte-macrophage colony-stimulating factor in matched endometriosis and endometrial tissues. Am J Obstet Gynecol 1994;171:740–745.

106. Ferrara N, Houck K, Jakeman L, et al. The vascular endothelial growth factor family of peptides. J Cell Biochem 1991;47:211–218.

107. D'Angelo G, Struman I, Martial J, et al. Activation of mitogen-activated protein kinases by vascular endothelial growth factor and basic fibroblast growth factor in capillary endothelial cells is inhibited by the antiangiogenic factor 16-kDa-terminal fragment of prolactin. Proc Natl Acad Sci USA 1995;92:6374–6378.

108. Houck K, Leung D, Rowland A, et al. Dual regulation of vascular endothelial growth factor bioavailability by genetic and proteolytic mechanisms. J Biol Chem 1992;267:26031–26037.

109. Charnock-Jones D, Sharkey A, Rajput-Williams J, et al. Identification and localization of alternately spliced mRNAs for vascular endothelial growth factor in human uterus and estrogen regulation in endometrial carcinoma cell lines. Biol Reprod 1993;48:1120–1128.

110. Torry D, Holt V, Keenan J, et al. Vascular endothelial growth factor expression in cycling human endometrium. Fertil Steril 1996;66:72–80.

111. Shifren J, Tseng J, Zaloudek C, et al. Ovarian steroid regulation of vascular endothelial growth factor in the human endometrium: implications for angiogenesis during the menstrual cycle and in the pathogenesis of endometriosis. J Clin Endocrinol Metab 1996;81:3112–3118.

112. Li X, Gregory J, Ahmed A. Immunolocalization of vascular endothelial growth factor in human endometrium. Growth Factors 1994;11:277–282.

113. Cullinan-Bove K, Koos R. Vascular endothelial growth factor/vascular permeability factor expression in the rat uterus: rapid stimulation by estrogen correlates with estrogen-induced increases in uterine capillary permeability and growth. Endocrinology 1993;133:829–837.

114. Shweiki D, Itin A, Neufeld G, et al. Patterns of expression of vascular endothelial growth factor (VEGF) and VEGF receptors in mice suggest a role in hormonally regulated angiogenesis. J Clin Invest 1993;91:2235–2243.

115. Liu Y, Cox S, Morita T, et al. Hypoxia regulates vascular endothelial growth factor gene expression in endothelial cells. Identification of a 5' enhancer. Circ Res 1995;77:638–643.

116. Li J, Perrella M, Tsai J, et al. Induction of vascular endothelial growth factor gene expression by interleukin-1 beta in rat aortic smooth muscle cells. J Biol Chem 1995;270:308–312.

117. Brogi E, Wu T, Namiki A, et al. Indirect angiogenic cytokines upregulate VEGF and bFGF gene expression in vascular smooth muscle cells, whereas hypoxia upregulates VEGF expression only. Circulation 1994;90:649–652.

118. Goldman C, Kim J, Wong W, et al. Epidermal growth factor stimulates vascular endothelial growth factor production by human malignant glioma cells: a model of glioblastoma multiforme pathophysiology. Mol Biol Cell 1993;4:121–133.

119. Ben-Av P, Crofford L, Wilder R, et al. Induction of vascular endothelial growth factor expression in synovial fibroblasts by prostaglandin E and interleukin-1: a potential mechanism for inflammatory angiogenesis. FEBS Lett 1995;372:83–87.

120. Dvorak H, Senger D, Dvorak A, et al. Regulation of extravascular coagulation by microvascular permeability. Science 1985;227:1059–1061.

121. Nisolle M, Casanas-Roux F, Anaf V, et al. Morphometric study of the stromal vascularization in peritoneal endometriosis. Fertil Steril 1993;59:681–684.

122. McLaren J, Prentice A, Charnock-Jones D, et al. Vascular endothelial growth factor (VEGF) concentrations are elevated in peritoneal fluid of women with endometriosis. Human Reprod 1996;11:220–223.

123. McLaren J, Prentice A, Charnock-Jones D, et al. Vascular endothelial growth factor is produced by peritoneal fluid macrophages in endometriosis and is regulated by ovarian steroids. J Clin Invest 1996;98:482–489.

124. Cordon-Cardo C, Vlodavsky I, Haimovitz-Friedman A, et al. Expression of basic fibroblast growth factor in normal human tissues. Lab Invest 1990;63:832–840.

125. Rusnati M, Casarotti G, Pecorelli S, et al. Basic fibroblast growth factor in ovulatory cycle and postmenopausal human endometrium. Growth Factors 1990;3:299–307.

126. Salat-Baroux J, Romain S, Alvarez S, et al. Biochemical and immunohistochemical multiparametric analysis of steroid receptors and growth factor receptors in human normal endometrium in spontaneous cycles and after the induction of ovulation. Human Reprod 1994;9:200–208.

127. Pekonen F, Nyman T, Rutanen E. Differential expression of keratinocyte growth factor and its receptor in the human uterus. Mol Cell Endocrinol 1993;95:43–49.

128. Huang J, Papasakelariou C, Dawood M. Epidermal growth factor and basic fibroblast growth factor in peritoneal fluid of women with endometriosis. Fertil Steril 1996;65:931–934.

129. Nicosia R, Nicosia S, Smith M. Vascular endothelial growth factor, platelet-derived growth factor, and insulin-like growth factor-1 promote rat aortic angiogenesis in vitro. Am J Pathol 1994;145:1023–1029.

130. Heldin C, Westermark B, Wasteson A. Platelet-derived growth factor: purification and partial characterization. Proc Natl Acad Sci USA 1979;76:3722–3726.

131. Antoniades H, Scher C, Stiles C. Purification of human platelet-derived growth factor. Proc Natl Acad Sci USA 1979;76:1809–1813.

132. Shimokado K, Raines E, Madtes D, et al. A significant part of macrophage-derived growth factor consists of at least two forms of PDGF. Cell 1985;43:277–286.

133. Hart C, Bailey M, Curtis D, et al. Purification of PDGF-AB and PDGF-BB from human platelet extracts and identification of all three PDGF dimers in human platelets. Biochemistry 1990;29:166–172.

134. Khachigian L, Chesterman C. Platelet-derived growth factor and alternative splicing: a review. Pathology 1992;24:280–290.

135. Heldin C, Backstrom G, Ostman A, et al. Binding of different dimeric forms of PDGF to human fibroblasts: evidence for two separate receptor types. EMBO J 1988;7:1387–1393.

136. Williams L. Signal transduction by the platelet-derived growth factor receptor. Science 1989;243:1564–1570.

137. Chegini N, Rossi M, Masterson B. Platelet-derived growth factor (PDGF), epidermal growth factor (EGF), and EGF and PDGF beta-receptors in human endometrial tissue: localization and in vitro action. Endocrinology 1992;130:2373–2385.

138. Boehm K, Daimon M, Gorodeski I, et al. Expression of the insulin-like and platelet-derived growth factor genes in human uterine tissues. Mol Reprod Dev 1990;27:93–101.

139. Surrey E, Halme J. Effect of platelet-derived growth factor on endometrial stromal cell proliferation in vitro: a model for endometriosis? Fertil Steril 1991;56:672–679.

140. Munson L, Upadhyaya N, Van Meter S. Platelet-derived growth factor promotes endometrial epithelial cell proliferation. Am J Obstet Gynecol 1995;173:1820–1825.

141. Halme J, White C, Kauma S, et al. Peritoneal macrophages from patients with endometriosis release growth factor activity in vitro. J Clin Endocrinol Metab 1988; 66:1044–1049.

142. Olive D, Montoya I, Riehl R, et al. Macrophage-conditioned media enhance endometrial stromal cell proliferation in vitro. Am J Obstet Gynecol 1991;164:953–958.

143. Massagué J, Cheifetz S, Boyd F, et al. TGF-beta receptors and TGF-beta binding proteoglycans: recent progress in identifying their functional properties. Ann NY Acad Sci 1990;593:59–72.

144. Hooper W. The role of transforming growth factor-beta in hematopoiesis. A review. Leuk Res 1991;15:179–184.

145. Kauma S, Matt D, Strom S, et al. Interleukin-1 beta, human leukocyte antigen HLA-DR alpha, and transforming growth factor-beta expression in endometrium, placenta, and placental membranes. Am J Obstet Gynecol 1990;163:1430–1437.

146. Tang X, Zhao Y, Rossi M, et al. Expression of transforming growth factor-beta (TGF beta) isoforms and TGF beta type II receptor messenger ribonucleic acid and protein, and the effect of TGF betas on endometrial stromal cell growth and protein degradation in vitro. Endocrinology 1994;135:4450–4459.

147. Arici A, MacDonald P, Casey M. Modulation of the levels of transforming growth factor beta messenger ribonucleic acids in human endometrial stromal cells. Biol Reprod 1996;54:463–469.

148. Dumont N, O'Connor-McCourt M, Philip A. Transforming growth factor-beta receptors on human endometrial cells: identification of the type I, II, and III receptors and glycosyl-phosphatidylinositol anchored TGF-beta binding proteins. Mol Cell Endocrinol 1995;111:57–66.

149. Bruner K, Rodgers W, Gold L, et al. Transforming growth factor beta mediates the progesterone suppression of an epithelial metalloproteinase by adjacent stroma in the human endometrium. Proc Natl Acad Sci USA 1995;92:7362–7366.

150. Hammond M, Oh S, Anners J, et al. The effect of growth factors on the proliferation of human endometrial stromal cells in culture. Am J Obstet Gynecol 1993;168:1131–1137.

151. Moulton B. Transforming growth factor-beta stimulates endometrial stromal apoptosis in vitro. Endocrinology 1994;134:1055–1060.

152. Oosterlynck D, Meuleman C, Waer M, et al. Transforming growth factor-beta activity is increased in peritoneal fluid from women with endometriosis. Obstet Gynecol 1994;83:287–292.

153. Le Roith D. Insulin-like growth factor receptors and binding proteins. Baillieres Clin Endocrinol Metab 1996;10:49–73.

154. Baker J, Liu J, Robertson E, et al. Role of insulin-like growth factors in embryonic and postnatal growth. Cell 1993;75:73–82.

155. Giudice L, Dsupin B, Gargosky S, et al. The insulin-like growth factor system in human peritoneal fluid: its effects on endometrial stromal cells and its potential relevance to endometriosis. J Clin Endocrinol Metab 1994;79:1284–1293.

156. Giudice L, Dsupin B, Jin I, et al. Differential expression of messenger ribonucleic acids encoding insulin-like growth factors and their receptors in human uterine endometrium and decidua. J Clin Endocrinol Metab 1993;76:1115–1122.

157. Zhou J, Dsupin B, Giudice L, et al. Insulin-like growth factor system gene expression in human endometrium during the menstrual cycle. J Clin Endocrinol Metab 1994;79:1723–1734.

158. Tang X, Rossi M, Masterson B, et al. Insulin-like growth factor I (IGF-I), IGF-I receptors, and IGF binding proteins 1-4 in human uterine tissue: tissue localization and IGF-I action in endometrial stromal and myometrial smooth muscle cells in vitro. Biol Reprod 1994;50:1113–1125.

159. Koutsilieris M, Akoum A, Lazure C, et al. N-terminal truncated forms of insulin-like growth factor binding protein-3 in the peritoneal fluid of women without laparoscopic evidence of endometriosis. Fertil Steril 1995;63:314–321.

160. Cohen S, Carpenter G. Human epidermal growth factor: isolation and chemical and biological properties. Proc Natl Acad Sci USA 1975;72:1317–1321.

161. Massagué J. Transforming growth factor-alpha. A model for membrane-anchored growth factors. J Biol Chem 1990;265:21393–21396.

162. Curtis S, Washburn T, Sewall C, et al. Physiological coupling of growth factor and steroid receptor signaling pathways: estrogen receptor knockout mice lack estrogen-like response to epidermal growth factor. Proc Natl Acad Sci USA 1996;93:12626–12630.

163. Giudice L. Growth factors and growth modulators in human uterine endometrium: their potential relevance to reproductive medicine. Fertil Steril 1994;61:1–17.

164. Haining R, Cameron I, Papendorp C, et al. Epidermal growth factor in human endometrium: proliferative effects in culture and immunocytochemical localization in normal and endometriotic tissues. Human Reprod 1991;6:1200–1205.

165. Huang J, Yeh J. Quantitative analysis of epidermal growth factor receptor gene expression in endometriosis. J Clin Endocrinol Metab 1994;79:1097–1101.

166. Mellor S, Thomas E. The actions of estradiol and epidermal growth factor in endometrial and endometriotic stroma in vitro. Fertil Steril 1994;62:507–513.

167. De Leon F, Vijayakumar R, Brown M, et al. Peritoneal fluid volume, estrogen, progesterone, prostaglandin, and epidermal growth factor concentrations in patients with and without endometriosis. Obstet Gynecol 1986;68:189–194.

168. Vercellini P, Trespidi L, De Giorgi O, et al. Endometriosis and pelvic pain: relation to disease stage and localization. Fertil Steril 1996;65:299–304.

169. Stovall D, Bowser L, Archer D, et al. Endometriosis-associated pelvic pain: Evidence for an association between stage of disease and persistence of chronic pelvic pain. American Society for Reproductive Medicine 1995 Meeting Program 1995:S157[abstract].

170. Yeh J, Seibel M. Artificial insemination with donor sperm: a review of 108 patients. Obstet Gynecol 1987;70:3413–3416.

171. Collins J, Wrixon W, Janes L, et al. Treatment-independent pregnancy among infertile couples. N Engl J Med 1983;309:1201–1206.

172. Callard R, Gearing A. The Cytokine Facts Book. London: Academic Press, 1994.

13

ONCOGENES AND GROWTH FACTORS IN GYNECOLOGIC ONCOLOGY

Oliver Dorigo and Jonathan S. Berek

UCLA School of Medicine, Los Angeles, California

The discovery of cancer causing mechanisms has provided opportunities to begin to understand the molecular pathology of gynecologic malignancies (1). This chapter summarizes current knowledge about the role of oncogenes and growth factors in gynecologic malignancies. Furthermore, currently ongoing efforts to inhibit oncogenesis, for example, by interrupting growth factor pathways or targeting the overexpression of oncogenes using molecular techniques, are described.

ONCOGENES

An oncogene is any gene that encodes a protein able to transform cells in culture or to induce cancer in animals. The word stems from the Greek "onkos," meaning a bulk or mass. Most oncogenes derive from genes whose products play a role in normal cellular growth-controlling pathways (2).

Cytokines in Human Reproduction, Edited by Joseph A. Hill
ISBN 0-471-35242-X Copyright © 2000 Wiley-Liss, Inc.

The first oncogenes were found as genetic material of oncogenic viruses that were capable of transforming normal fibroblast cell lines. Later, tumor DNA was found to have transforming characteristics. Among the many genes described as having oncogenic potential are HER-2/neu, myc, and ras. The overexpression of the oncogene HER-2/neu in ovarian cancer characterizes a group of patients with unfavorable tumor biology and a significantly worse prognosis (3). In addition, some proto-oncogenes such as the epidermal growth factor receptor (EGF-R) and the macrophage colony stimulating factor receptor (fms) are expressed along with their respective ligands in some gynecologic malignancies.

Either oncoproteins are mutant forms of the protein products of the corresponding proto-oncogenes, or products of an oncogene and its proto-oncogene are the same. The oncoprotein causes cancer either by being present where it normally is absent, or by being expressed at a level much higher than normal. In these cases, the mutation creating the oncogene changes transcriptional control rather than protein structure.

Her2-Neu

The HER-2/neu proto-oncogene, also known as c-erbB-2, neu, and HER2, is located on the long arm of chromosome 17 and encodes a 185 kDa transmembrane glycoprotein with intrinsic tyrosine kinase activity and similarity to the receptor for epidermal growth factor (3, 4). HER-2/neu protein overexpression occurs in gynecologic malignancies including those of the ovary, endometrium, fallopian tube, and cervix. Overexpression is secondary to gene amplification and/or overexpression of the HER-2/neu related p185 protein. No specific ligand has been identified yet. However, HER-2/neu has complex activation pathways and can form both homodimeric and heterodimeric associations with other related receptor proteins. Serum HER-2/neu levels may be used as a tumor marker in a subset of patients with tumors that overexpress the HER-2/neu receptor. Modulation of HER-2/neu overexpression is currently being studied as a novel therapeutic approach and includes the use of receptor antibodies, antisense DNA, antigen-activated cytotoxic lymphocytes, and adenovirus mediated E1A delivery to HER-2/neu overexpressing tumor cells.

Expression of HER2/neu. A number of groups have studied the expression of HER2/neu in gynecologic malignancies. It is difficult to compare these studies, because they differ in various aspects, including the origin and number of specimens studied, the methods used to determine HER2/neu and p185 expression, and the statistical analysis of that data. Although HER-2/neu, neu, and c-erbB-2 both describe the same proto-oncogene, the terminology chosen by the authors of the summarized original studies have been maintained in the following.

Overexpression of c-erb-B2 in ovarian cancer may be able to identify a group of patients with unfavorable tumor biology and a significantly worse prognosis. In a study by Meden et al., 51 of 275 ovarian cancer cases (19%) showed p185 overexpression dependent on the histological subtype (5). Correlation with tumor stage and the degree of histological differentiation was not observed. Patients with p185-positive tumors had a significantly worse prognosis with median survival of 20 months compared with 33 months for p185-negative tumors. p185 overexpression was iden-tified as an independent prognostically relevant factor in this study. The same group of investigators determined p185 in sera from 57 previously untreated ovarian cancer patients (6). The mean serum value for the normal controls was 1,203 human neu unit (HNU)/ml, with a range of 595–1,947 HNU/mL. The ovarian cancer patients showed serum levels ranging from 526 to 16,332 HNU/mL. Again, there was no association between serum oncoprotein levels and tumor stage, histological type, or grading. In a study by McKenzie et al., serum and tissue levels of HER-2/neu were correlated. El-evated serum levels (> 2050 HNU/mL) of circulating Her-2/neu determinants were detected in sera from 15% of 48 patients (7). Of 17 specimen with immunohisto-chemical Her-2/neu overexpression, serum neu levels were elevated in 5 (29%). Among the 28 patients with normal to moderate tissue expression of neu, only 2 (7%) had elevated serum neu levels.

Rubin found strong membrane staining for HER-2/neu in 25 specimen of 105 ovarian cancer patients (24%); the other tumor specimens showed weaker membrane staining or no immunoreactivity (8). There was no correlation of HER-2/neu expres-sion with any of a variety of clinical factors, including stage, grade, cell type, and residual tumor. Multivariate analysis showed that HER-2/neu overexpression con-ferred a marginal worsening of survival for the subgroup of patients with surgically confirmed tumor residual after chemotherapy. Excluding tumors of low malignant potential, Singleton et al. found c-erbB-2 oncogene overexpression in 10 of the 56 ovarian cancer specimen, but expression did not correlate with histological type, grade, stage, or prognosis (9). In 79 primary carcinomas analyzed by Tanner et al., 20% showed strong expression, 17% weak expression, 5% very weak expression, and 58% no expression of c-erb-B2 (10). Kaplan-Meier analysis revealed no significant association between strong expression of c-erbB-2 and survival. Only a subgroup of patients with stage III and IV disease with strong expression of c-erbB-2 showed a significantly shorter median survival time. Fluorescence in situ hybridization (FISH) was used to demonstrate moderate to high amplification of HER-2/neu in ovarian cancer cells in 10 of 43 samples by Young et al. (11). In some cells, the amplified HER2/neu was dispersed throughout the nucleus, whereas in other cells, clusters of oncogene amplification were observed.

The levels of p185 detected by immunohistochemistry are not necessarily related to the amplification of the HER-2/neu gene. In 75 samples of ovarian cancer studied by Morali, the erbB2 gene was amplified in only one case and a marked increase in erbB2 mRNA was found only in the same case (12). Staining for p185, however, was positive in 18.5% of all specimen. The staining was always confined to the cytoplasm except in the case that showed amplification of erbB2 in which p185 was localized in the membrane. It is possible that p185 protein had a longer half-life in the positive cases, this might explain the discrepancy between lack of gene amplification and pro-tein staining in this study.

In early ovarian cancer, HER-2/neu overexpression seems to occur only infre-quently, making it unlikely that such overexpression is an early event in ovarian car-cinogenesis. Gadducci et al. found positive immunostaining for p185 in primary ovarian cancer in none of 6 stage I, but in 23% of 22 stage III-IV tumors (13). Rubin et al. analyzed the expression of HER-2/neu on frozen tumor specimens from 40 patients with early epithelial ovarian cancer (14). HER-2/neu expression did not appear to be a strong prognostic marker in early epithelial ovarian cancer. No statistically significant relationship was found between HER-2/neu expression and survival, stage, or grade.

Expression of HER-2/neu does not seem to be correlated with clinical parameters in ovarian tumors of low malignant potential. Dean et al. studied 20 serous tumors of low malignant potential (STLMP) and 19 serous carcinomas in stages I and II (15). Two of four stage I STLMP in patients with disease progression showed positive staining for the gene product, whereas none of seven stage I nonprogressive STLMP showed positive staining. Five of the six stage III nonprogressive STLMP showed positive staining, whereas none of three stage III STLMP with clinical progression showed positive staining.

Interestingly, immunohistochemically detected HER-2/neu expression was found to occur more frequently in familial ovarian carcinomas than has been reported in sporadic ovarian carcinomas in a study by Auranen et al. (16). From a population-based study of 559 patients with epithelial ovarian carcinoma, Auranen identified 27 families with two or more ovarian carcinoma cases occurring in first-degree relatives. The percentage of aneuploid tumors was 46%, and that of HER-2/neu positive tumors was 69%.

Goff et al. studied a series of ovarian cancers for expression of multiple oncogenes (17). HER-2/neu was overexpressed in 7 cases (11%), EGF-R in 12 cases (19%), and Ki-67 and TNF-α in all but one case. Comparison by histological grade only revealed a significant correlation between EGF-R and histologically grade 3 tumors. No recognizable pattern of oncogene overexpression could be observed.

In 24 normal endometrial samples studied by Berchuck et al., light to moderate staining for HER-2/neu was seen in the glands, and there was no variation in staining intensity during the menstrual cycle (18). Among 95 endometrial adenocarcinomas, nine were found to have stronger staining for HER-2/neu when compared to the normal endometrium. High expression of HER-2/neu was significantly higher in patients with metastatic disease (27%) compared to patients with disease confined to the uterus (4%) (18). In 100 endometrial cancers examined by Kohlberger et al., the HER-2/neu oncoprotein was expressed in the tumors of 21 patients (19). HER-2/neu oncoprotein expression was associated with poor overall survival.

In 71 patients with surgical stage I endometrioid carcinoma studied by Nazeer et al., HER-2/neu expression was correlated with outcome independent of other factors (20). Saffari et al. found 47 of 90 (52%) endometrial cancers staining positive for HER-2/neu. HER-2/neu gene amplification was detected in 17 of 81 (21%) cases (21). Endometrial cancer with HER-2/neu gene amplification conferred a significantly shorter overall survival. Furthermore, tumors with moderate or strong HER-2/neu immunostaining were associated with a lower cumulative overall survival than tumors with low immunostaining. Determination of HER-2/neu by immunostaining in 100 primary endometrial cancers by Lukes et al. showed that HER-2/neu was predictive of the presence of persistent or recurrent disease by univariante but not in the multivariable analysis (22).

In a study by Wang et al., 22 of 34 patients (64.7%) with endometrial tumors had c-erbB-2 protein-positive and EGF-R-negative tumors, and eight (23.5%) had tumors positive for both proteins (23). Although immunostaining for c-erbB-2 protein was not correlated with the stage or grade of differentiation, the expression of EGF-R in addition to c-erbB-2 protein was more frequently observed with advanced stage of disease and was inversely correlated with the grade of differentiation and with the expression of estrogen and progesterone receptors on the tumor. An analysis of 247 patients with endometrial cancer by Hetzel identified overexpression of HER-2/neu as strong in 37 patients (15%), mild in 144 (58%), and none in 66 (27%) (24). The strong and the mild staining groups were distinct from the nonstaining group in predicting progression-free survival. Strong overexpression was associated with a poor overall survival.

Among 192 specimens from patients with stage III squamous cell carcinoma of the cervix treated with radiation therapy alone, Oka et al. found that 143 specimens were negative for c-erbB-2 oncoprotein, 12 were weakly positive or ambiguous, 31 were positive, and 6 were strongly positive (25). The 5-year survival rate of the 155 patients, who tested c-erbB-2 negative or weakly positive, was significantly better than that of the 37 patients with positive or strongly positive expression (61% versus 41%). In a study by Mitra et al., 14% of 50 primary, untreated squamous cell carcinomas of the uterine cervix were found to be c-erbB-2 positive (26). Amplification of c-erbB-2 ranged from 5 to 68 copies. In addition, two tumors with c-erbB-2 amplification showed additional restriction fragments, suggesting possible mutation or rearrangement of the gene.

In 44 cases of cervical adenocarcinoma studied by Kihana et al., the expression of c-erbB-2 protein was detected in 34 cases (77%) with strong expression on cell membranes in 11 cases (25%) associated with amplification of the c-erbB-2 gene (27). Expression of the protein on cell membranes was significantly more frequent in clinical stage II or III (9 of 23) than at stage 0 or 1 (2 of 21), and was associated with poorer prognosis. C-erb B-2 oncoprotein expression was observed in 42% of all cervical cancer specimen and increased significantly with stage progression in a study by Nakano et al. (28). The 5-year survival rates of c-erbB-2 positive patients and c-erbB-2 negative patients were 45% and 75%, respectively, indicating that c-erbB-2 positive patients showed significantly poorer survival.

Modulation of HER-2 neu Expression.

Modulation of HER-2 neu Expression.   Different approaches have been used to modulate the expression of HER-2/neu in vitro and in vivo. Downregulation of HER-2/neu in general seems to confer reduced tumorigenicity and has shown promising preclinical and clinical evidence for possible novel therapeutic approaches in various HER-2/neu overexpressing cancers.

Modulation of HER-2/neu expression by interferon-gamma (IFN-γ) might represent a mechanism by which IFNs inhibit cell proliferation. Studies by Doppler et al. and Marth et al. showed that IFN-γ mediated reduction in HER-2 expression in ovarian carcinoma cell lines (29, 30). Reduction of HER-2/neu was paralleled by decreased cell proliferation. Furthermore, IFN-α, -γ, -ω and all reduced HER-2 specific protein and RNA levels in ovarian carcinoma cell lines (31). Treatment with IFN-γ markedly enhanced the sensitivity of HER2/neu-overexpressing ovarian tumor cells to lysis by lymphokine activated killer cells (LAK) in a study by Fady et al. (32). Increased sensitivity to lysis was associated with an increase in effector–target conjugate formation, the induction of target cell intercellular adhesion molecule 1 (ICAM-1) expression, and the downregulation of HER2/neu expression.

An interesting observation was made by Gercel-Taylor and Taylor (33). The treatment of ovarian cancer cells with lipids derived from human ovarian cancer ascites produced increased cell proliferation that was correlated with increased cellular expression of the proto-oncogene product c-fos and c-erbB2 in all three ovarian tumor cell lines studied. When specific fatty acids were tested, 14:0, 16:1, and 18:1 were principally responsible for the observed enhancement of c-erbB2 levels, whereas the fatty acids 18:0 and 20:4 produced the greatest increase in c-fos expression. It is possible that ovarian cancer ascites contains a lipid based factor that may promote the loss of normal growth regulation.

The adenovirus 5 E1A gene product was found to suppress transformation and metastatic properties induced by mutation activated rat neu oncogene in mouse embryo fibroblast cells. Yu et al. introduced the E1A gene into the ovarian cancer cell line SKOV3.ip1, which overexpresses c-erbB-2/neu (34). E1A-expressing ovarian cancer cell lines had decreased c-erbB-2/neu-encoded p185 expression and reduced tumorigenicity in nu/nu mice. Xing et al. showed that the K1 mutant of the SV40 large T antigen inhibited human HER-2/neu promoter in human ovarian cancer cells (35). Treatment of ovarian tumor bearing mice using liposome mediated K1 gene transfer decreased the p185 protein level by K1 expression in these cancer cells and significantly prolonged mice survival.

MDX-210 is a bispecific antibody that recognizes both the Fc γ R1 on monocytes and macrophages as well as the cell surface product of the HER-2/neu oncogene. It has been used in a number of clinical trials to treat patients with HER-2/neu expressing tumors of the breast and ovary (36). Rodriguez used unconjugated monoclonal antibodies and an immunotoxin (TA-1-ricin) reactive with this HER-2/neu to inhibit cell proliferation significantly in several ovarian cancer cell lines (37). A single-chain antibody–exotoxin A fusion protein was shown to inhibit protein synthesis and elicit cytotoxicity in erbB-2 expressing tumor cells by Wels et al. (38). In athymic nude mice, administration of this fusion protein inhibited the growth of erbB-2-overexpressing human ovarian carcinoma cells.

Pietras et al. used a combination of anti HER-2/neu receptor antibody and cisplatin treatment of ovarian cancer cell lines demonstrating a synergistic decrease in cell growth (39). In addition, antibody mediated an increased sensitivity to cisplatin in drug-resistant ovarian carcinoma cells containing multiple copies of HER-2/neu gene. Therapy with antibodies to HER-2/neu receptor led to a 35% to 40% reduction in repair of cisplatin-DNA adducts after cisplatin exposure and promoted drug-induced killing in target cells. This phenomenon was termed receptor enhanced chemosensitivity.

Deshane et al. demonstrated that downregulation of erbB-2 expression is possible using an anti-erbB-2 single-chain immunoglobulin (sFv) gene to direct expression of intracellular anti-erbB-2 antibody (40). Transient expression of this gene in the human ovarian carcinoma cell line SKOV-3 resulted in complete downregulation of erbB-2 expression. The intracellular anti-erbB-2 antibody exerted a marked anti-neoplastic effect on the SKOV3 cell line resulting in an arrest of anchorage-independent growth. SKOV-3 cells transfected with the anti-erbB-2 antibody gene failed to grow into tumors in animals. Furthermore, the expression of erbB-2 in SKOV-3 cells could be downregulated in vivo by injecting tumor bearing mice with the anti-erbB-2 antibody gene attached to a DNA/polylysine complex for transfection of cells. The effectiveness of this novel approach to treat ovarian cancer patients with erbB-2 positive tumors is being investigated under a clinical protocol.

Glucocorticoid regulation of HER-2/neu expression was investigated using the SKOV-3 ovarian cancer cell line by Karlan et al. (41). Cells cultured in the presence of dexamethasone or hydrocortisone displayed a dose-dependent increase in HER-2/neu mRNA. Cells treated with actinomycin D showed prolongation of the half-life of existing HER-2/neu transcripts in the presence of dexamethasone. No concomitant increase in the p185HER-2/neu receptor protein in response to dexamethasone could be demonstrated by western blot or immunohistochemical analyses. Cellular proliferation was inhibited approximately 20% by the presence of dexamethasone. These data suggest that post-transcriptional regulatory mechanisms may play a role in modulating some of the biologic effects of the HER-2/neu oncogene.

Immune Responses to HER-2/neu. HER-2/neu has been shown to represent a target for immune effector cells, particularly cytotoxic T-lymphocytes (CTL). Targeting of HER-2/neu by T cells may prove useful for understanding the mechanisms of recognition, tolerance, and therapeutic use of human tumor reactive T cells. Ioannides et al. showed that CTLs, expanded from tumor associated lymphocytes with HER-2/neu positive ovarian tumors, can specifically recognize synthetic peptides corresponding to amino acids 971-980 of HER-2/neu protein (42). Fisk et al. showed that oligopeptides analogues of HER-2/neu isolated from a target area of T cells can induce an anti-tumor CTL response (43). CTLs, generated in the presence of these peptides in vitro, lysed HER-2/neu positive ovarian tumors but not natural killer target K562 cells.

Yoshino et al. found that ovarian cancer cell clones with high expression of HER-2/neu displayed a significantly higher sensitivity to CTL killing as compared with low expressing clones (44). Treatment of ovarian cancer cells with IFN-γ decreased the expression of HER2/neu but significantly increased the expression of HLA class I molecules. Interestingly, despite the increase in HLA class I molecules on the cell surface, CTL-mediated cytolysis of both the high and low HER-2/neu expressing ovarian cancer cell lines was significantly decreased. It is possible that the sensitivity of ovarian epithelial tumor cells to CTL-mediated lysis is associated with the level of HER2/neu expression.

Epidermal Growth Factor

Epidermal growth factor (EGF) was originally discovered in crude preparations of nerve growth factor prepared from mouse submaxillary glands. Human EGF was isolated from urine and based on its inhibitory effect on gastric secretion named urogastrone, accordingly (45). EGF belongs to a family of growth factors that are characterized by the presence of at least one EGF structural unit in their extracellular domain, defined by the presence of a conserved six cysteine motif that forms three disulfide bonds. EGF is initially synthesized as a 130 kDa precursor transmembrane protein containing nine EGF units (46). The membrane EGF precursor is capable of binding to the EGF receptor (EGF-R) and was reported to be biologically active. In vitro, EGF predominantly stimulates proliferation and differentiation of mesenchymal and epithelial cells. In vivo, EGF induces epithelial development, promotes angiogenesis, and inhibits gastric acid secretion.

Expression of EGF and EGF-R has not been demonstrated to have a significant impact on growth of ovarian cancer. Bauknecht et al. documented elevated levels of EGF and of EGF-like factors in crude cellular extracts of ovarian tumors compared to nonmalignant tissue (47). "Jennings et al found no significant differences in EGF-R expression in peritoneal biopies from gynecologic cancer patients compared to pentoneal biopies from patients with benign disease" (48). In 266 ovarian cancers, Meden et al. detected EGF-R in 13% and c-erbB-2 oncogene product p185 in 18% of primary tumors (4). EGF-R had no significant influence on survival time, whereas c-erbB-2 oncogene product p185 positive patients had a significantly worse prognosis compared to p185 negative cases. Ottensmeier et al. found no evidence for constitutive tyrosine phosphorylation of the p170 EGF-R in eight epithelial ovarian cancer cell lines tested, although each line demonstrated inducible phosphorylation in response to exogenous EGF (49). Media conditioned by five ovarian cancer cell lines, as well as malignant ascites obtained from 12 different ovarian cancer patients, were not capable of stimulating EGF-R phosphorylation. Finally, the proliferation of ovarian cancer cell lines was not significantly inhibited in the presence of neutralizing anti-EGF receptor antibody. Rodriguez et al. demonstrated the presence of EGF-R in normal ovarian epithelial cells and ovarian cancer cell lines (50). The number and affinity of receptors was similar in the normal epithelium and cancer cell lines, but there was no relationship between EGF-R number and responsiveness to EGF.

Recent data suggest that a signal through the EGF-R may be involved in regulating the CA 125 secretion from human ovarian carcinomas. Kurachi et al. demonstrated that pre-therapeutic serum CA 125 levels were significantly greater in patients with EGF-R-expressing carcinomas (51). Furthermore, TGF-α increased CA 125 secretion from an ovarian cancer cell line in vitro.

EGF-R expression was observed in one of eight cases with classical endometrioid adenocarcinoma, in 10 of 11 cases with endometrial adenocarcinoma and benign squamous metaplasia, and in 6 of 17 with adenosquamous carcinoma by Jasonni et al. (52). In mucinous and serous papillary adenocarcinoma, EGF-R immunostaining was not observed. EGF-R protein levels in 23 nonmalignant uteri ranged from undetectable to 50 fmol/mg membrane protein compared with EGF-R in 76 endometrial cancers ranging from undetectable to 7674 fmol/mg in a study by Sanfilippo et al. (53). In an analysis of 34 endometrial cancers by Wang et al., 22 (64.7%) had c-erbB-2 protein-positive and EGF-R-negative tumors, and 8 (23.5%) had tumors positive for both proteins (54). Expression of EGF-R in addition to c-erbB-2 protein was more frequently observed with advancing stage of disease and was inversely correlated with the grade of differentiation.

A number of studies suggest a significant paracrine role of EGF on proliferation of endometrial cancer cells. Malignant endometrial cells increased thymidine incorporation when incubated with EGF (+20.75%), TGF-α (+19.8%), or IGF-1 (+32.8%) compared to untreated control cells in a study by Reynolds et al. (55). In contrast, normal endometrial cells were inhibited by EGF (–24.9%), TGF-α (–25.6%), and IGF-1 (-31.9%). It is possible that endometrial cancer cells have lost responsiveness to factors that inhibit proliferation in normal endometrial cells. EGF-R was seen in all normal uteri and in 27 uteri with adenocarcinoma in a study by Zarcone et al. (56). It was absent in 11 patients with cancer. No correlation was found between the intensity of immunohistochemical staining and histological grade, depth of myometrial invasion, and clinical stage.

Kristensen et al. found overexpression of EGF-R in 25.8% of 132 cervical cancer specimen from patients with stage IB disease (57). The disease free survival was shorter for patients with tumors overexpressing EGF-R. In a multivariate analysis, EGF-R was found to be an independent prognostic factor. Kim et al. demonstrated overexpression of EGF-R in 29 of 40 (72.5%) invasive cervical cancers and in 5 of 20 (25%) CIN patients (58). In this study, the EGF-R levels in invasive cervical cancer were not correlated with clinical outcome.

Increased expression of EGF-R in vulvar malignancies seems to be correlated with lymph node metastasis and decreased patient survival. In a study by Johnson analyzing the expression of EGF-R in squamous vulvar malignancies, a significant increase in mean EGF-R levels was demonstrated in the primary tumor (67%) versus benign vulvar epithelium (31%) (59). The likelihood of lymph node metastasis was significantly elevated in those patients with a low tissue EGF-R level and in those patients with a primary tumor EGF-R level. Disease-free survival in those patients with high EGF-R levels in the primary tumor was 25%, contrasting with a disease-free survival of 54% in those patients with low EGF-R levels.

c-myc

Chromosomal translocations are common features of tumor cells and can be responsible for the overexpression of certain proto-oncogenes. For example, human Burkitt lymphomas and mouse plasmocytomas harbor a specific translocation involving the chromosomal bands of the c-myc proto-oncogene and the genes encoding immunoglobulin proteins (60). This chromosomal translocation places the regulation of c-myc expression under the influence of the immunoglobulin locus without altering the structure of the protein. Transgenic mice that express the c-myc gene under immunoglobulin control develop lymphomas.

Constitutive c-myc expression blocks the differentiation of murine erythroleukemia cells, which is consistent with the block in differentiation associated with many tumor cells (61). The transforming activity of c-myc derives from its ability to bind specifically to DNA and subsequently induce a set of cellular target genes (62).

The c-myc oncogene has been implicated in malignant progression in a variety of human tumors. In many instances, amplification and/or elevated expression of the c-myc gene have been associated with poor prognosis or decreased survival. In other cases, correlations have been demonstrated between c-myc activation and specific parameters of advanced neoplastic stage such as hormone independence or invasiveness (63). The tumor types exhibiting c-myc include breast, colon, small cell lung carcinoma, lymphomas, and ovarian and squamous cell carcinomas (64).

In 22 cases of ovarian cancer, amplification of c-myc was found in 54.5%, N-ras in 64.1%, and c-erb B in 31.8% in a study by Xin (65). Frequency of amplification of more than two of theses oncogenes at the same time was found in 40.9%. Relationships between the incidence of metastatic spread, microvessel density, and expression of proto-oncogene products were investigated in human ovarian carcinomas by Volm et al. (66). Ovarian carcinomas with a high microvessel density showed a significantly increased formation of metastases. Tumors with positive immunoreactivity of c-jun and c-myc products had a higher metastatic spread. A marginally significant correlation existed between the expression of erbB1 and metastatic spread. Five of 17 ovarian cancer tumor samples demonstrated amplification of the myc oncogene in a study by Baker et al. (67).

The increase in proliferation of the human ovarian cancer cell line NIH:OVCAR-3 after treatment with estradiol was paralleled by a fourfold increase in c-myc mRNA expression (68). Antisense oligonucleotide to c-myc specifically inhibited estrogen stimulated c-myc protein expression as well as the growth of NIH:OVCAR-3 cells. These results suggest that transcriptional induction of c-myc expression by estrogen plays a critical role in the proliferation of NIH:OVCAR-3 cells.

Overexpression of c-myc was seen in 6 of 12 leiomyomas, 11 of 23 leiomyosarcomas, and 9 of 9 malignant mixed mullerian tumors in a study by Jeffers et al. (69). There was no significant difference in mitotic rate or in survival between c-myc positive and negative cases of leiomyosarcoma. Overexpression of c-myc did not correlate with survival. Expression of c-myc mRNA was observed in all of 10 cases of endometrial carcinoma by Sato et al. (70).

Wu found c-myc to be overexpressed in 17 of 48 cases (35%) of cervical cancer (71). Relapse was observed in 7 of 15 cases (47%) with overexpression of c-myc, whereas relapse was observed in only 3 of 30 cases (10%) that did not overexpress c–myc. The 5-year survival rate was significantly lower in the cases overexpressing c-myc. No correlation between lymph node metastasis, cervical stromal invasion, and c–myc overexpression was found.

Seven of 9 cervical carcinomas exhibited elevated c-myb transcriptional activity in a study by Nurnberg et al. (72). In contrast to malignant cervical neoplasias, only 3 of 15 condylomata accuminata expressed a sparse signal for c-myb mRNA. The authors furthermore demonstrated that c-myb stimulated HPV-derived oncoprotein expression via transcriptional activation. In a study by Devictor et al., positive c-myc protein staining was observed in microinvasive cervical carcinomas in 70% and CIN 3 lesions in 19% (73). Varying levels of c-myc overexpression were observed in 12 of 23 cervical carcinomas (52%) by Cromme et al. (74).

Ras

The ras genes acquire transforming activity either by enhanced expression or by a single point mutation. A single base-pair mutation at specific sites within ras genes confers the capacity to transform certain cell lines in vitro (75). The predominant sites of K-ras mutations in ovarian tumors are at codons 12 and 13.

In 28 tissue specimens of human ovarian cancer examined by Chien and Chow, one specimen was found with a c-Ha-ras point mutation at codon 12, two had a c-Ki-ras mutation at codon 12, and one had a c-Ki-ras mutation at codon 13 (76). Ki-ras mutations were found in one of 20 ovarian cystadenomas, 6 of 20 low malignant potential tumors of the ovary, and one of 23 ovarian carcinomas by Teneriello et al. (77). All except one of the Ki-ras mutations identified were GGT to GAT transversions at codon 12. The presence of Ki-ras mutations was associated with advanced stage disease. In 35 patients with ovarian tumors studied by Fujimoto et al., five disclosed K-ras point mutations at codon 12 with transition from GGT to GAT in all cases (78). Only one case with K-ras oncogene amplification was found and no c-myc or erbB-2 amplification was detected. These mutations were mainly observed in early clinical disease stages, suggesting that mutations of K-ras may be an early event in the development of ovarian cancer.

In general, mucinous ovarian neoplasms display a higher incidence of K-ras mutations than serous ovarian tumors. Cuatrecasas et al. studied K-ras point mutations at codons 12 and 13 in 95 mucinous ovarian neoplasms (79). The overall frequency of codon 12/13 ras gene mutations was 68%. A higher incidence of K-ras mutations in mucinous tumors compared to serous ones was also observed in a series of 57 mucinous and 47 serous ovarian tumors by Ichikawa et al. (80). Mutations were detected in 4 of 30 mucinous adenomas (13%), in 4 of 12 mucinous tumors of borderline malignancy (33%), and in 7 of 15 mucinous carcinomas (46%). Only 1 of 17 serous carcinomas had a mutation of K-ras. All mutations identified were in codon 12. In a series of 37 ovarian tumors analyzed by Enomoto et al., the overall frequency of ras gene mutations was 27% (81). K-ras mutations occurred again more frequently in mucinous tumors (6 of 8) than in serous carcinomas (2 of 10) or in all nonmucinous types of epithelial ovarian tumors combined (3, 22). Mok et al. detected mutations of the K-ras proto-oncogene in 21 of 44 cases (48%) of borderline ovarian epithelial tumors, with 20 of the 21 mutations identified at codon 12 (82). Mutation of K-ras was detected at a higher frequency in mucinous borderline tumor (identified in 12 of 19 cases) compared to serous borderline tumor (identified in 9 of 25 cases). In a study by Fujita et al., K-ras mutations were found in 12 of 17 (71%) mucinous tumors and occurred more frequently than in serous carcinomas (4/31, 13%) or in all nonmucinous types of ovarian epithelial tumors combined (7/53, 13%) (83).

The frequency and intensity of ras p21 staining were observed to increase with the degree of malignancy in ovarian cancer patients in a study by Yaginuma et al. (84). There was no significant difference in ras p21 expression between early and late stages of ovarian tumors arising from the coelomic epithelium. With respect to prognosis, no differences were observed between the ras p21-positive and -negative ovarian tumors. Normal ovarian and ovarian cancer tissues from 35 patients were tested for LDH-A-ras protein complex formation, and for the expression of ras and LDH-A genes by Chow et al. (85). Elevated levels of c-Ki-ras and LDH-A mRNA transcripts were noted by northern blot analysis in 49% (17/35) and 40% (14/35) of ovarian cancers, respectively. Concurrent high expression of both genes was demonstrated in 11 cases (31%). Tyrosylphosphorylation of LDH-A was demonstrated in normal and malignant ovarian tissues, and the extent of phosphorylation correlated with the stage of ovarian cancer.

Scambia et al. studied the expression of p21/ras oncoprotein in a group of 14 normal and cystic ovaries, six benign tumors, 42 primary ovarian cancers, and 15 omental metastases (86). Levels of p21 were similar in normal and cystic ovaries and in benign tumors, whereas they were significantly higher in malignant tumors than in control tissues, and in omental metastases than in primary ovarian carcinomas. Estrogen and progesterone receptor-positive tumors expressed higher p21 levels than did estrogen and progesterone receptor-negative tumors. Survival in p21 positive tumors was significantly worse. Studies by Zachos et al. suggest that steroid hormone receptor binding could directly activate the H-ras oncogenic potency in human endometrial and ovarian lesions (87). This study reported increased binding of the glucocorticoid receptor to the H-ras GR element in more than 90% of endometrial tumors and in all ovarian tumors tested. The authors also found elevated binding of the estrogen receptor in the H-ras ER element in ovarian tumors compared to normal tissue.

C-Ki-ras activation appears to be an early oncogenic event in endometrial cancer, because it is homogeneously present in premalignant and malignant endometrial tissues. Duggan et al. identified c-Ki-ras mutations in nine of 60 (15%) endometrial cancer specimens (88). In eight tumors, c-Ki-ras mutations were uniformly present in the cancerous tissue. One tumor exhibited heterogeneous mutational activation, with mutant c-Ki-ras alleles detected in only grade 2 carcinoma cells but not grade 1 carcinoma cells. C-Ki-ras mutations were present in adjacent hyperplasia with atypia but absent from hyperplasia without atypia. Of 19 endometrial adenocarcinomas, point mutations in ras genes were found in seven tumors by Enomoto et al. (89). All mutations were localized in codon 12 and were predominantly found in tumors with a more aggressive histological pattern. In endometrial hyperplasia, K-ras mutations were found in 2 of 16 hyperplasias with atypia but not in adenomatous or in serous hyperplasias. C-Ki-ras mutations were detected in 24 of 110 (22%) endometrial adenocarcinoma cases in a study by Tsuda et al. (90). Mutations were more frequent in tumors associated with endometrial hyperplasia (11 of 20, 55%) than in those without hyperplasia (10 of 73, 14%). In addition, the frequency of mutations was significantly higher in tumors showing an infiltrative growth pattern accompanied by a stromal response consisting of edematous fibrous tissue (19 of 58, 33%), than in those which revealed an expansive growth pattern without such a stromal reaction (5 of 52, 10%).

In 112 carcinomas of the endometrium studied by Caduff et al., Ki-ras codon 12 mutations were observed in 13 (91). None of 17 papillary serous-clear cell carcinomas contained Ki-ras codon 12 mutations. Mizuuchi et al. reported mutations in codon 12 or 13 of K-ras in 6 of 49 cases (12.2%) of endometrial cancer (92). In this study, K-ras activation appeared to be an independent risk factor when compared by multivariate analysis with clinical stage, depth of myometrial invasion, and patient age. In 10 of 45 (22.2%) endometrial carcinomas studied by Fujimoto et al., K-ras point mutations were found at codon 12 (93). Transition from GGT to GAT was most frequent (41.7%). Double point mutations (GAT/GCT) were detected in two cases. The positive rate of lymph node metastasis tended to be higher in the group with positive mutations. In a series of 221 cases of endometrioid endometrial carcinoma, Ito et al. found that K-ras mutations were significantly associated with the presence of lymph node metastases (94). Furthermore, in the postmenopausal age group (>60 years), the presence of K-ras mutations was higher in patients who died or experienced recurrence (41.2% vs 13.0%).

Estrogen was found by Fujimoto et al. to increase c-Ha-ras expression and tyrosine kinase (TK) activity in uterine endometrial fibroblasts and the Ishikawa endometrial cancer cell line (95). In contrast, progesterone diminished c-Ha-ras expression and TK activity induced by estradiol in the fibroblasts, but not in Ishikawa cells, which persistently overexpressed c-Ha-ras.

The major peptide product of the c-ras oncogene is a 21 kDa peptide (p21), but other larger "ras-related" peptides have been described in urine obtained from patients with several types of cancers. Ras peptides were not detected in proliferative or secretory endometrium or in benign adenomatous hyperplasia in a study by Long et al. (96). In contrast, 95% of the grade 2 and 3 endometrial adenocarcinoma studied contained detectable ras peptides within neoplastic cells. In contrast to other studies, ras peptides were found within stromal cells of high-grade endometrial carcinomas.

Expression of p21 protein was investigated in 18 normal endometrial tissues and in 37 human primary endometrial carcinomas by Scambia et al. (97). In contrast to the described studies by Long, p21 levels were detected in normal endometrium and were significantly higher in secretory than in proliferative endometrium. However, primary endometrial carcinomas had a significantly higher p21 expression than normal proliferative tissues. Immunohistochemical analysis showed that most of the tumor cells expressed p21 oncoprotein whereas the stromal component was unreactive. Interestingly, estrogen receptor positive tumors expressed higher p21 levels than did ER-negative tumors (77% vs. 33%).

In 170 squamous cell carcinomas of the uterine cervix of different histologic types, overexpression of p21 was noted in 57.1% of keratinizing type and 54.2% of large cell nonkeratinizing type, but in only 38.7% of small cell type (98). Tenti found K-ras mutations in 15 of 88 cervical cancer specimens (99). Mutations were more frequent in mucin secreting than in nonmucin secreting tumors. Clinicopathological parameters of the disease and the overall survival were independent of K-ras mutations. Among 25 cervical adenocarcinomas studied by Jiko et al., c-Ki-ras gene mutations were detected in only 4% of cases (100).

Adenocarcinoma of the fallopian tube is a rare tumor with a poor prognosis. Few studies regarding the molecular pathogenesis of these tumors have been reported. In one study by Mizuuchi, K-ras point mutations were detected at codon 12 in seven of eight tumors (101). K-ras mutations occurred with high frequency in this series of eight patients with fallopian tube carcinoma, suggesting that mutations of this proto-oncogene could play an important role in the molecular pathogenesis of fallopian tube carcinoma.

Human Papilloma Virus

A large number of studies have investigated the pathophysiological mechanisms potentially involved in human papilloma viruses (HPV) associated in gynecologic malignancies. Most of these studies have concentrated on cervical cancer, where the prevalence of HPV infection is far greater than in other gynecologic cancers. The mechanisms by which the HPVs function in malignant progression appear to be related to the activity of the two viral oncoproteins E6 and E7, which form complexes with several cell proteins normally involved in controlling cell growth (102).

HPV in Cervical Cancer. Cervical cancer develops from well defined precursor lesions referred to as either cervical intraepithelial neoplasia (CIN) or squamous intraepithelial lesions (103). Specific types of HPV are now known to be the principal etiologic agents for both cervical cancer and its precursors. Chen et al. demonstrated that expression of oncogenic proteins of HPV-16 can cause tumor metastasis in nude mice (104). Although HPV-16 plays an important role regarding the progression of HPV-associated cervical cancers, the development of cervical cancer is a multistep process that cannot be explained simply by infection with specific types of HPV (103, 105). One additional event that appears to play a role in tumor progression is integration of HPV DNA into the host genome. Integration of HPV DNA frequently disrupts the E2 open reading frames, resulting in overexpression of the E6 and E7 oncoproteins, possibly causing genomic instability. Additional co-factors and mutational events may be important in the pathogenesis of invasive cervical cancers and may include chromosomal rearrangements, loss of constitutional heterozygosity, and proto-oncogene activation.

Approximately 90% of cervical cancers contain HPV DNA, particularly the HPV serotypes 16 and 18 (105). HPV persistence and the development of high-grade cervical intraepithelial neoplasia (HGSIL) were reported to be closely associated with HPV16 in a longitudinal study of 42 women by Londesborough et al. (106). 56% of HPV16 isolates were persistent compared to 7% of other HPV types, and all four subsequent CIN 3 lesions were found in women with persistent infection. Interestingly, 10 of 12 women with a variant of HPV16 bearing a base change at nucleotide 350 had persistent infection, compared to only 1 of 16 women infected with the HPV16 prototype. This observation indicates that certain variants within a HPV serotype might confer a higher risk of cervical epithelial cell transformation.

Different HPV serotypes may lead to predominance of certain histological changes in the cervical epithelium. In a study by Iwasawa et al., HPV DNA was detected in 324 of 352 squamous cell carcinomas (92%) and 81 of 108 adenocarcinomas (75%) (107). HPV 16 was detected in 78% of squamous cell carcinomas, but only in 17% of adenocarcinomas. In contrast, only 16% of squamous cell carcinomas but 56% of adenocarcinomas contained HPV18 DNA. In many cervical cancers, HPV-16 DNA genomes are found to be integrated into the host chromosome. Jeon et al. demonstrated that integration of HPV-16 DNA leads to increased steady-state levels of mRNAs encoding the viral oncogenes E6 and E7 (108).

The presence of HPV E6 mRNAs in peripheral blood of stage IVb cervical cancer patients with metastasis to distant organs was demonstrated in a study by Pao et al. (109). Thirteen of 15 (86.7%) cervical cancer tissues from the same number of patients were found to contain HPV type 16 DNA. Peripheral-blood specimens from 12 of 13 cervical HPV positive patients were found to contain HPV-specific mRNA detectable by reverse transcription and PCR. None of the cervical tissues from all 12 normal controls as well as peripheral blood specimens from two cervical HPV-negative cancer patients contained detectable amounts of HPV type 16 mRNA. HPV E6 mRNAs in peripheral blood may be a sensitive indicator of circulating cervical cancer cells with potential clinical applications in the treatment of cervical cancer.

Immune Responses to HPV. HPV infection stimulates humoral and cellular immune responses. Viscidi et al. detected serum antibodies to HPV-16 E6 and E7 proteins in cervical cancer patients in 56% and 43%, respectively, compared to 0.7% and 4.1% of controls (110). Antibodies to either protein were detected in 72% of sera from invasive cases and 5.8% of sera from controls. 37 newly diagnosed cervical cancer patients were studied for evidence of HPV infection by Fisher et al. (111). Elevated antibody titers to HPV 16 E6 and E7 were detected in 16.8% and 32.8% of the women, respectively. Although no difference across disease stage was detected for E6 antibody titers, increasing proportions of positivity to E7 antibody titers with stage of disease were detected.

Strickler et al. screened 59 women with LGSIL and 38 with high HGSIL for serologic markers of HPV infection (112). The combination of IgG to an epitope in the E6 protein of HPV 16 and IgA to HPV 16 virus-like particles (VLPs) was detected in 53% of LGSILs and 65% of HGSILs but only 9% of controls. Sera from 95 women with CIN, 95 age-matched female blood donors, and 155 children between 1 and 12 years of age were tested for levels of serum IgG to HPV peptides in a study by Marais et al. (113). In women with CIN, an increase in HPV-16 seropositivity suggested a possible role of antibodies against HPV-16 as an important marker of CIN in women over 40 years of age. Interestingly, children's sera antibodies were detected to HPV-16 in 44.5% and HPV-18 in 18.7%, indicating infection with either HPV-16 or a related virus. This observation might have important implications for the use of prophylactic vaccines against HPV infection that are theoretically most effective in preventing HPV infection.

CTL responses to HPV type 16 E6 and E7 proteins were measured in 20 women with HPV by Nakagawa et al. (114). CTL responses to E6 and E7 were detected in six of eight and five of nine HPV-16-positive women without CIN, respectively. Responses to E6 or E7 were each detected in only 2 of 7 HPV-16-positive women with CIN. The authors suggest that CTL responses may play a role in disease protection, because CTL responses to E6 or E7 were more commonly detected in HPV-16-positive women without CIN than in HPV-16-positive women with CIN. However, the number of study individuals was too small to reach statistical significance. Alexander et al. demonstrated that novel CTLs, capable of recognizing a HPV type 16 E7 epitope, can be generated by using peripheral blood mononuclear cells from irradiated patients with cervical cancer (115). In a study by Ressing et al., patients with HPV16 positive lesions were found to have memory CTLs against a HPV16 E7-encoded epitope (116). These data suggest that natural cellular immunity against HPV16 occurs in patients with cervical lesions.

Immunosuppression by HPV. Despite a number of studies demonstrating the immunogenicity of HPV related peptides, immune responses against HPV infection may also be suppressed with increased cervical epithelial changes. The production of cytokines that serve to enhance potentially protective cell mediated immunity may be defective in women with extended HPV infection.

Clerici et al. observed a pronounced shift from type 1 to type 2 cytokine responses in peripheral blood lymphocytes (PBLs) from patients with extensive HPV infection of the lower genital tract (117). The interleukin-2 (IL-2) response of PBLs in vitro to overlapping peptides from HPV-16 E6 and E7 oncoproteins was compared with the degree of cervical cytological abnormality among 140 women in a cross-sectional study by Tsukui et al. (118). Cytologically normal women had the highest rate of IL-2 production against HPV-16 peptides (35%). A decline of IL-2 production was observed with increasing disease severity from LGSIL (20% of normal controls), HGSIL (17%), and cancer patients (7%).

Proliferative T cell responses to peptides representing the HPV-16 E7 protein were measured using short-term T cell lines derived from peripheral blood by Luxton et al. (119). Proliferative T cell responses to both HPV-16 E7 and L1 were reduced in women with cervical carcinoma in comparison to responses in women with cervical dysplasia and from healthy controls. These observations may reflect downregulation of immune responses to HPV-16 E7 in women with cervical dysplasia and cervical carcinoma. Ellis et al. found in HLA-B7 individuals that a consistent variation in the HPV16 E6 oncoprotein sequence is capable of altering an HLA-B7 peptide binding epitope in a way likely to influence immune recognition by CTLs (120). These results illustrate a biologically relevant potential mechanism for escape from immune surveillance of HPV16 in HLA-B7 individuals.

HPV Vaccines. The presence and consistent expression of the genes encoding the HPV E6 and E7 proteins in the great majority of cervical cancers has led to the development of vaccines against HPV infection. Modified forms of the E6 and E7 proteins from HPV16 and HPV18 have, for example, been expressed in recombinant vaccinia virus. Studies in mice using recombinant virus for vaccination of animals showed induction of HPV-specific CTL responses (121). Alternatively, virus like particles (VLP) are attractive subunit vaccine candidates because they lack potentially oncogenic papilloma virus DNA and express the conformationally dependent epitopes necessary to induce high-titer neutralizing antibodies (122). VLP are highly favored as immunogens for human vaccine trials to prevent genital HPV infection. Another vaccine approach employed the TraT protein, known as ISCAR (immunostimulatory carrier), as carrier molecule for HPV E7 proteins. Immunization of animals with the ISCAR conjugate was able to elicit specific antibody and CTL responses that killed both E7 peptide-pulsed and whole E7 gene-transfected tumor target cells (123)

A live recombinant vaccinia virus expressing the E6 and E7 proteins of HPV 16 and 18, was used in a phase I/II trial in eight patients with late stage cervical cancer by Borysiewicz et al. (124). Vaccination resulted in no significant clinical side effects. All patients developed an antivaccinia antibody response and three of eight patients showed HPV-specific antibody responses due to the vaccination. HPV-specific CTLs were detected in one of three evaluated patients. Although the use of HPV vaccines might be useful in preventing or even treating cervical cancer, further studies are needed to optimize this strategy and to investigate the clinical efficacy of this approach.

Downregulation of HPV. Several investigators have attempted to block the expression of HPV proteins. Hamada et al. introduced an antisense transcript to HPV16 E6 and E7 RNA into HPV 16 positive cervical cancer cells using a recombinant adenoviral vector (125). The growth of the HPV antisense transfected cervical cancer cells was significantly suppressed and tumorigenicity in mice was completely abrogated. Inhibition of HPV related protein expression has also been accomplished using antisense oligonucleotides delivered by liposomes into cervical cancer cells (126). Other investigators have used hammerhead ribozymes to bind and cleave RNA transcripts derived from the E6 and E7 genes of human papillomavirus HPV-18. HPV RNA from the HeLa cervical cancer cell line was cleaved effectively by three different ribozymes used in a study by Chen et al. (127). Using antisense phosphorothioate oligonucleotides against the E6 and E7 proteins, Tan and Ting demonstrated growth inhibition of the cervical cell lines CaSki and SiHa. In nude mice, treatment with antisense oligonucleotides against E6 and E7 led to substantially smaller tumors (128).

HPV and Co-factors. Other factors that might act synergistically with HPV in the development of cervical cancer, have been investigated. Simons et al. studied cervical DNA adduct levels and the prevalence of HPV 16 in women with normal cervical cytology who had a history of smoking (129). No significant difference in smoking related DNA damage between HPV-positive and HPV-negative smokers could be detected. Chen et al. reported that herpes virus 6 (HHV-6) was capable of infecting human cervical epithelial cells and altering expression of HPV genes (130). HHV-6 infection of immortalized cervical epithelial cell lines showed enhanced expression of HPV RNAs encoding the viral oncoproteins E6 and E7. Cervical carcinoma cells infected with HHV-6 induced more rapid development of tumors in mice than did noninfected cells. It is possible that HHV-6 contains transactivation signals, which induce transcription of HPV transforming genes.

Jun/Fos

The jun genes (c-jun, jun-B, and jun-D) play a role in critical cell functions such as proliferation, differentiation, and apoptosis. Neyns documented expression of c-jun, jun-B, and jun-D in almost all 28 human ovarian cancer tissues tested (131). In cultured ovarian cancer cells, c-jun and jun-B expression was found to be inducible by serum. High jun-B expression relates to a more malignant phenotype both in vitro and in vivo. In contrast, the jun-D gene was suppressed in ovarian cancer cells compared to normal ovarian surface epithelial cells. Downregulation of jun-D might therefore be part of the malignant ovarian epithelial cell phenotype.

Analysis of EGF-R, TGF-α, c-myc, and c-jun expression in 33 stage III/IV and 2 stage I/II ovarian carcinomas showed a correlation between the mRNA and protein levels of EGF-R and TGF-α for tumors with low or high rates of expression (132).

High expression rates of EGF-R, TGF-α, and c-myc were detected in 6, 7, and 10 of 35 ovarian carcinomas, respectively. C-jun mRNA was detected in 18 of 19 cases studied.

Overexpression of cellular oncogenes c-fos and jun-B in the uterine endometrial epithelium may contribute to the molecular mechanism underlying the uterine toxicity associated with chronic tamoxifen treatment. In a study by Nephew et al., treatment of castrated rats with tamoxifen resulted in uterine luminal and glandular epithelial hypertrophy and basally located nuclei by 36 h (133). Expression of c-fos and jun-B messenger RNA was first detected in luminal and glandular epithelial cells at 12-36 h post tamoxifen injection persisted for 7 days.

Bcl-2

The presence of the bcl-2 protein, a marker for inhibition of programmed cell death, has been studied by a number of investigators. Uehara et al. examined 259 cervical squamous cell carcinoma specimens and found 85 (33%) positive for bcl-2 (134). No significant difference in survival at 5 years was noted between patients with negative (78%) and positive (82%) tumors. However, when bcl-2 positive tumors were divided into partially stained (62 of 85, 73%) and diffusely stained (23 of 85, 27%) groups, the patients with partial staining had a significantly better prognosis than those with diffuse or negative staining.

Harmsel Ter et al. found that bcl-2 was strongly expressed in the basal cell compartment of normal ectocervical squamous epithelium and in nearly all reserve cells, whereas in endocervical columnar cells it was only moderately expressed (135). In immature squamous metaplastic epithelium, bcl-2 expression varied. Bcl-2 could be detected in all premalignant lesions, showing a striking increase in the number of positive cells with increasing severity of CIN, in combination with a mild increase in staining intensity. All adenocarcinomas were positive ($n = 5$), whereas five of eight squamous cell carcinomas expressed bcl-2. The increase in bcl-2 expression in higher grades of CIN and invasive cancers might imply an increased protection of these neoplastic conditions against programmed cell death. This protection might facilitate the induction of genetic instability in dysplastic epithelial cells and confer the capacity of high grade CIN lesions to evolve into cervical carcinoma.

Nakamura et al. examined the expression of bcl-2 oncoprotein in the uterine cervix and endometrium (136). Endocervix with glandular dysplasia and endometrium with endometrial hyperplasia showed intense immunoreactivity for bcl-2 in 87.5% and 65.4%, respectively. Fewer than 30% of adenocarcinomas in these tissues had no or weak bcl-2 expression. Conversely, most of both squamous intraepithelial neoplasia and squamous cell carcinoma of the uterine cervix showed weak or no bcl-2 expression. These results suggest that upregulation of bcl-2 in premalignant lesions and downregulation after malignant change may be a mechanism more common in glandular uterine epithelium than in squamous epithelium. It is possible that bcl-2 plays an important role in the early stages of multistep carcinogenesis in glandular tissue, conferring a growth advantage for premalignant cells and allowing accumulation of gene abnormalities.

Observations made by Saegusa et al. support the role of bcl-2 in early cervical cancer development. Bcl-2 immunoreactivity was found in 17 of 46 (37%) CIN I/II, 48 of 75 (64%) CIN III, and 12 of 60 (20%) invasive squamous cervical cancers, providing evidence for the possible impact of bcl-2 on sequential cervical epithelial transformation (137). In a series by Tjalma et al., 48 of 76 (63%) cervical carcinomas were found to be bcl-2 positive (138). Bc1-2 immunoreactivity did not correlate with tumor histology, stage, presence of lymph node metastases, or involvement of the lymphovascular space. Interestingly, the 5 year survival rate for patients with bcl-2 negative tumors was 34% compared to 71% for patients with bcl-2 positive tumors. Bcl-2 expression and vascular permeation were independent predictors of overall survival in their study.

In another study by McCluggage et al., bcl-2 was found to be overexpressed in 9 of 33 cases of adenocarcinoma of the cervix (139). Frequent expression of bcl-2 proteins in cervical HPV associated epithelial lesions was described by Kurvinen et al., but was not useful for predicting clinical outcome (140).

Cyclins

Cyclin D1, a cell-cycle control gene, has recently been shown to be identical to an oncogene alternatively known as BCL-1 and PRAD1, which are implicated in lymphomas and parathyroid adenomas, respectively. PRAD1 complexes to the product of the retinoblastoma (Rb) tumor suppressor gene, an event followed by Rb inactivation.

Kurzrock et al. found abnormalities of PRAD1 in seven of 13 squamous cell lines of gynecologic origin (141). These abnormalities included amplification and rearrangement of DNA and overexpression of mRNA. The role of PRAD1 as a cell-cycle regulatory gene and its interactions with the Rb tumor suppressor gene suggests that PRAD1 deregulation may be a significant molecular event in the evolution of these tumors.

Homology between cyclin D1 and HPV E7 binding sites for the retinoblastoma tumor suppressor protein suggests that HPV oncoproteins, cyclin D1, and other cell cycle regulatory proteins may act through a common mechanism in the pathogenesis of human cervical squamous cell carcinoma. Nichols et al. examined 48 cases of cervical neoplasia for cyclin D1 protein expression (142). In normal squamous epithelium and LGSIL, constitutively low expression of cyclin D1 was observed. In situ hybridization demonstrated cyclin D1 mRNA overexpression in three of five cases of LGSIL, one of eight cases of HGSIL, 14 of 18 cases of invasive squamous cell carcinoma, two of five cases of adenocarcinoma in situ, one of seven cases of invasive adenocarcinoma, and two of five cases of small cell undifferentiated carcinoma. The authors of this study suggested a limited role for cyclin D1 protein in the pathogenesis of HPV-associated invasive cervical squamous carcinoma.

MDM2

The MDM2 oncogene, which forms an autoregulatory loop with the wild-type p53 protein, has been reported to be amplified in a high percentage of human sarcomas, thus abolishing the antiproliferative function of p53. Only a limited number of studies have described the role of MDM2 in gynecologic malignancies. Two missense point mutations, one nucleotide sequence polymorphism, and one amplification of the MDM2 gene were observed in 1 of 53 cervical cancer specimens examined by Ikenberg et al. (143). Amplification of the MDM2 gene was found in 2.8% of 179 ovarian tumors analyzed by Courjal et al. (144). Amplification occurred preferentially in stage 3 tumors and correlated with Erb-B-2 amplification. These findings suggest that MDM2 amplifications may represent a late event in ovarian cancer development.

Other Oncogenes

The MET oncogene encodes the receptor for hepatocyte growth factor/scatter factor, a unique growth factor that induces not only proliferation of epithelial cells, but also enhances cell motility and invasiveness. DNA level and expression of the Met/HGF receptor gene were examined in human ovary, benign ovarian tumors, and epithelial ovarian carcinomas (145). The Met/HGF receptor was detectable in the surface epithelium of normal ovary. The level of expression was unchanged in benign ovarian tumors of various origins. Fourteen of 67 malignant carcinomas (20%) showed a 3- to 10-fold increase in Met/HGF expression. In five additional cases, the Met/HGF protein was overexpressed 50-fold. Overexpressing tumors belonged to different histological variants, but had a well differentiated phenotype. Overexpression was associated clinically with disease and significantly correlated with premenopausal status of patients.

Eleven ovarian neoplasms including two benign tumors were analyzed for the amplification of fgfr4 and fgfr3 genes and for int2 and hst1 oncogenes (146). The fgfr4 gene was found to be amplified in two ovarian tumors. Amplification of hst1 was found in one benign ovarian tumor. Estimation of FGF-3 oncogene amplification in DNA samples extracted from paraffin embedded sections of 136 ovarian cancer samples was performed by Rosen et al. (147). A weakly positive correlation between preoperative CA 125 serum levels and the degree of amplification of the FGF-3 gene was reported. The association between clinical stage and FGF-3 copy number was statistically significant. However, no correlation was found between FGF-3 amplification and overall survival.

GROWTH FACTORS

A number of growth factors have been suggested to play a role in the development and growth of gynecologic tumors (148). Ascites fluid from ovarian cancer patients, for example, contains a variety of factors that confer mitogenic activity in vitro and in vivo for both primary cultures and established human ovarian cancer cell lines. These factors include tumor necrosis factor α (TNF-α), transforming growth factor α and ß (TGF-α, TGF-ß) epidermal growth factor (EGF), interleukin-1 (IL-1), granulocyte macrophage colony stimulating factor (GM-CSF), interleukin-6 (IL-6), and interleukin-10.

Cytokines are peptide molecules that share some specific characteristics. They mediate a variety of different biologic functions, depending on the target cell type or the maturational status of the target cell. They were originally divided into lymphokines (produced by lymphocytes), interleukins (produced by leukocytes), monokines (originating from monocytes), interferons, and colony stimulating factors. Cytokines are mainly involved in immunity and inflammation, are produced transiently and locally, are extremely potent, and interact with high-affinity cellular receptors. The cell-surface binding of cytokines by specific receptors ultimately leads to a change in the cellular proliferation and/or in the pattern of RNA and protein synthesis, resulting in altered cell behavior.

Interleukin-1

Interleukin-1 (IL-1) comprises several polypeptides with a wide range of biologic activities, including direct effects on several cells involved in immune responses (149). IL-1 plays important roles as a mediator of host innate and adaptive immune responses. In addition to its effects as a lymphocyte activating factor, IL-1 induces fever, is highly inflammatory, stimulates the production of acute-phase reactants, induces proliferative responses in a variety of tissues, and causes resorption of cartilage and bone (150). There are two defined forms of IL-1: IL-1-α and IL-1-ß. These molecules have similar biologic functions, but show only about 25% amino acid homology. The primary sources of IL-1 are monocytes and macrophages.

IL-1 has been found to be expressed in ovarian tumors (151). IL-1 can induce TNF expression in primary cultures of ovarian cancer cells (152). IL-1-α and IL-6 were found to enhance growth of cervical cancer cells in vitro by Castrilli et al. (153). In a study by Woodworth and Simpson, normal cervical cells constitutively secreted IL-1 α, IL-1 ß, IL-1 receptor antagonist, IL-6, IL-8, TNF-α, and GM-CSF (154). In contrast, four cervical cell lines immortalized by HPV DNAs and three carcinoma lines secreted selected lymphokines at significantly reduced levels. Kawakami found that the messenger RNA for IL-1 α was expressed in six and IL-1 ß in four out of eight ovarian cancer cell lines (155). Two cell lines secreted a high amount of IL-1 α, but none secreted IL-1 ß. The growth of these cells was significantly stimulated by the addition of recombinant IL-1 α. These cells expressed two classes of IL-1 binding receptors on their surface. The results indicate that IL-1 α is an autocrine growth stimulator for some ovarian cancer cells and suggest that IL-1 α plays an important role in the progression of this disease.

Interleukin-6

IL-6 is a 20 to 25 kDa pleiotropic factor that—among other effects—can induce B cell differentiation to immunoglobulin-secreting cells (156). It furthermore induces thymocyte proliferation and production of acute-phase reactants by hepatocytes. IL-6 has activity as a colony stimulating factor for hematopoietic progenitor cells (157). Interleukin-6 is produced primarily by activated monocytes and macrophages, although T and B cells can produce this lymphokine. Several types of tumor cells produce IL-6, and IL-6 has been proposed to act as an autocrine growth factor for different types of neoplasms.

Using a cutoff of 6 pg/mL based on a survey in normal healthy women, Scambia et al. found elevated levels of serum IL-6 in 53% of 45 patients with primary epithelial ovarian cancer and less frequently in patients with endometrial and cervical cancer (37% and 10%, respectively) (158). In cancer patients, increased IL-6 serum levels were related to the presence of the tumor, for all postoperative patients exhibited a marked decrease. In patients with advanced ovarian cancer, postoperative levels of IL-6 correlated with residual disease. Very high levels of IL-6 were observed in the ascitic fluid of nine ovarian cancer patients, but IL-6 mRNA was not detected in tumor cells. This suggests that the increased production of IL-6 observed in ovarian cancer is probably reactive and possibly a result of cytokine network responses.

In order to determine whether IL-6 can function as an autocrine growth factor, the endogenous production of IL-6 in 4 ovarian cancer cell lines was inhibited in vitro using antisense oligonucleotides by Watson et al. (159). Cells treated with IL-6 oligonucleotides showed reduced IL-6 production and an 80% to 85% decrease in proliferation. These data indicate that IL-6 is an important autocrine growth factor in ovarian cancer cells. Watson et al. found, furthermore, that the epithelial ovarian cancer cell lines CAOV-3, OVCAR-3, and SKOV-3 constitutively produced biologically active IL-6 (160). The addition of either exogenous IL-6 or antibodies to IL-6 did not affect the cellular proliferation of the cell lines. Significant levels of IL-6 were found in ascitic fluids of ovarian cancer patients and in the supernatants of primary cultures from freshly excised ovarian tumors. Lidor et al. demonstrated constitutive production of macrophage colony stimulating factor and IL-6 by human ovarian surface epithelial cells (161).

In another study by Ferdeghini et al., IL-6 was detected in 9% in sera of patients with benign uterine diseases, 11% of patients with CIN, 44% of patients with cervical cancer, and 11% of patients with endometrial cancer (162). In patients with cervical cancer, serum IL-6 levels > 3 pg/ml were found in 36% of 25 patients with stage Ib–IIa disease and in 64% of 11 patients with stage IIb–IV disease. In endometrial cancer patients, serum detectable IL-6 levels were observed in none of 30 patients with stage I–II disease and in 57% of 7 patients with stage III–IV disease.

IL-6 may play a role in the pathogenesis of carcinoma of the uterine cervix because its increased expression is associated with advanced neoplastic cervical lesions. Both IL-6 and its soluble receptor significantly stimulated growth of three immortal and four cervical carcinoma-derived cell lines analyzed in a study by Iglesias et al. (163). IL-6-mediated proliferation was accompanied by increased expression of RNAs encoding TGF-α and amphiregulin, two epidermal growth factor receptor ligands.

Tartour et al. demonstrated a significant increase in the expression of the IL-6 gene in invasive cervical carcinoma as compared to cervical intraepithelial neoplasia and normal cervix (164). Immunohistochemical analysis identified IL-6 protein only on stroma cells, which, based on morphological criteria, most likely belong to the macrophage lineage. This was reinforced by the correlation observed between IL-6 gene expression and macrophage tumor infiltration. No IL-6 immunostaining of cervical tumor cells was shown. In contrast to in vitro studies, the stromal origin of IL-6 suggests that this cytokine may modulate tumor cell proliferation by a paracrine rather than an autocrine mechanism.

Takano et al. found that four of eight well differentiated squamous cell carcinomas of the cervix secreted a large amount (> 1500 pg/48 h/10^6 cells) of IL-6 in nude mice (165). In contrast, poorly differentiated squamous cell carcinomas and all of the seven adenocarcinoma cell lines secreted a small amount (< 500 pg/48 h/10^6 cells of IL-6). About one-third of patients with squamous cell carcinomas had a raised serum IL-6 value.

Granulocyte Macrophage Colony Stimulating Factor

Granulocyte macrophage colony stimulating factor (GM-CSF) was initially characterized as a growth factor that can stimulate the growth of granulocyte macrophage progenitors (166). GM-CSF is also a growth factor for erythroid, megakaryocyte, and eosinophil progenitors (167). It is produced by a number of different cell types including activated T cells, B cells, macrophages, mast cells, endothelial cells, and fibroblasts in response to cytokine or immune and inflammatory stimuli. GM-CSF can also induce human endothelial cells to migrate and proliferate, as well as stimulate the proliferation of a number of tumor cell lines, including adenocarcinoma cell lines. GM-CSF exerts its biologic effects through binding to specific cell surface receptors. The high-affinity receptors, required for human GM-CSF signal transduction, have been shown to be heterodimers consisting of a GM-CSF-specific α chain and a common ß chain that is shared by the high-affinity receptors for IL-3 and IL-5. G-CSF showed no growth-stimulating effects in any of the four established ovarian cancer cell lines tested by Connor et al. (168). In five primary cultures treated with G-CSF, only one demonstrated statistically significant increases in growth in a dose-dependent manner. It is possible that G-CSF may act as growth factors in some but not all ovarian cancer cells.

Macrophage Colony Stimulating Factor

Human macrophage colony stimulating factor (M-CSF), was originally described as a factor that can stimulate the formation of macrophage colonies from bone marrow hematopoietic progenitor cells (169). M-CSF can be produced by, for example, fibroblasts, activated macrophages, or secretory epithelial cells of the endometrium. M-CSF effects include stimulation of macrophage proliferation and cytotoxic activity and regulation of release of cytokines and other inflammatory modulators from macrophages.

All four ovarian cancer cell lines studied by Suzuki et al. expressed mRNA for c-fms, the M-CSF receptor protein, whereas three secreted M-CSF into the culture medium (170). The exogenous administration of M-CSF caused no significant enhancement of cellular proliferation in any cell line. It is possible that the simultaneous production of M-CSF and c-fms by ovarian cancer cells represents an autocrine mechanism that may modulate cellular proliferation.

M-CSF and its receptor c-fms protein were found to be significantly overexpressed in endometrial cancers by Leiserowitz et al. (171). C-fms overexpression in endometrial cancer was positively correlated with abnormal DNA ploidy, high-grade lesions, and possibly extrauterine metastases. Ishikawa endometrial cancer cells expressed M-CSF and c-fms transcripts in a study by Takeda et al. (172). These cells are constitutively stimulated by M-CSF. Expression of a dominant negative, mutant c-fms gene in Ishikawa cells partially inhibited proliferation of these cells in vitro, suggesting that M-CSF/receptor regulation may be an important mechanism in endometrial cancer that aberrantly express M-CSF and fms genes.

Insulin-like Growth Factor

Insulin-like growth factor I and II (IGF) belong to the family of growth factors that are structurally homologous to proinsulin (173). Mature IGF-I and IGF-II share approximately 70% sequence identity. IGF-I is a potent mitogenic growth factor that among other functions mediates the growth-promoting activities of growth hormone postnatally. The biologic actions of IGFs are modulated by specific binding proteins (insulin growth factor binding proteins (IGFBP), which may either inhibit or enhance the effects of IGF at the cellular level. Two cell surface receptors have been identified: type I with structural similarities to the insulin receptor, and IGF receptor type II.

It is possible that the IGF/IGF-I receptor model represents another loop of autocrine growth regulation in ovarian cancer. Both IGF and IGF receptors are present in ovarian cancer tissue (174). Yun et al. found that IGF-II was significantly expressed in ovaries and ovarian cancers (175). Of 10 ovarian cancer cell lines studied by Yee et al., three expressed IGF-I mRNA (176). RNA extracted from primary and metastatic ovarian cancer tissues also expressed IGF-I mRNAs. Type I IGF receptor mRNA was found in all 10 ovarian cancer cell lines and all seven primary or metastatic ovarian cancer tissues. IGF-I was found to be a mitogen for OVCAR-3, demonstrating the presence of a functional type IGF-I/ IGF-I receptor mediated autocrine loop expressed by ovarian cancer cells.

The IGF system is thought to function as a mediator of steroid hormone actions in the endometrium. In the endometrium, IGFBP-1 gene expression is stimulated by progesterone and inhibited by insulin, whereas IGFBP-1 inhibits the mitogenic action of IGF-I. In endometrial cancer tissues, IGFBP-1 mRNA was undetectable or minimally expressed when studied by RT-PCR (177). The mean levels of IGFBP-2 and IGFBP-4,and IGFBP-5 mRNAs in endometrial cancer tissues did not differ from those in normal endometrium, in which no cyclic variation was observed, suggesting that the genes encoding IGFBP-2, IGFBP-4, and IGFBP-5 are not hormonally regulated in the endometrium. It is possible that continuous stimulation of the endometrial epithelial cells by IGFs with suppressed IGFBP-1 expression may lead to an imbalance in the IGF system of the endometrium and trigger an uncontrolled cell proliferation, ultimately resulting in malignant transformation.

Transforming Growth Factor α

Transforming growth factor α (TGF-α) is a member of the EGF family of cytokines. The soluble forms of these cytokines are released from the transmembrane protein by proteolytic cleavage. Membrane bound proTGF-α is biologically active and plays a role in mediation of cell adhesion and in paracrine stimulation of adjacent cells. Expression of TGF-α is found in a variety of tumor cell lines, but also in normal tissues during embryogenesis and in adult tissues, including pituitary, brain, keratinocytes, and macrophages. TGF-α binds to the EGF receptor and activates the receptor tyrosine kinase. It shows a similar potency to EGF as a mitogen for fibroblasts and acts as an inducer of epithelial development and angiogenesis in vivo.

TGF-α may represent an autocrine growth factor for cell lines derived from ovarian cancers of epithelial origin. All 17 ovarian cancer cell lines examined by Stromberg et al. expressed the EGF-R and 16 cell lines concomitantly secreted TGF-α (178). The growth of eight ovarian cell lines was stimulated in a dose-dependent manner when grown in the presence of exogenous TGF-α. Growth in four of five cell lines capable of serumfree propagation was inhibited from 28% to 56% when cultured in medium containing a TGF-α-neutralizing monoclonal antibody. Zhou and Leung showed that EGF/TGF-α stimulated cell growth and DNA synthesis in the human ovarian cancer cell line OVCAR-3, but inhibited cell proliferation and DNA synthesis in CAOV-3 cells (179). TGF-ß 1 invariably inhibited cell proliferation and DNA synthesis in both cell lines. Both cell lines expressed TGF-α, TGF-ß 1, and EGF receptors.

Transforming Growth Factor ß

Transforming growth factor ß (TGF-ß) is a multifunctional polypeptide growth factor (180). Specific TGF-ß receptors have been found on almost all mammalian cell types. Although the effects of TGF-ß vary according to the cell line and in vitro conditions, it is generally stimulatory for cells of mesenchymal origin and inhibitory for cells of epithelial or neuroectodermal origin (181). A number of more closely related proteins exist that are designated TGF-ß 1, TGF-ß 1.2, TGF-ß 2, TGF-ß 3, TGF-ß 4, and TGF-ß 5. TGF-ß 1 and TGF-ß 2 have been found in the highest concentration in human platelets and mammalian bone, but are produced by many cell types in smaller amounts. TGF-ß 1, TGF-ß 2, and TGF-ß 1.2 have similar biologic activities, although differences in binding to certain types of receptors and differential responses to TGF-ß 1 and TGF-ß 2 have been reported.

Henriksen et al. examined tissue samples of normal ovary and benign as well as malignant ovarian neoplasms for expression of the different TGF-ß isoforms, the latent TGF-ß binding protein (LTBP), TGF-ß type I (TGF-ß R-II) receptors, and endoglin by immunohistochemistry and in situ hybridization (182). Expression of all ligands was significantly increased in tumor cells compared with the normal epithelial cells. In contrast, LTBP immunoreactivity was detected significantly more often in normal epithelium than in tumor cells. In the blood vessels of malignant tumors, significantly increased TGF-ß 1 reactivity and decreased TGF-ß 2 reactivity were found when compared to those of normal ovaries and benign tumors. Patients with malignant tumors expressing TGF-ß 1, TGF-ß R-I, or endoglin in blood vessels demonstrated longer survival than those having negatively stained tumors. In contrast, positive endoglin staining in tumor cells correlated with decreased survival even in advanced disease or in patients with residual tumor bulk after surgery.

It is possible that loss of the TGF-ß pathway may play a role in the development of some ovarian cancers. Berchuck et al. found that proliferation of normal ovarian epithelial cells was inhibited by TGF-ß (> 40%) (183). Among the ovarian cancer cell lines, proliferation of one was markedly inhibited (> 95%), two were only modestly inhibited (< 20%), and two were unaffected. In addition, all of the normal ovarian epithelial cells and four of five ovarian cancer cell lines produced TGF-ß. TGF-ß significantly inhibited proliferation in 19 of 20 ovarian cancer cell cultures obtained from ascites as demonstrated by Hurteau et al. (184). Among five immortalized ovarian cancer cell lines, only one cell line was markedly growth inhibited by TGF-ß and showed DNA fragmentation characteristic of apoptosis in a study by Havrilesky et al. (185). TGF-ß inhibited growth of all 10 primary ovarian cancers, but only 3 of 10 were found to undergo apoptosis when treated with TGF-ß.

The influence of TGF-ß and EGF on the endometrial cancer cell line HEC-1-A was investigated by Bergman et al. (186). EGF-stimulated proliferation was inhibited by TGF-ß in a dose- and time-dependent manner. TGF-ß also reversibly decreased EGF-induced c-fos mRNA expression in a dose- and time-dependent manner. These results show that TGF-ß negatively modulates EGF-induced c-fos expression, which may be related to the observed inhibition of carcinoma cell proliferation.

Loss of responsiveness to TGF-ß 1 or loss of TGF-ß 1 production may also be important in the progression of CIN to invasive cervical carcinoma. Comerci et al. found 100% positive staining for the intracellular form of TGF-ß 1 in normal cervical epithelium (187). In CIN, TGF-ß 1 was positive in 73.3%, and invasive carcinomas stained positive in only 44.1%. In contrast, percent positive staining for the extracellular form of TGF-ß 1 was 63.6% for stroma underlying normal epithelium, 60% for stroma associated with CIN, and 94.1% for stroma surrounding invasive cancer. These findings indicate that tumor progression in cervical cancer may be indirectly promoted by TGF-ß 1 secreted into or produced by supporting stromal elements.

Tumor Necrosis Factor α

Tumor necrosis factor α (TNF-α) and TNF-ß are two related proteins that bind to the same cell surface receptors (TNF RI and TNF RII) and produce a variety of similar effects (188). An important effect is the ability to kill certain tumor cells directly (189). TNF is expressed in activated T and B lymphocytes. In addition to its cytotoxic action on tumor cells, TNF has been shown to be a mediator of inflammation and autoimmune function (190).

Gotlieb et al. found that TNF-α induced a significant upregulation of p53 mRNA levels in ovarian cancer cells grown in nude mice and in vitro (191). The maximum level of induction was 8 h, and the upregulation of p53 was dose-dependent. In addition, TNF-α induced a dose-dependent increase in DNA fragmentation. In studies by Wu et al., TNF-α was found to stimulate the proliferation of OVCA 432 cells (152). Furthermore, IL-1 was able to increase the endogenous production of TNF-α and thus indirectly stimulate tumor growth via an autocrine pathway. When the production of TNF-α in OVCA 432 cells was inhibited using antisense technology, the IL-1-induced endogenous expression of TNF-α was significantly downregulated and the described growth stimulation by IL-1 was abrogated. This study shows that strategies to block TNF-α production might provide a therapeutic approach in ovarian cancer patients with tumors found to be growth stimulated by TNF-α.

Interferon

The interferons IFN-α, IFN-ß, and IFN-γ interfere with viral production. These factors have a variety of effects on the immune system and direct antitumor effects (192). For example, IFN-γ is a T cell–produced lymphokine with direct effects on immune function. IFN-γ is a potent inducer of the expression of MHC Class II molecules on monocytes and macrophages (193). Because of this activity, it has been implicated as an important factor in enhancing the activity of antigen-presenting cells. IFN-γ acts as a positive feedback signal for T cell activation and effects on B cell activation and differentiation.

Pao et al. found significantly reduced transcription of the IFN-γ gene in CIN and cervical cancer tissue as compared to normal cervix (194). There was no change of IL-1 α, IL-6, and TNF-α gene expression in either CIN or cervical cancer tissues. IFN-γ decreased proliferation of four ovarian cancer cell lines by 30% to 40%, whereas EGF-R expression was upregulated by IFN-γ as shown by Boente et al. (195). In contrast, IFN-γ treatment of normal ovarian epithelial cells affected neither proliferation nor EGF-R levels.

Fibroblast Growth Factor

Basic fibroblast growth factor (bFGF) has both angiogenic and mitogenic activity and has been found in a variety of other neoplasms. Ovarian cancer cell lines are capable of producing bFGF as well as other members of the FGF family of genes and have the ability to respond to bFGF (196). Addition of bFGF to three ovarian cancer cell lines resulted in a statistically significant increase in cell number. Immunohistochemical staining for bFGF demonstrated a cytoplasmic distribution of bFGF in the three cell lines. Both high- and low-affinity binding sites for human recombinant bFGF were expressed by all three lines. Di Blasio et al. showed that a bFGF-like protein was present in seven ovarian epithelial neoplasms and in primary cultures of dispersed ovarian cancer cells (197).

The expression of acidic FGF-1 and basic FGF-2 was found to increase with dedifferentiation, myometrial invasion, and staging in endometrial cancers (198). Endometrial cancers might mainly secrete FGF-1 and -2, which leads to neovascularization and subsequently accelerated growth, invasion, and metastasis. Sliutz et al. examined 105 serum samples from 20 patients with cervical cancer for levels of bFGF (199). Basic FGF reached a sensitivity of 65.7% at a specificity of 91.5% when applying a cutoff level of 15 pg/mL. A continuous increase of bFGF serum levels before the clinical detection of relapse was seen in two cases with a mean time of 4 months. Preoperative serum levels were not of prognostic value and showed no correlation with pelvic lymph node metastasis. These data suggest that in cervical cancer patients, soluble bFGF may be useful in early detection of primary tumors, recurrences, and monitoring of therapy. The levels of bFGF and its mRNA were significantly higher in advanced uterine cancers in a study by Fujimoto (200).

Steroid Hormones and Growth Factors

Steroid hormones can regulate the expression of the transforming growth factors and epidermal growth factor receptors in endometrial cancer cells in culture. It is also possible to demonstrate that these growth factors function in an autocrine fashion to regulate proliferation of, for example, endometrial cancer cells in vitro. Constitutive expression or overexpression of such factors and their receptors may be important in the growth progression of endometrial neoplasia. For example, the presence of a direct extrapituitary action of gonadotropin-releasing hormone (GnRH) via specific receptors in endometrial cancer has been suggested as an explanation for the therapeutic effect of GnRH analogue in recurrent disease. GnRH mRNA transcripts were detected in two endometrial cancer cell lines, a choriocarcinoma cell line, and tissues from endometrium and placenta by Chatzaki et al. (201). However, secretion of immunoreactive GnRH could be detected by RIA in only 1 of 10 endometrial cancer tissues in primary culture, and in none of the cell lines. Furthermore, no high-affinity GnRH binding sites could be found in either endometrial cancer cell lines or tissue.

VEGF

Angiogenesis, the induction of new capillaries and venules, has been associated with tumor growth. Increased tumor size and new vessel growth may enhance the capability of tumor cells to enter the circulation and potentiate metastatic disease.

Twenty-nine of 66 ovarian cancer tumor samples were found to overexpress VEGF in a study by Paley et al. (202). Median disease free survival for the VEGF positive group was 22 months, compared with >108 months for the VEGF negative group. In a multivariate analysis, only elevated VEGF expression was associated with poorer survival. mRNA encoding VEGF was detected in all ovarian and endometrial cancers studied by Doldi et al. (203). VEGF was more densely expressed in endometrial carcinoma. VEGF expression was also identified in cells obtained from ovarian and endometrial ascitic fluid.

Evidence for increased vascularity in squamous cell carcinoma specimen of the cervix was found by Wiggins et al. (204). Microvessel counts in patients with squamous cell carcinoma were significantly different from those of control. Furthermore, microvessel count was significantly correlated with vascular space involvement. Microvessel density was also significantly correlated with levels of VEGF in a series of vulvar intraepithelial neoplasia (VIN) studied by Bancher-Todesca et al. (205). For both microvessel density and VEGF expression, the differences between VIN I and VIN III and between VIN II and VIN III were statistically significant. Guidi et al. evaluated 66 cervical biopsy specimens for expression of VEGF (206). VEGF mRNA expression, epithelial-stromal vascular cuffing, and microvessel density counts were significantly increased in invasive carcinoma and in HGSIL lesions as compared with LGSIL and benign squamous epithelium.

Expression of VEGF was detected in all tissues of human vulvar neoplastic and nonneoplastic tissues in a study by Chopra et al. (207). VEGF mRNA was highly expressed in VIN associated with HPV infection and minimally expressed in invasive squamous cells carcinoma of the vulva. Nonneoplastic lesions, such as chronic inflammation, lichen sclerosus, lichen planus, squamous hyperplasia, and squamous papilloma showed no significant differences in VEGF mRNA expression.

Vascular permeability factor (VPF), also known as vascular endothelial growth factor, is a homodimeric glycoprotein that acts on vascular endothelium as a potent permeability inducing agent and mitogen. Abundant levels of VPF have been identified by an immunoassay in the ascites of patients with epithelial ovarian cancer (208). Olson et al. identified the malignant epithelium as one source of VPF in the ascites of ovarian tumor patients (209). The two secreted isoforms, VPF121 and VPF165, were found to be expressed in normal and neoplastic ovaries. VPF may be an important mediator of ascites formation and tumor metastasis observed in neoplastic conditions of the ovary.

Platelet Derived Growth Factor

Platelet derived growth factor (PDGF) is a megakaryocyte derived polypeptide growth factor. It stimulates proliferation of both epithelial and endothelial cells in an autocrine fashion (210). The growth factor has three isoforms and binds to two defined receptors (termed PDGFRα and PDGFRß) (211). PDGF expression is common (70% to 100%) in ovarian cancer tissue and in cell lines, but undetectable in normal ovarian tissue (212). Berchuck et al. failed to demonstrate that exogenous PDGF stimulates proliferation of ovarian cancer cells, consistent with the lack of expression of PDGF (213). It is possible that PDGF has a paracrine effect in ovarian tumors, for example, mediating connective tissue stroma formation (214). PDGF and its receptors have been identified in the endometrium. Sources of PDGF include macrophages and platelets at sites of ectopic endometrial growth. All isoforms of PDGF tested were potent mitogens for two endometrial epithelial cell lines in a study by Munson et al. (215).

SUMMARY

A large variety of oncogenes and growth factors that influence the growth of gynecologic cancers in vitro and in vivo have been identified in the last decade. Increased knowledge about the oncogenic pathways will provide new diagnostic and therapeutic approaches. However, an unknown array of pathways important for malignant transformation still must be identified to account for the complexity of malignant cell growth. It also remains to be determined which alterations of oncogene and growth factor expression are most important in different malignancies. The development of novel molecular techniques such as gene transfer will make the application in patients feasible. Undergoing efforts in gene therapy for cancer will define the parameters for in vitro and in vivo gene manipulation either to block the suppression of oncogenes and growth factors or to redirect the immune system against the cancer disease.

REFERENCES

1. Berchuck A, Kohler MF, Bast RC Jr. Oncogenes in ovarian cancer. Hematol Oncol Clin North Am 1992;(4):813–827.

2. Varmus H. Oncogenes and the Molecular Origins of Cancer. New York: Cold Spring Harbor Press, 1989:3–44.

3. Meden H, Kuhn W. Overexpression of the oncogene c-erbB-2 (HER2/neu) in ovarian cancer: a new prognostic factor. Eur J Obstet Gynecol Reprod Biol 1997;71(2):173–179.

4. Meden H, Marx D, Raab T, Kron M, Schauer A, Kuhn W. EGF-R and overexpression of the oncogene c-erbB-2 in ovarian cancer: immunohistochemical findings and prognostic value. J Obstet Gynaecol 1995;21(2):167–178.

5. Meden H, Marx D, Rath W, Kron M, Fattahi-Meibodi A, Hinney B, Kuhn W, Schauer A. Overexpression of the oncogene c-erb B2 in primary ovarian cancer: evaluation of the prognostic value in a Cox proportional hazards multiple regression. Int J Gynecol Pathol 1994;Jan;13(1):45–53.

6. Meden H, Marx D, Fattahi A, Rath W, Kron M, Wuttke W, Schauer A, Kuhn W. Elevated serum levels of a c-erbB-2 oncogene product in ovarian cancer patients and in pregnancy. J Cancer Res Clin Oncol 1994;120(6):378–381.

7. McKenzie SJ, DeSombre KA, Bast BS, Hollis DR, Whitaker RS, Berchuck A, Boyer CM, Bast RC Jr. Serum levels of HER-2 neu (C-erbB-2) correlate with overexpression of p185neu in human ovarian cancer. Cancer 1993;71(12):3942–3946.

8. Rubin SC, Finstad CL, Wong GY, Almadrones L, Plante M, Lloyd KO. Prognostic significance of HER-2/neu expression in advanced epithelial ovarian cancer: a multivariate analysis. Am J Obstet Gynecol 1993;168(1 Pt 1):162–169.

9. Singleton TP, Perrone T, Oakley G, Niehans GA, Carson L, Cha SS, Strickler JG. Activation of c-erbB-2 and prognosis in ovarian carcinoma. Cancer 1994;73(5):1460–1466.

10. Tanner B, Kreutz E, Weikel W, Meinert R, Oesch F, Knapstein PG, Becker R. Prognostic significance of c-erB-2 mRNA in ovarian carcinoma. Gynecol Oncol 1996;62(2):268–277.

11. Young SR, Liu WH, Brock JA, Smith ST. ERBB2 and chromosome 17 centromere studies of ovarian cancer by fluorescence in situ hybridization. Genes Chromosomes Cancer 1996;16(2):130–137.

12. Morali F, Cattabeni M, Tagliabue E, Campiglio M, Menard S, Marzola M, Lucchini V, Colombo N, Mangioni C, Redaelli L. Overexpression of p185 is not related to erbB2 amplification in ovarian cancer. Ann Oncol 1993;4(9):775–799.

13. Gadducci A, Ciancia EM, Campani D, Malagnino G, De Luca F, Facchini V, Pingitore R, Fioretti P. Immunohistochemical detection of p185 product, p21 product, and proliferating cell nuclear antigen (PCNA) in formalin-fixed, paraffin-embedded tissues from ovarian carcinomas. Preliminary data. Eur J Gynaecol Oncol 1994;15(5):359–368.

14. Rubin SC, Finstad CL, Federici MG, Scheiner L, Lloyd KO, Hoskins WJ. Prevalence and significance of HER-2/neu expression in early epithelial ovarian cancer. Cancer 1994;73(5):1456–1459.

15. Dean CJ, Allan S, Eccles S, McFarlane C, Styles J, Valeri M, Sandle J, Bakir A, Sacks N. The product of the c-erbB-2 proto-oncogene as a target for diagnosis and therapy in breast cancer. Cancer 1992;70(12):2857–2860.

16. Auranen A, Grenman S, Kleml PJ. Immunohistochemically detected p53 and HER-2/neu expression and nuclear DNA content in familial epithelial ovarian carcinomas. Cancer 1997;79(11):2147–2153.

17. Goff BA, Shy K, Greer BE, Muntz HG, Skelly M, Gown AM. Overexpression and relationships of HER-2/neu, epidermal growth factor receptor, p53, Ki-67, and tumor necrosis factor alpha in epithelial ovarian cancer. Eur J Gynaecol Oncol 1996;17(6):487–492.

18. Berchuck A, Rodriguez G, Kinney RB, Soper JT, Dodge RK, Clarke-Pearson DL, Bast RC, Jr. Overexpression of HER-2/neu in endometrial cancer is associated with advanced stage disease. Am J Obstet Gynecol 1991;164(1)15–21.

19. Kohlberger P, Loesch A, Koelbl H, Breitenecker G, Kainz C, Gitsch G. Prognostic value of immunohistochemically detected HER-2/neu oncoprotein in endometrial cancer. Cancer Lett 1996;98(2):151–155.

20. Nazeer T, Ballouk F, Malfetano JH, Figge H, Ambros RA. Multivariate survival analysis of clinicopathologic features in surgical stage I endometrioid carcinoma including analysis of HER-2/neu expression. Am J Obstet Gynecol 1995;173(6):1829–1834.

21. Saffari B, Jones LA, el-Naggar A, Felix JC, George J, Press MF. Amplification and overexpression of HER-2/neu (c-erbB2) in endometrial cancers: correlation with overall survival. Cancer Res 1995;55(23):5693–5698.

22. Lukes AS, Kohler MF, Pieper CF, Kerns BJ, Bentley R, Rodriguez GC, Soper JT, Clarke-Pearson DL, Bast RC Jr, Berchuck A. Multivariable analysis of DNA ploidy, p53, and HER-2/neu as prognostic factors in endometrial cancer. Cancer 1994;73(9):2380–2385.

23. Wang D, Konishi I, Koshiyama M, Mandai M, Nanbu Y, Ishikawa Y, Mori T, Fujii S. Expression of c-erbB-2 protein and epidermal growth receptor in endometrial carcinomas. Correlation with clinicopathologic and sex steroid receptor status. Cancer 1993;72(9):2628–2637.

24. Hetzel DJ, Wilson TO, Keeney GL, Roche PC, Cha SS, Podratz. HER-2/neu expression: a major prognostic factor in endometrial cancer. Gynecol Oncol 1992;47(2):179–185.

25. Oka K, Nakano T, Arai T. c-erbB-2 Oncoprotein expression is associated with poor prognosis in squamous cell carcinoma of the cervix. Cancer 1994;73(3):664–671.

26. Mitra AB, Murty VV, Pratap M, Sodhani P, Chaganti RS. ERBB2 (HER2/neu) oncogene is frequently amplified in squamous cell carcinoma of the uterine cervix. Cancer Res 1994;54(3):637–639.

27. Kihana T, Tsuda H, Teshima S, Nomoto K, Tsugane S, Sonoda T, Matsuura S, Hirohashi S. Prognostic significance of the overexpression of c-erbB-2 protein in adenocarcinoma of the uterine cervix. Cancer 1994;73(1):148–153.

28. Nakano T, Oka K, Ishikawa A, Morita S. Correlation of cervical carcinoma c-erb B-2 oncogene with cell proliferation parameters in patients treated with radiation therapy for cervical carcinoma. Cancer 1997;79(3):513–520.

29. Doppler W, Ofner D, Ullrich A, Daxenbichler G. Effects of interferons on the expression of the proto-oncogene HER-2 in human ovarian carcinoma cells. Int J Cancer 1992;50(1):64–68.

30. Marth C, Muller-Holzner E, Zeimet AG, Greiter E, Cronauer MV, Doppler W, Eibl B, Hynes NE, Daxenbichler G. [Interferon-gamma suppresses expression of the HER-2 oncogene in ovarian cancer cells] Gynakol Geburtshilfliche Rundsch 1992;32(1):31–34.

31. Marth C, Cronauer MV, Doppler W, Ofner D, Ullrich A, Daxenbichler G. Effects of interferons on the expression of the proto-oncogene HER-2 in human ovarian carcinoma cells. Int J Cancer 1992;50(1):64–68.

32. Fady C, Gardner AM, Gera JF, Lichtenstein A. Interferon-induced increase in sensitivity of ovarian cancer targets to lysis by lymphokine-activated killer cells: selective effects on HER2/neu-overexpressing cells. Cancer Res 1992;52(4):764–769.

33. Gercel-Taylor C, Taylor DD. Effect of patient-derived lipids on in vitro expression of oncogenes by ovarian tumor cells. Gynecol Obstet Invest 1996;42(1):42–48.

34. Yu D, Wolf JK, Scanlon M, Price JE, Hung MC. Enhanced c-erbB-2/neu expression in human ovarian cancer cells correlates with more severe malignancy that can be suppressed by E1A. Cancer Res 1993;53(4):891–898.

35. Xing X, Matin A, Yu D, Xia W, Sorgi F, Huang L, Hung MC. Mutant SV40 large T antigen as a therapeutic agent for HER-2/neu-overexpressing ovarian cancer. Cancer Gene Ther 1996;(3):168–174.

36. Valone FH, Kaufman PA, Guyre PM, Lewis LD, Memoli V, Ernstoff MS, Wells W, Barth R, Deo Y, Fisher J, et al. Clinical trials of bispecific antibody MDX-210 in women with advanced breast or ovarian cancer that overexpresses HER-2/neu. J Hematother 1995;4(5):471–475.

37. Rodriguez GC, Boente MP, Berchuck A, Whitaker RS, O'Briant KC, Xu F, Bast RC Jr. The effect of antibodies and immunotoxins reactive with HER-2/neu on growth of ovarian and breast cancer cell lines. Am J Obstet Gynecol 1993;168:228–232.

38. Wels W, Harwerth IM, Mueller M, Groner B, Hynes NE. Selective inhibition of tumor cell growth by a recombinant single-chain antibody-toxin specific for the erbB-2 receptor. Cancer Res 1992;52(22):6310–6376.

39. Pietras RJ, Fendly BM, Chazin VR, Pegram MD, Howell SB, Slamon DJ. Antibody to HER-2/neu receptor blocks DNA repair after cisplatin in human breast and ovarian cancer cells. Oncogene 1994;9(7):1829–1838.

40. Deshane J, Cabrera G, Grim JE, Siegal GP, Pike J, Alvarez RD, Curiel DT. Targeted eradication of ovarian cancer mediated by intracellular expression of anti-erbB-2 single-chain antibody [see comments]. Gynecologic Oncol 1995;59(1):8–14.

41. Karlan BY, Jones J, Slamon DJ, Lagasse LD. Glucocorticoids stabilize HER-2/neu messenger RNA in human epithelial ovarian carcinoma cells. Gynecol Oncol 1994;53(1):70–77.

42. Ioannides CG, Fisk B, Fan D, Biddison WE, Wharton JT, O'Brian CA. Cytotoxic T cells isolated from ovarian malignant ascites recognize a peptide derived from the HER-2/neu proto-oncogene. Cell Immunol 1993;151(1):225–234.

43. Fisk B, Chesak B, Pollack MS, Wharton JT, Ioannides CG. Oligopeptide induction of a cytotoxic T lymphocyte response to HER-2/neu proto-oncogene in vitro. Cell Immunol 1994;157(2):415–427.

44. Yoshino I, Peoples GE, Goedegebuure PS, Maziarz R, Eberlein TJ. Association of HER2/neu expression with sensitivity to tumor-specific CTL in human ovarian cancer. J Immunol 1994;152(5):2393–2400.

45. Gregory H. Isolation and structure of urogastrone and its relationship to epidermal growth factor. Nature 1975;257(5524):325–327.

46. Scott J, Urdea M, Quiroga M, Sanchez-Pescador R, Fong N, Selby M, Rutter WJ, Bell GI. Structure of a mouse submaxillary messenger RNA encoding epidermal growth factor and seven related proteins. Science 1983;221(4607):236–240.

47. Bauknecht T, Kiechle M, Bauer G, Siebers, J.W. Characterization of growth factors in human ovarian carcinomas. Cancer Res 1986;46:2614–2618.

48. Jennings TS, Dottino PR, Mandeli JP, Segna RA, Kelliher K, Cohen CJ. Growth factor expression in normal peritoneum of patients with gynecologic carcinoma. Gynecol Oncol 1994;55(2):190–197.

49. Ottensmeier C, Swanson L, Strobel T, Druker B, Niloff J, Cannistra SA. Absence of constitutive EGF receptor activation in ovarian cancer cell lines. Br J Cancer 1996;74(3):446–452.

50. Rodriguez GC, Berchuck A, Whitaker RS, Schlossman D, Clarke-Pearson DL, Bast RC Jr. Epidermal growth factor receptor expression in normal ovarian epithelium and ovarian cancer. II. Relationship between receptor expression and response to epidermal growth factor. Am J Obstet Gynecol 1991;164(3):745–750.

51. Kurachi H, Adachi H, Morishige K, Adachi K, Takeda T, Homma H, Yamamoto T, Miyake A. Transforming growth factor-alpha promotes tumor markers secretion from human ovarian cancers in vitro. Cancer 1996;78(5):1049–1054.

52. Jasonni VM, Amadori A, Santini D, Ceccarelli C, Naldi S, Flamigni C. Epidermal growth factor receptor (EGF-R) and transforming growth factor alpha (TGFA) expression in different endometrial cancers. Anticancer Res 1995;15(4):1327–1332.

53. Sanfilippo JS, Miseljic S, Yang AR, Doering DL, Shaheen RM, Wittliff JL. Quantitative analyses of epidermal growth factor receptors, HER-2/neu oncoprotein and cathepsin D in nonmalignant and malignant uteri. Cancer 1996;77(4):710–716.

54. Wang D, Konishi I, Koshiyama M, Mandai M, Nanbu Y, Ishikawa Y, Mori T, Fujii S. Expression of c-erbB-2 protein and epidermal growth receptor in endometrial carcinomas. Correlation with clinicopathologic and sex steroid receptor status. Cancer 1993;72(9):2628–2637.

55. Reynolds RK, Owens CA, Roberts JA. Cultured endometrial cancer cells exhibit autocrine growth factor stimulation that is not observed in cultured normal endometrial cells. Gynecol Oncol 1996;60(3):380–386.

56. Zarcone R, Bellini P, Cardone G, Vicinanza G, Cardone A. Epidermal growth factor receptor expression: is it the same in normal and malignant endometria? Clin Exp Obst Gynecol 1995;22(4):298–300.

57. Kristensen GB, Holm R, Abeler VM, Trope CG. Evaluation of the prognostic significance of cathepsin D, epidermal growth factor receptor, and c-erbB-2 in early cervical squamous cell carcinoma. An immunohistochemical study. Cancer 1996;78(3):433–440.

58. Kim JW, Kim YT, Kim DK, Song CH, Lee JW. Expression of epidermal growth factor receptor in carcinoma of the cervix. Gynecol Oncol 1996;60(2):283–287.

59. Johnson GA, Mannel R, Khalifa M, Walker JL, Wren M, Min KW, Benbrook DM. Epidermal growth factor receptor in vulvar malignancies and its relationship to metastasis and patient survival. Gynecol Oncol 1997;65(3):425–429.

60. Evan G: Cancer—a matter of life and cell death. Int J Cancer 1997;71(5):709–711.

61. Coppola JA, Parker JM, Schuler GD, Cole MD. Continued withdrawal from the cell cycle and regulation of cellular genes in mouse erythroleukemia cells blocked in differentiation by the c-myc oncogene. Mol Cell Biol 1989;9(4):1714–1720.

62. Hann SR, Dixit M, Sears RC, Sealy L. The alternatively initiated c-Myc proteins differentially regulate transcription through a noncanonical DNA-binding site. Genes Dev 1994;8(20):2441–2452.

63. Garte SJ. The c-myc oncogene in tumor progression. Crit Rev Oncog 1993;4(4):435–449.

64. Bonilla M, Ramirez M, Lopez-Cueto J, Gariglio P. In vivo amplification and rearrangement of c-myc oncogene in human breast tumors. J Natl Cancer Inst 1988;80(9):665–671.

65. Xin XY. [The amplification of c-myc, N-ras, c-erb B oncogenes in ovarian malignancies] Chung Hua Fu Chan Ko Tsa Chih 1993;28(7):405–407, 442.

66. Volm M, Koomagi R, Kaufmann M, Mattern J, Stammler G. Microvessel density, expres-

sion of proto-oncogenes, resistance-related proteins and incidence of metastases in primary ovarian carcinomas. Clin Exp Metastasis 1996;14(3):209–214.

67. Baker VV, Borst MP, Dixon D, Hatch KD, Shingleton HM, Miller D. c-myc amplification in ovarian cancer. Gynecol Oncol 1990;38(3):340–342.

68. Chien CH, Wang FF, Hamilton TC. Transcriptional activation of c-myc proto-oncogene by estrogen in human ovarian cancer cells. Mol Cell Endocrinol 1994;99(1):11–19.

69. Jeffers MD, Richmond JA, Macaulay EM. Overexpression of the c-myc proto-oncogene occurs frequently in uterine sarcomas. Mod Pathol, 1995;8(7):701–704.

70. Sato S, Jiko K, Ito K, Ozawa N, Yajima A, Miyazaki S, Sasano H. Expression of c-myc mRNA and protein in human endometrial carcinoma; simultaneous study of in situ hybridization and immunohistochemistry. Tohoku J Exp Med 1993;170(4):229–234.

71. Wu HJ. [The expression of c-myc protein in uterine cervical cancer: a possible prognostic indicator]. Nippon Sanka Fujinka Gakkai Zasshi. Acta Obstet Gynaecol Jap 1996;48(7):515–521.

72. Nurnberg W, Artuc M, Nawrath M, Lovric J, Stuting S, Moelling K, Czarnetzki BM, Schadendorf D. Human c-myb is expressed in cervical carcinomas and transactivates the HPV-promoter. Cancer Res 1995;55(19):4432–4437.

73. Devictor B, Bonnier P, Piana L, Andrac L, Lavaut MN, Allasia C, Charpin C. c-myc protein and Ki-67 antigen immunodetection in patients with uterine cervix neoplasia: correlation of microcytophotometric analysis and histological data. Gynecol Oncol, 1993;49(3):284–290.

74. Cromme FV, Snijders PJ, van den Brule AJ, Kenemans P, Meijer CJ, Walboomers JM. MHC class I expression in HPV 16 positive cervical carcinomas is post-transcriptionally controlled and independent from c-myc overexpression. Oncogene 1993;8(11):2969–2975.

75. de Vries JE, ten Kate J, Bosman FT. p21ras in carcinogenesis. Pathol Res Pract 1996;192(7):658–668.

76. Chien CH, Chow SN. Point mutation of the ras oncogene in human ovarian cancer. DNA Cell Biol 1993;12(7):623–627.

77. Teneriello MG, Ebina M, Linnoila RI, Henry M, Nash JD, Park RC, Birrer MJ. p53 and Ki-ras gene mutations in epithelial ovarian neoplasms. Cancer Res 1993;53(13):3103–3108.

78. Fujimoto I, Shimizu Y, Umezawa S, Katase K, Hirai Y, Yamauchi K, Hasumi K. [Studies on the point mutation of ras oncogene in ovarian tumor] Nippon Sanka Fujinka Gakkai Zasshi 1993;45(11):1289–1296.

79. Cuatrecasas M, Villanueva A, Matias-Guiu X, Prat J. K-ras mutations in mucinous ovarian tumors: a clinicopathologic and molecular study of 95 cases. Cancer 1997;79(8):1581–1586.

80. Ichikawa Y, Nishida M, Suzuki H, Yoshida S, Tsunoda H, Kubo T, Uchida K, Miwa M. Mutation of K-ras protooncogene is associated with histological subtypes in human mucinous ovarian tumors. Cancer Res 1994;54(1):33–35.

81. Enomoto T, Weghorst CM, Inoue M, Tanizawa O, Rice JM. K-ras activation occurs frequently in mucinous adenocarcinomas and rarely in other common epithelial tumors of the human ovary. Am J Pathol 1991;139(4):777–785.

82. Mok SC, Bell DA, Knapp RC, Fishbaugh PM, Welch WR, Muto MG, Berkowitz RS, Tsao SW. Mutation of K-ras protooncogene in human ovarian epithelial tumors of borderline malignancy Cancer Res 1993;53(7):1489–1492.

83. Fujita M, Enomoto T, Inoue M, Tanizawa O, Ozaki M, Rice JM, Nomura T. Alteration of the p53 tumor suppressor gene occurs independently of K-ras activation and more fre-

quently in serous adenocarcinomas than in other common epithelial tumors of the human ovary. Jpn J Cancer Res 1994;85(12):1247–1256.

84. Yaginuma Y, Yamashita K, Kuzumaki N, Fujita M, Shimizu T. ras oncogene product p21 expression and prognosis of human ovarian tumors. Gynecol Oncol 1992;46(1),45–50.

85. Chow SN, Lin JK, Li SS, Chien CH. Identification of LDH-ras p21 protein complex and expression of these genes in human ovarian cancer. Gynecol Oncol 1997;64(1),114–120.

86. Scambia G, Catozzi L, Panici PB, Ferrandina G, Coronetta F, Barozzi R, Baiocchi G, Uccelli L, Piffanelli A, Mancuso S. Expression of ras oncogene p21 protein in normal and neoplastic ovarian tissues: correlation with histopathologic features and receptors for estrogen, progesterone, and epidermal growth factor. Am J Obstet Gynecol 1993;168(1 Pt 1):71–87.

87. Zachos G, Varras M, Koffa M, Ergazaki M, Spandidos DA. Glucocorticoid and estrogen receptors have elevated activity in human endometrial and ovarian tumors as compared to the adjacent normal tissues and recognize sequence elements of the H-ras proto-oncogene. Jpn J Cancer Res 1996;87(9):916–922.

88. Duggan BD, Felix JC, Muderspach LI, Tsao JL, Shibata DK. Early mutational activation of the c-Ki-ras oncogene in endometrial carcinoma. Cancer Res 1994;54(6):1604–1607.

89. Enomoto T, Inoue M, Perantoni AO, Buzard GS, Miki H, Tanizawa O, Rice JM. K-ras activation in premalignant and malignant epithelial lesions of the human uterus Cancer Res 1991;51(19);5308–5314.

90. Tsuda H, Jiko K, Yajima M, Yamada T, Tanemura K, Tsunematsu R, Ohmi K, Sonoda T, Hirohashi S. Frequent occurrence of c-Ki-ras gene mutations in well differentiated endometrial adenocarcinoma showing infiltrative local growth with fibrosing stromal response. Int J Gynecol Pathol 1995;14(3):255–259.

91. Caduff RF, Johnston CM, Frank TS. Mutations of the Ki-ras oncogene in carcinoma of the endometrium. Am J Pathol 1995;146(1):182–188.

92. Mizuuchi H, Nasim S, Kudo R, Silverberg SG, Greenhouse S, Garrett CT. Clinical implications of K-ras mutations in malignant epithelial tumors of the endometrium. Cancer Res 1992;52(10):2777–2781.

93. Fujimoto I, Shimizu Y, Hirai Y, Chen JT, Teshima H, Hasumi K, Masubuchi K, Takahashi M. Studies on ras oncogene activation in endometrial carcinoma. Gynecol Oncol 1993;48(2):196–202.

94. Ito K, Watanabe K, Nasim S, Sasano H, Sato S, Yajima A, Silverberg SG, Garrett CT. K-ras point mutations in endometrial carcinoma: effect on outcome is dependent on age of patient. Gynecol Oncol 1996;63(2):238–246.

95. Fujimoto J, Ichigo S, Hori M, Morishita S, Tamaya T. Estrogen induces c-Ha-ras expression via activation of tyrosine kinase in uterine endometrial fibroblasts and cancer cells. Steroid Biochem Mol Biol 1995;55(1):25–33.

96. Long CA, O'Brien TJ, Sanders MM, Bard DS, Quirk JG Jr. ras oncogene is expressed in adenocarcinoma of the endometrium. Am J Obstet Gynecol 1988;159(6):1512–1516.

97. Scambia G, Catozzi L, Benedetti-Panici P, Ferrandina G, Battaglia F, Giovannini G, Distefano M, Pellizzola D, Piffanelli A, Mancuso S. Expression of ras p21 oncoprotein in normal and neoplastic human endometrium. Gynecol Oncol 1993;50(3):339–346.

98. Sagae S, Kuzumaki N, Hisada T, Mugikura Y, Kudo R, Hashimoto M. ras oncogene expression and prognosis of invasive squamous cell carcinomas of the uterine cervix. Cancer 1989;63(8): 1577–1582.

99. Tenti P, Romagnoli S, Silini E, Pellegata NS, Zappatore R, Spinillo A, Zara C, Ranzani

GN, Carnevali L. Analysis and clinical implications of K-ras gene mutations and infection with human papillomavirus types 16 and 18 in primary adenocarcinoma of the uterine cervix. Int J Cancer, 1995;64(1):9–13.

100. Jiko K, Tsuda H, Sato S, Hirohashi S. Pathogenetic significance of p53 and c-Ki-ras gene mutations and human papillomavirus DNA integration in adenocarcinoma of the uterine cervix and uterine isthmus. Int J Cancer 1994;59(5),601–606.

101. Mizuuchi H, Mori Y, Sato K, Kamiya H, Okamura N, Nasim S, Garrett CT, Kudo R. High incidence of point mutation in K-ras codon 12 in carcinoma of the fallopian tube. Cancer 1995;76(1):86–90.

102. Vousden K. Interactions of human papillomavirus transforming proteins with the products of tumor suppressor genes. FASEB J 1993;7(10):872–879.

103. Park TW, Fujiwara H, Wright TC. Molecular biology of cervical cancer and its precursors. Cancer, 1995;76(10 Suppl.):1902–1913.

104. Chen L, Ashe S, Singhal MC, Galloway DA, Hellstrom I, Hellstrom KE. Metastatic conversion of cells by expression of human papillomavirus type 16 E6 and E7 genes. Proc Natl Acad Sci, 1993;90(14):6523–6527.

105. Munoz N, Bosch FX. The causal link between HPV and cervical cancer and its implications for prevention of cervical cancer. Bulle Pan Am Health Org 1996;30(4):362–377.

106. Londesborough P, Ho L, Terry G, Cuzick J, Wheeler C, Singer A. Human papillomavirus genotype as a predictor of persistence and development of high-grade lesions in women with minor cervical abnormalities. Int J Cancer, 1996;69(5):364–368.

107. Iwasawa A, Nieminen P, Lehtinen M, Paavonen J. Human papillomavirus DNA in uterine cervix squamous cell carcinoma and adenocarcinoma detected by polymerase chain reaction. Cancer, 1996;77(11):2275–2279.

108. Jeon S, Lambert PF. Integration of human papillomavirus type 16 DNA into the human genome leads to increased stability of E6 and E7 mRNAs: implications for cervical carcinogenesis. Proc Natl Acad Sci 1995;92(5):1654–1658.

109. Pao CC, Hor JJ, Yang FP, Lin CY, Tseng CJ. Detection of human papillomavirus mRNA and cervical cancer cells in peripheral blood of cervical cancer patients with metastasis. J Clin Oncol 1997;15(3):1008–1012.

110. Viscidi RP, Sun Y, Tsuzaki B, Bosch FX, Munoz N, Shah KV. Serologic response in human papillomavirus-associated invasive cervical cancer. Int J Cancer 1993;55(5):780–784.

111. Fisher SG, Benitez-Bribiesca L, Nindl I, Stockfleth E, Muller M, Wolf H, Perez-Garcia F, Guzman-Gaona J, Gutierrez-Delgado F, Irivin W, et al. The association of human papilloma virus type 16 E6 and E7 antibodies with stage of cervical cancer. Gynecol Oncol, 1996;61(1):73–78.

112. Strickler HD, Schiffman MH, Eklund C, Glass AG, Scott DR, Sherman ME, Wacholder S, Kurman RJ, Manos MM, Schiller JT, et al. Evidence for at least two distinct groups of humoral immune reactions to papillomavirus antigens in women with squamous intraepithelial lesions. Cancer Epid Biom Prev 1997;6(3):183–188.

113. Marais D, Rose RC, Williamson AL. Age distribution of antibodies to human papillomavirus in children, women with cervical intraepithelial neoplasia and blood donors from. S Africa J Med Virol 1997;51(2):126–131.

114. Nakagawa M, Stites DP, Farhat S, Sisler JR, Moss B, Kong F, Moscicki AB, Palefsky JM. Cytotoxic T lymphocyte responses to E6 and E7 proteins of human papillomavirus type 16: relationship to cervical intraepithelial neoplasia. J Inf Dis 1997;175(4):927–931.

115. Alexander M, Salgaller ML, Celis E, Sette A, Barnes WA, Rosenberg SA, Steller MA.

Generation of tumor-specific cytolytic T lymphocytes from peripheral blood of cervical cancer patients by in vitro stimulation with a synthetic human papillomavirus type 16 E7 epitope. Am J Obstet Gynecol 1996;175(6):1586–1593.

116. Ressing ME, van Driel WJ, Celis E, Sette A, Brandt MP, Hartman M, Anholts JD, Schreuder GM, ter Harmsel WB, Fleuren GJ, et al. Occasional memory cytotoxic T-cell responses of patients with human papillomavirus type 16-positive cervical lesions against a human leukocyte antigen-A *0201-restricted E7-encoded epitope. Cancer Res 1996;56(3):582–588.

117. Clerici M, Merola M, Ferrario E, Trabattoni D, Villa ML, Stefanon B, Venzon DJ, Shearer GM, De Palo G, Clerici E. Cytokine production patterns in cervical intraepithelial neoplasia: association with human papillomavirus infection [see comments]. J Nat Cancer Inst, 1997;89(3):245–250.

118. Tsukui T, Hildesheim A, Schiffman MH, Lucci J 3rd, Contois D, Lawler P, Rush BB, Lorincz AT, Corrigan A, Burk RD, et al. Interleukin 2 production in vitro by peripheral lymphocytes in response to human papillomavirus-derived peptides: correlation with cervical pathology. Cancer Res 1996;56(17):3967–3974.

119. Luxton JC, Rowe AJ, Cridland JC, Coletart T, Wilson P, Shepherd PS. Proliferative T cell responses to the human papillomavirus type 16 E7 protein in women with cervical dysplasia and cervical carcinoma and in healthy individuals. J Gen Virol 1996;77 (Pt 7):1585–1593.

120. Ellis JR, Keating PJ, Baird J, Hounsell EF, Renouf DV, Rowe M, Hopkins D, Duggan-Keen MF, Bartholomew JS, Young LS, et al. The association of an HPV16 oncogene variant with HLA-B7 has implications for vaccine design in cervical cancer. Nature Med 1995;1(5):464–470.

121. Boursnell ME, Rutherford E, Hickling JK, Rollinson EA, Munro AJ, Rolley N, McLean CS, Borysiewicz LK, Vousden K, Inglis SC. Construction and characterisation of a recombinant vaccinia virus expressing human papillomavirus proteins for immunotherapy of cervical cancer. Vaccine 1996;14(16):1485–1494.

122. Kirnbauer R. Papillomavirus-like particles for serology and vaccine development. Intervirology 1996;39(1–2):54–61.

123. Tindle RW, Croft S, Herd K, Malcolm K, Geczy AF, Stewart T, Fernando GJ. A vaccine conjugate of 'ISCAR' immunocarrier and peptide epitopes of the E7 cervical cancer-associated protein of human papillomavirus type 16 elicits specific Th1- and Th2-type responses in immunized mice in the absence of oil-based adjuvants. Clin Exp Immunol 1995;101(2):265–271.

124. Borysiewicz LK, Fiander A, Nimako M, Man S, Wilkinson GW, Westmoreland D, Evans AS, Adams M, Stacey SN, Boursnell ME, et al. A recombinant vaccinia virus encoding human papillomavirus types 16 and 18, E6 and E7 proteins as immunotherapy for cervical cancer [see comments]. Lancet 1996;347(9014):1523–1527.

125. Hamada K, Sakaue M, Alemany R, Zhang WW, Horio Y, Roth JA, Mitchell MF. Adenovirus-mediated transfer of HPV 16 E6/E7 antisense RNA to human cervical cancer cells. Gynecol Oncol 1996;63(2):219–227.

126. Lappalainen K, Pirila L, Jaaskelainen I, Syrjanen K, Syrjanen S. Effects of liposomal antisense oligonucleotides on mRNA and protein levels of the HPV 16 E7 oncogene. Anticancer Res 1996;16(5A):2485–2492.

127. Chen Z, Kamath P, Zhang S, Weil MM, Shillitoe EJ. Effectiveness of three ribozymes for cleavage of an RNA transcript from human papillomavirus type 18. Cancer Gene Ther 1995;2(4):263–271.

128. Tan TM, Ting RC. In vitro and in vivo inhibition of human papillomavirus type 16 E6 and E7 genes. Cancer Res 1995;55(20):4599–4605.

129. Simons AM, Mugica van Herckenrode C, Rodriguez JA, Maitland N, Anderson M, Phillips DH, Coleman DV. Demonstration of smoking-related DNA damage in cervical epithelium and correlation with human papillomavirus type 16, using exfoliated cervical cells. Br J Cancer 1995;71(2):246–249.

130. Chen M, Popescu N, Woodworth C, Berneman Z, Corbellino M, Lusso P, Ablashi DV, Di-Paolo JA. Human herpesvirus 6 infects cervical epithelial cells and transactivates human papillomavirus gene expression. J Virol 1994;68(2):1173–1178.

131. Neyns B, Katesuwanasing, Vermeij J, Bourgain C, Vandamme B, Amfo K, Lissens W, DeSutter P, Hooghe-Peters E, DeGreve J. Expression of the jun family of genes in human ovarian cancer and normal ovarian surface epithelium. Oncogene 1996;12(6):1247–1257.

132. Kommoss F, Bauknecht T, Birmelin G, Kohler M, Tesch H, Pfleiderer A. Oncogene and growth factor expression in ovarian cancer. Acta Obstet Gynecol Scand Suppl 1992;155:19–24.

133. Nephew KP, Polek TC, Khan SA. Tamoxifen-induced proto-oncogene expression persists in uterine endometrial epithelium. Endocrinol 1996;137(1):219–224.

134. Uehara T, Kuwashima Y, Izumo T, Kishi K, Shiromizu K, Matsuzawa M. Expression of the proto-oncogene bcl-2 in uterine cervical squamous cell carcinoma: its relationship to clinical outcome. Eur J Gynaecol Oncol, 1995;16(6):453–460.

135. Ter Harmsel B, Smedts F, Kuijpers J, Jeunink M, Trimbos B, Ramaekers F. BCL-2 immunoreactivity increases with severity of CIN: a study of normal cervical epithelia, CIN, and cervical carcinoma. J Pathol 1996;179(1):26–30.

136. Nakamura T, Nomura S, Sakai T, Nariya S. Expression of bcl-2 oncoprotein in gastrointestinal and uterine carcinomas and their premalignant lesions. Human Pathol 1997;28(3):309–315.

137. Saegusa M, Takano Y, Hashimura M, Shoji Y, Okayasu I. The possible role of bcl-2 expression in the progression of tumors of the uterine cervix. Cancer 1995;76(11):2297–2303.

138. Tjalma W, Weyler J, Goovaerts G, De Pooter C, Van Marck E, van Dam P. Prognostic value of bcl-2 expression in patients with operable carcinoma of the uterine cervix. J Clin Pathol 1997;50(1):33–36.

139. McCluggage G, McBride H, Maxwell P, Bharucha H. Immunohistochemical detection of p53 and bcl-2 proteins in neoplastic and non-neoplastic endocervical glandular lesions. Int J Gynecol Pathol 1997;16(1):22–27.

140. Kurvinen K, Syrjanen K, Syrjanen S. p53 and bcl-2 proteins as prognostic markers in human papillomavirus-associated cervical lesions. J Clin Oncol 1996;14(7):2120–2130.

141. Kurzrock R, Ku S, Talpaz M. Abnormalities in the PRAD1 (CYCLIN D1/BCL-1) oncogene are frequent in cervical and vulvar squamous cell carcinoma cell lines. Cancer 1995;75(2):584–590.

142. Nichols GE, Williams ME, Gaffey MJ, Stoler MH. Cyclin D1 gene expression in human cervical neoplasia. Mod Pathol 1996;9(4):418–425.

143. Ikenberg H, Matthay K, Schmitt B, Bauknecht T, Kiechle-Schwarz M, Goppinger A, Pfleiderer A. p53 mutation and MDM2 amplification are rare even in human papillomavirus-negative cervical carcinomas. Cancer, 1995;76(1):57–66.

144. Courjal F, Cuny M, Rodriguez C, Louason G, Speiser P, Katsaros D, Tanner MM,

Zeillinger R, Theillet C. DNA amplifications at 20q13 and MDM2 define distinct subsets of evolved breast and ovarian tumours. Br J Cancer 1996;74(12):1984–1989.

145. Di Renzo MF, Olivero M, Katsaros D, Crepaldi T, Gaglia P, Zola P, Sismondi P, Comoglio PM. Overexpression of the MET/HGF receptor in ovarian cancer. Int J Cancer 1994;58(5):658–662.

146. Jaakkola S, Salmikangas P, Nylund S, Partanen J, Armstrong E, Pyrhonen S, Lehtovirta P, Nevanlinna H. Amplification of fgfr4 gene in human breast and gynecological cancers. Int J Cancer 1993;54(3):378–382.

147. Rosen A, Sevelda P, Klein M, Dobianer K, Hruza C, Czerwenka K, Hanak H, Vavra N, Salzer H, Leodolter S, et al. First experience with FGF-3 (INT-2) amplification in women with epithelial ovarian cancer. Br J Cancer 1993;67(5):1122–1125.

148. Merogi AJ, Marrogi AJ, Ramesh R, Robinson WR, Fermin CD, Freeman SM. Tumor-host interaction: analysis of cytokines, growth factors, and tumor-infiltrating lymphocytes in ovarian carcinomas. Human Pathol 1997;28(3):321–331.

149. Di Giovine FS, Duff GW. Interleukin 1: The first interleukin. Immunol Today 1990;11:13.

150. Smith KA. Lymphokine regulation of T cell and B cell function. In: Paul WE, ed. Fundamental Immunology. New York: Raven Press, 1984:559.

151. Malik, S. & Balkwill, F. Epithelial ovarian cancer: a cytokine propelled disease? Br J Cancer 1991;64:617–620.

152. Wu S, Meeker WA, Wiener JR, Berchuck A, Bast RC Jr, Boyer CM. Transfection of ovarian cancer cells with tumor necrosis factor-alpha (TNF-alpha) antisense mRNA abolishes the proliferative response to interleukin-1 (IL-1) but not TNF-alpha. Gynecol Oncol 1994;53:59–63.

153. Castrilli G, Tatone D, Diodoro MG, Rosini S, Piantelli M, Musiani P. Interleukin 1alpha and interleukin 6 promote the in vitro growth of both normal and neoplastic human cervical epithelial cells. Br J Cancer 1997;75(6):855–859.

154. Woodworth CD, Simpson S. Comparative lymphokine secretion by cultured normal human cervical keratinocytes, papillomavirus-immortalized, and carcinoma cell lines. Am J Pathol 1993;142(5):1544–1555.

155. Kawakami Y, Nagai N, Ota S, Ohama K, Yamashita U Interleukin-1 as an autocrine stimulator in the growth of human ovarian cancer cells. Hiroshima J Med Sci 1997;46(1):51–59.

156. Wong GG, Clark SC. Multiple actions of interleukin 6 within a cytokine network. Immunol Today 1988;9(5):137–139.

157. Wong GG, Witek-Giannotti J, Hewick RM, Clark SC, Ogawa M. Interleukin 6: identification as a hematopoietic colony-stimulating factor. Behring Institute Mitteilungen, 1988;83:40–47.

158. Scambia G, Testa U, Panici PB, Martucci R, Foti E, Petrini M, Amoroso M, Masciullo V, Peschle C, Mancuso S. Interleukin-6 serum levels in patients with gynecological tumors. Int J Cancer 1994;57(3):318–323.

159. Watson JM, Berek JS, Martinez-Maza O. Growth inhibition of ovarian cancer cells induced by antisense IL-6 oligonucleotides. Gynecol Oncol 1993;49:8–12.

160. Watson JM, Sensintaffar JL, Berek JS, Martinez-Maza O. Constitutive production of interleukin 6 by ovarian cancer cell lines and by primary ovarian tumor cultures. Cancer Res 1990;50(21):6959–6965.

161. Lidor Y J, Xu F I, Martinez-Maza O, et al. Constitutive production of macrophage colony

stimulating factor and IL-6 by human ovarian sudace epithelial cells. Exp Cell Res 1993;207:332–339.

162. Ferdeghini M, Gadducci A, Prontera C, Bonuccelli A, Annicchiarico C, Fanucchi A, Facchini V, Bianchi R. Serum interleukin-6 levels in uterine malignancies. Preliminary data. Anticancer Res 1994;14(2B):735–737.

163. Iglesias M, Plowman GD, Woodworth CD. Interleukin-6 and interleukin-6 soluble receptor regulate proliferation of normal, human papillomavirus-immortalized, and carcinoma-derived cervical cells in vitro. Am J Pathol 1995;146(4):944–952.

164. Tartour E, Gey A, Sastre-Garau X, Pannetier C, Mosseri V, Kourilsky P, Fridman WH. Analysis of interleukin 6 gene expression in cervical neoplasia using a quantitative polymerase chain reaction assay: evidence for enhanced interleukin 6 gene expression in invasive carcinoma. Cancer Res 1994;54(23):6243–6248.

165. Takano H, Harigaya K, Ishii G, Sugaya Y, Soeta S, Nunoyama T, Shirasawa H, Shimizu K, Tokita H, Simizu B, Mikata A, Sekiya S. Interleukin-6 (IL-6) production in carcinoma of the cervix. Arch Gynecol Obstet 1996;258(1):25–33.

166. Gasson JC, Weisbart RH, Kaufman SE, Clark SC, Hewick RM, Wong GG, Golde DW. Purified human granulocyte-macrophage colony-stimulating factor: direct action on neutrophils. Science 1984;226(4680):1339–1342.

167. Souza LM, Boone TC, Gabrilove J, Lai PH, Zsebo KM, Murdock DC, Chazin VR, Bruszewski J, Lu H, Chen KK, et al. Recombinant human granulocyte colony-stimulating factor: effects on normal and leukemic myeloid cells. Science 1986;232(4746):61–65.

168. Connor JP, Squatrito RC, Terrell KL, Antisdel BJ, Buller RE. In vitro growth effects of colony-stimulating factors in ovarian cancer. Gynecol Oncol 1994;52(3):347–352.

169. Metcalf D. Multi-CSF-dependent colony formation by cells of a murine hemopoietic cell line: specificity and action of multi-CSF. Blood 1985;65(2):357–362.

170. Suzuki M, Sekiguchi I, Ohwada M, Sato I, Matsui T, Tanabe T, Hashimoto S, Yamada M. Expression of c-fms proto-oncogene product by ovarian cancer cell lines with effects of macrophage colony-stimulating factor on proliferation. Oncology 1996;53(2):99–103.

171. Leiserowitz GS, Harris SA, Subramaniam M, Keeney GL, Podratz KC, Spelsberg TC. The proto-oncogene c-fms is overexpressed in endometrial cancer. Gynecol Oncol 1993;49(2):190–196.

172. Takeda S, Soutter WP, Dibb NJ, White JO. Biological activity of the receptor for macrophage colony-stimulating factor in the human endometrial cancer cell line Ishikawa. Br J Cancer 1996;73(5):615–619.

173. Zapf J, Froesch ER. Insulin-like growth factors/somatomedins: structure, secretion, biological actions and physiological role. Hormone Res 1986;24(2–3):121–130.

174. Beck EP, Russo P, Gliozzo B, Jaeger W, Papa V, Wildt L, Pezzino V, Lang N. Identification of insulin and insulin-like growth factor I (IGF I) receptors in ovarian cancer tissue. Gynecol Oncol 1994;53(2):196–201.

175. Yun K, Fukumoto M, Jinno Y Monoallelic expression of the insulin-like growth factor-2 gene in ovarian cancer. Am J Pathol 1996;148(4):1081–1087.

176. Yee D, Morales FR, Hamilton TC, Von Hoff DD. Expression of insulin-like growth factor I, its binding proteins, and its receptor in ovarian cancer. Cancer Res 1991;51(19):5107–5112.

177. Rutanen EM, Nyman T, Lehtovirta P, Ammala M, Pekonen F. Suppressed expression of insulin-like growth factor binding protein-1 mRNA in the endometrium: a molecular

mechanism associating endometrial cancer with its risk factors. Int J Cancer 1994;59(3):307–312.

178. Stromberg K, Collins TJ 4th, Gordon AW, Jackson CL, Johnson GR. Transforming growth factor-alpha acts as an autocrine growth factor in ovarian carcinoma cell lines Cancer Res 1992;52(2):341–347.

179. Zhou L, Leung BS. Growth regulation of ovarian cancer cells by epidermal growth factor and transforming growth factors alpha and ß 1. Biochim Biophys Acta 1992;1180(2):130–136.

180. Lawrence DA. Transforming growth factor-ß: a general review. Eur Cytokine Network 1996;7(3):363–374.

181. Kehrl JH. Transforming growth factor-ß: an important mediator of immunoregulation. Int J Cell Cloning 1991;9(5):438–450.

182. Henriksen R, Gobl A, Wilander E, Oberg K, Miyazono K, Funa K. Expression and prognostic significance of TGF-ß isotypes, latent TGF-ß 1 binding protein, TGF-ß type I and type II receptors, and endoglin in normal ovary and ovarian neoplasms. Lab Invest 1995;73(2):213–220.

183. Berchuck A, Rodriguez G, Olt G, Whitaker R, Boente MP, Arrick BA, Clarke-Pearson DL, Bast RC Jr. Regulation of growth of normal ovarian epithelial cells and ovarian cancer cell lines by transforming growth factor-ß. Am J Obstet Gynecol 1992;166(2):676–684.

184. Hurteau J, Rodriguez GC, Whitaker RS, Shah S, Mills G, Bast RC, Berchuck A. Transforming growth factor-ß inhibits proliferation of human ovarian cancer cells obtained from ascites. Cancer 1994;74(1):93–99.

185. Havrilesky LJ, Hurteau JA, Whitaker RS, Elbendary A, Wu S, Rodriguez GC, Bast RC Jr, Berchuck A. Regulation of apoptosis in normal and malignant ovarian epithelial cells by transforming growth factor ß. Cancer Res 1995;55(4):944–948.

186. Bergman CA, Talavera F, Christman GM, Baker VV, Roberts JA, Menon KM. Transforming growth factor-ß negatively modulates proliferation and c-fos expression of the human endometrial adenocarcinoma cell line HEC-1-A. Gynecol Oncol 1997;65(1):63–68.

187. Comerci JT Jr, Runowicz CD, Flanders KC, De Victoria C, Fields AL, Kadish AS, Goldberg GL. Altered expression of transforming growth factor-ß 1 in cervical neoplasia as an early biomarker in carcinogenesis of the uterine cervix. Cancer 1996;77(6):1107–1114.

188. Hill CM, Lunec J. The TNF-ligand and receptor superfamilies: controllers of immunity and the Trojan horses of autoimmune disease? Mol Aspects Med 1996;17(5):455–509.

189. Rink L, Kirchner H. Recent progress in the tumor necrosis factor-alpha field. Int Arch Allergy Immunol 1996;111(3):199–209.

190. Kunkel SL, Remick DG, Strieter RM, Larrick JW. Mechanisms that regulate the production and effects of tumor necrosis factor-alpha. Crit Rev Immunol 1989;9(2):93–117.

191. Gotlieb WH, Watson JM, Rezai A, Johnson M, Martinez-Maza O, Berek JS. Cytokine-induced modulation of tumor suppressor gene expression in ovarian cancer cells: up-regulation of p53 gene expression and induction of apoptosis by tumor necrosis factor-alpha. Am J Obstet Gynecol 1994;170(4):1121–1128.

192. Golub SH. Immunological and therapeutic effects of interferon treatment of cancer patients. Clin Immunol Allergy 1984;4:377.

193. Nathan CF, Murray HW, Wiebe ME, Rubin BY. Identification of γ-interferon as the lymphokine that activates human macrophage oxidative metabolism and antimicrobial activity. J Exp Med 1983;158:670.

194. Pao CC, Lin CY, Yao DS, Tseng CJ. Differential expression of cytokine genes in cervical cancer tissues. Biochem Biophys Res Commun 1995;214(3):1146–1151.

195. Boente MP, Berchuck A, Rodriguez GC, Davidoff A, Whitaker R, Xu FJ, Marks J, Clarke-Pearson DL, Bast RC Jr. The effect of interferon gamma on epidermal growth factor receptor expression in normal and malignant ovarian epithelial cells. Am J Obstet Gynecol 1992;167(6):1877–1882.

196. Crickard K, Gross JL, Crickard U, Yoonessi M, Lele S, Herblin WF, Eidsvoog K. Basic fibroblast growth factor and receptor expression in human ovarian cancer. Gynecol Oncol 1994;55(2):277–284.

197. Di Blasio AM, Carniti C, Vigano P, Vignali M. Basic fibroblast growth factor and ovarian cancer. J Steroid Biochem Mol Biol 1995;53(1–6):375–379.

198. Fujimoto J, Hori M, Ichigo S, Tamaya T. Expressions of the fibroblast growth factor family (FGF-1, 2 and 4) mRNA in endometrial cancers. Tumour Biol 1996;17(4):226–233.

199. Sliutz G, Tempfer C, Obermair A, Reinthaller A, Gitsch G, Kainz C. Serum evaluation of basic fibroblast growth factor in cervical cancer patients. Cancer Lett 1995;94(2):227–231.

200. Fujimoto J, Ichigo S, Hori M, Hirose R, Sakaguchi H, Tamaya T. Expression of basic fibroblast growth factor and its mRNA in advanced uterine cervical cancers. Cancer Lett 1997;111(1–2):21–26.

201. Chatzaki E, Bax CM, Eidne KA, Anderson L, Grudzinskas JG, Gallagher CJ. The expression of gonadotropin-releasing hormone and its receptor in endometrial cancer, and its relevance as an autocrine growth factor. Cancer Res 1996;56(9):2059–2065.

202. Paley PJ, Staskus KA, Gebhard K, Mohanraj D, Twiggs LB, Carson LF, Ramakrishnan S. Vascular endothelial growth factor expression in early stage ovarian carcinoma. Cancer 1997;80(1):98–106.

203. Doldi N, Bassan M, Gulisano M, Broccoli V, Boncinelli E, Ferrari A. Vascular endothelial growth factor messenger ribonucleic acid expression in human ovarian and endometrial cancer. Gynecol Endocrinol 1996;10(6):375–382.

204. Wiggins DL, Granai CO, Steinhoff MM, Calabresi P. Tumor angiogenesis as a prognostic factor in cervical carcinoma. Gynecol Oncol 1995;56(3):353–356.

205. Bancher-Todesca D, Obermair A, Bilgi S, Kohlberger P, Kainz C, Breitenecker G, Leodolter S, Gitsch G. Angiogenesis in vulvar intraepithelial neoplasia. Gynecol Oncol 1997;64(3):496–500.

206. Guidi AJ, Abu-Jawdeh G, Berse B, Jackman RW, Tognazzi K, Dvorak HF, Brown LF. Vascular permeability factor (vascular endothelial growth factor) expression and angiogenesis in cervical neoplasia. J Natl Cancer Inst 1995;87(16):1237–1245.

207. Chopra V, Dinh TV, Hannigan EV. Angiogenin, interleukins, and growth-factor levels in serum of patients with ovarian cancer: correlation with angiogenesis. Cancer J Sci Am 1996;2(5):279.

208. Yea KT, Wang HH, Nagy JA, Sioussat TM, Ledbetter SR, Hoogewerf AN, Zhou Y, Masse EM, Senger DR, Dvorak HF, et al. Vascular permeability factor (vascular endothelial growth factor) in guinea pig and human tumor and inflammatory effusions. Cancer Res 1993;53:2912–2918.

209. Olson TA, Mohanraj D, Carson LF, Ramakrishnan S. Vascular permeability factor gene expression in normal and neoplastic human ovaries. Cancer Res 1994;54(1):276–280.

210. Ross R, Raines EW, Bowen-Pope, DF. The biology of platelet-derived growth factor. Cell 1986;46:155–169.

211. Westermark B, Heldin C-H. Platelet-derived growth factor in autocrine transformation. Cancer Res 1991;51:5087–5092.

212. Versnel MA, Haarbrink M, Langerak AW, De Laat RAJM, Hagemeijer A, Van der Kwast, TH. Human ovarian tumors of epithelial origin express PDGF in vitro and in vivo. Cancer Genet Cytogenet 1994;73:60–64.

213. Berchuck A, Olt GJ, Everitt L, Soisson AR, Bast RC, Boyer CM. The role of peptide growth factors in epithelial ovarian cancer. Obstet Gynecol 1990;75:255–262.

214. Golombick T, Dajee D, Bezwoda WR. Extracellular matrix interactions 2: extracellular matrix structure is important for growth factor localization and function. In Vitro Cell Dev Biol 1995;31:396–403.

215. Munson L, Upadhyaya NB, Van Meter S. Platelet-derived growth factor promotes endometrial epithelial cell proliferation. Am J Obstet Gynecol 1995;173(6):1820–1825.

INDEX

Acetylcholine, stress and, 5
Acquired immunity, 161–162
Activin, 27
Acute inflammation, 120
Adaptive immunity, 171–172
Adoption, 3
Adrenocroticotrophic hormone (ACTH), 2, 7
Affinity binding, 113
Amniotic fluid (AF), 178, 180–181, 184, 209
Androgen-induced growth factor (AIGF), 104
Androgens
  biosynthesis, 53
  immunosuppressive, 24
Angiogenesis, 103–106
Antechinus stuartii, 24
Antibodies, antisperm, 54
Antibody dependent cellular cytotoxicity (ADCC), 164
Anti-inflammatory cytokines
  characteristics of, 174, 211
  hormonal regulation of, 214
  in placentas, synthesis and potential functions, 212–213
Antigen-antibody complexes, 163
Antigens
  autologous sperm, 25
  early pregnancy and, 161–162
  HLA class II, 54, 223
  immunity response and, 171–172
  MHC class II, 26, 62, 65
  orchitogenic, 25
  in peritoneal environment, 242–243
  Simian virus 40 T, 134
Antithrombin III, 101
Anxiety, infertility and, 3

Apoptosis, *see specific types of cells*
Atretic follicles, 45–46
Autoantibody production, 163
Autocrine growth factors, 94
Autoimmune disease, 5, 25–26

Bacteria, preterm labor and, 177–181
Bacterial infection, 83–84
B_2-adrenergic growth hormone, 6
Basic fibroblast growth factor (bFGF), 251
Basophils, 161
B cells, 7, 108–109, 162, 223
Bcl-2 protein, 304–305
Bioactive lipids, 213
Biosynthesis
  follicular development and, 62
  Leydig cell androgen, 31
  testosterone, 19
Bleeding, abnormal
  uterine, 120
  vaginal, 133
B lymphoctyes, 48, 52, 242, 263
Breast cancer, 296. *See also* Gynecologic oncology

Catecholamines, 2, 31
C-C chemokines, 85, 172–173, 175, 184, 244, 266
CCR3/CCR4/CCR5, 85
CD8+ T cells, 7, 48, 65, 207, 223–224
CD4+ T cells, 7, 25, 48, 109, 223
CD14+ macrophages, 207
Cell-cell binding, 205
Cell proliferation, 137–139
Central nervous system (CNS), 5–6, 8
Cervical cancer, HPV in, 300–301. *See also* Gynecologic oncology; Oncogenes